Everyday Technologies in Healthcare

Rehabilitation Science in Practice Series

Marcia J. Scherer
Institute for Matching Person & Technology, Webster, New York, USA

Dave J. Muller
University of Suffolk, United Kingdom

Everyday Technology in Healthcare
Christopher M. Hayre, Dave J. Muller, and Marcia Scherer

Enhancing Healthcare and Rehabilitation: The Impact
of Qualitative Research
Christopher M. Hayre and Dave Muller

Neurological Rehabilitation: Spasticity and Contractures
in Clinical Practice and Research
Anand D. Pandyan, Hermie J. Hermens, and Bernard A. Conway

Quality of Life Technology Handbook
Richard Schulz

Computer Systems Experiences of Users with and
Without Disabilities: An Evaluation Guide for Professionals
Simone Borsci, Masaaki Kurosu, Stefano Federici, and Maria Laura Mele

Assistive Technology Assessment Handbook - 2nd Edition
Stefano Federici and Marcia Scherer

Ambient Assisted Living
Nuno M. Garcia, Joel Jose P.C. Rodrigues

For more information about this series, please visit: https://www.crcpress.com/Rehabilitation-Science-in-Practice-Series/book-series/CRCPRESERIN

Everyday Technologies in Healthcare

Edited by

Dr Christopher M. Hayre
Assistant Professor: Medical Imaging
Visiting Senior Fellow: School of Health Sciences,
University of Suffolk, United Kingdom

&

Professor Dave J. Muller
Visiting Professor of Rehabilitation Psychology,
University of Suffolk, United Kingdom

&

Editor-in-Chief: Disability and Rehabilitation Journal.

Professor Marcia J. Scherer
President of the Institute for Matching Person and Technology
Editor-in-Chief: Disability & Rehabilitation:
Assistive Technology, United States

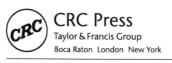

CRC Press is an imprint of the
Taylor & Francis Group, an **informa** business

CRC Press
Taylor & Francis Group
6000 Broken Sound Parkway NW, Suite 300
Boca Raton, FL 33487-2742

First issued in paperback 2023

ISBN 13: 978-1-032-65328-0 (pbk)
ISBN 13: 978-1-138-49170-0 (hbk)
ISBN 13: 978-1-351-03218-6 (ebk)

DOI: 10.1201/9781351032186

Library of Congress Cataloging-in-Publication Data

Names: Hayre, Christopher M., editor. | Mèuller, Dave J., editor. | Scherer, Marcia J. (Marcia Joslyn), 1948- editor.
Title: Everyday technology in healthcare / edited by Dr. Christopher M. Hayre, Professor Dave J. Muller, Professor Marcia J. Scherer.
Description: Boca Raton : Taylor & Francis, 2019. | Includes bibliographical references.
Identifiers: LCCN 2019010548| ISBN 9781138491700 (hardback : alk. paper) | ISBN 9781351032186 (ebook)
Subjects: | MESH: Biomedical Enhancement | Communication Aids for Disabled | Rehabilitation Research | Self-Help Devices | Disabled Persons—rehabilitation
Classification: LCC HV1569.5 | NLM W 82 | DDC 617/.033—dc23
LC record available at https://lccn.loc.gov/2019010548

Visit the Taylor & Francis Web site at
http://www.taylorandfrancis.com

and the CRC Press Web site at
http://www.crcpress.com

Dr Christopher M. Hayre would like to dedicate this book to his wife Charlotte for her ongoing support and commitment. He would also like to dedicate this book to his daughters Ayva, and the twins, Evelynn and Ellena. Love to all.

Professor Dave J. Muller would like to dedicate this to his extended family with love, Pam, Emily, Lucy, Tasha, Harlie, Toby, Edie, Kaya and Freya.

Professor Marcia J. Scherer would like to dedicate this to her husband and colleagues from whom she continues to learn so much. Further, she dedicates this to the users and providers of today and tomorrow in their quest to employ technologies wisely and in ways that add quality to life.

Collectively the editors congratulate one another for completing a worthwhile and enjoyable collaborative project.

Contents

Preface.. xi
Acknowledgements xiii
Editors... xv
Contributors... xvii

Section 1   Introductory Perspective

1. Everyday Technology in Healthcare: An Introduction........................... 3
   Christopher M. Hayre, Dave J. Muller, and Marcia J. Scherer

Section 2   Contemporary Applications in Healthcare

2. Therapy through Play: Advancing the Role of Robotics in
   Paediatric Rehabilitation 11
   S. Lindsay, L. Rampertab, and C.J. Curran

3. Alzheimer's and mHealth: Regulatory, Privacy and Ethical
   Considerations.. 31
   Bonnie Kaplan and Sofia Ranchordás

4. Exergaming for Health and Fitness Application............................... 53
   Maziah Mat Rosly, Hadi Mat Rosly, and Mark Halaki

5. Technology Solutions and Programs to Promote Leisure and
   Communication Activities with People with Intellectual and
   other Disabilities 71
   Giulio E. Lancioni, Nirbhay N. Singh, Mark F. O'Reilly, and Jeff Sigafoos

6. Using Digital Photography to Support the Communication of
   People with Aphasia, Dementia or Cognitive-Communication
   Deficits 89
   Karen Hux and Carly Dinnes

7. Common and Assistive Technology to Support People with Specific Learning Disabilities to Access Healthcare............................ 109
Dianne Chambers and Sharon Campbell

8. Pervasive and Emerging Technologies and Consumer Motivation... 123
David Banes

9. Feedback-Based Technologies for Adult Physical Rehabilitation.... 143
Leanne Hassett, Natalie Allen, and Maayken van den Berg

10. Engaging Young Children in Speech and Language Therapy via Videoconferencing 175
Stuart Ekberg, Sandra Houen, Belinda Fisher, Maryanne Theobald, and Susan Danby

11. Digital Communication and Social Media for People with Communicative and Cognitive Disabilities 193
Margret Buchholz, Ulrika Ferm, and Kristina Holmgren

12. Mobile Technology to Facilitate Self-Management and Independence among Adolescents and Young Adults with Disabilities – Best Practices and the State of the Science.................. 213
Michelle A. Meade and Marisa J. Perera

13. Principles and Practical Uses of Virtual Reality Games as a Physical Therapy Strategy 235
Lorena Cruz, Felipe Augusto dos Santos Mendes, Silvia Gonçalves Ricci Neri, and Rodrigo Luiz Carregaro

14. Project Career: The Matching Person and Technology Model and Everyday Technology in Action.. 259
Deborah Minton, Elaine Sampson, Amanda Nardone, and Callista Stauffer

15. Everyday Communication and Cognition Technologies.................... 271
Jerry K. Hoepner and Thomas W. Sather

16. Mobile Technology in Aphasia Rehabilitation: Current Trends and Lessons Learnt... 293
Caitlin Brandenburg and Emma Power

17. Technology Acceptance, Adoption, and Usability: Arriving at
Consistent Terminologies and Measurement Approaches 319
Lili Liu, Antonio Miguel Cruz, and Adriana Maria Rios Rincon

18. Artificial Intelligence 339
Hadi Mat Rosly and Maziah Mat Rosly

Index 355

Preface

This book presents the collaborative work of experienced researchers world-wide. It brings together an array of practitioners and researchers who are utilising everyday technology in order to enhance health and rehabilitative outcomes for patients. The studies demonstrate an array of opportunities that exist by utilising everyday technology within a number of contexts. Not only does this book present empiricism pertinent to health disciplines, but it also offers prospective researchers methodological insights and how these may resonate within other disciplines. Importantly, this book does not explore advancing technology and how this is impacting health outcomes, but examines technology that is readily accessible to consumers in society, which we term 'everyday'. By examining such works, it is anticipated that this text will have greater impact because the technology remains accessible to many.

This book examines the role of everyday technology throughout the life cycle in order to demonstrate the wide acceptance and impact of everyday technology and how it is facilitating both practitioners and patients in contemporary practices. In response, then, this text speaks to a number of audiences. Students writing for undergraduate and postgraduate dissertations/proposals will find the array of works insightful, supported with a vast number of references signposting to key texts. For academics, practitioners and prospective researchers this text offers key empirical and methodological insight that can help focus and uncover originality in their own field.

This proffered text begins with an introductory chapter by the editors. In this chapter, we detail the value of everyday technology in society. This sets the scene by demonstrating the upward trend of smart devices and how they already impact on our lives in general. Introducing the theoretical lens, actor-network theory (ANT), the editors feel this provides an overarching framework to the text, accepting that technology and a person remain equal and interconnected. Then, subsequent chapters from a number of internationally recognized scholars demonstrate pertinent empiricism by examining the role of everyday technology and how it enhances health conditions.

We anticipate that readers will find the collection of empirical examples useful for informing their own work, but also, it attempts to ignite new discussions and arguments regarding the application and use of everyday technology for enhancing health internationally.

Christopher M. Hayre

Dave J. Muller

Marcia J. Scherer

Acknowledgements

The editors would like to thank all contributing authors for sharing their innovative work on everyday technology. Your commitment to this book reflects the hard work undertaken, and it has been a pleasure for us to work with you and bring together this collection of sound work. The work demonstrated by the authors demonstrates the multifaceted application of technology, enhancing outcomes for individuals. This has been a thoroughly enjoyable and worthwhile project, which we hope readers will enjoy.

Editors

Dr Christopher M. Hayre is an assistant professor in Medical Imaging, positioned in the Institute of Applied Technology, Abu Dhabi, United Arab Emirates. After 10 years working clinically as a radiographer, he pursued a PhD exploring the impact of advancing technology and completed this in 2015. He has published an array of academic work in leading journals pertinent to medical imaging. In 2016, he founded the *Journal of Social Science & Allied Health Professions* and is now editor. He is currently involved in a number of scholarly projects involving dementia, virtual reality, everyday technology, personalized medicine, dose optimisation (X-rays) and artificial intelligence. He has recently been made editor of a CRC book series titled Medical Imaging Practices.

Professor Dave J. Muller is currently editor of the CRC series with Professor Marcia J. Scherer on Rehabilitation Science in Practice. He was founding editor of the journal *Aphasiology* and is currently editor in chief of the journal *Disability and Rehabilitation*. He has published over 40 refereed papers and has been involved either as series editor, editor or author of over 50 books. He is a visiting professor at the University of Suffolk, United Kingdom.

Dr. Marcia J. Scherer is president of the Institute for Matching Person & Technology as well as professor of Physical Medicine and Rehabilitation at the University of Rochester Medical Center in Rochester, New York. She is editor of the journal *Disability and Rehabilitation: Assistive Technology*. She is co-editor of the book series for CRC Press, *Rehabilitation Science in Practice Series*. Dr. Scherer has authored, edited, or co-edited eleven book titles and has published over 85 articles in peer-reviewed journals, 50 published proceedings papers and 35 book chapters on disability and technology.

Contributors

Natalie Allen
Discipline of Physiotherapy,
    Faculty of Health Sciences
The University of Sydney
Sydney, Australia

David Banes
David Banes Access and
    Inclusion Services Ltd
Milton Keynes, United
    Kingdom

Caitlin Brandenburg
Office for Research Governance
    and Development
Gold Coast Health
Queensland, Australia

Margret Buchholz
Department of Health and
    Rehabilitation
Institute of Neuroscience and
    Physiology, Sahlgrenska
    Academy, University of
    Gothenburg
and
DART Centre for AAC and
    AT, Queen Silvia Children's
    Hospital
Sahlgrenska University Hospital
Göteborg, Sweden

Sharon Campbell
La Trobe University
Melbourne, Australia

Rodrigo Luiz Carregaro
School of Physical Therapy
Universidade de Brasília (UnB),
    Campus UnB Ceilândia
and
Master's Programme in
    Rehabilitation Sciences
Universidade de Brasília (UnB)
Brasília, Brazil

Dianne Chambers
School of Education
University of Notre Dame Australia,
    Fremantle Campus
Fremantle, Australia

Antonio Miguel Cruz
Faculty of Rehabilitation Medicine
Department of Occupational
    Therapy
University of Alberta
and
Glenrose Rehabilitation Hospital
Edmonton, Alberta, Canada

Lorena Cruz
Centro Universitário do Planalto
    Central Apparecido dos Santos
    (UNICEPLAC)
Brasília, Brazil

C.J. Curran
Holland Bloorview Kids
    Rehabilitation Hospital
Toronto, Ontario, Canada

Susan Danby
School of Early Childhood &
  Inclusive Education
Queensland University of
  Technology
and
Centre for Children's Health
  Research
Brisbane, Australia

Carly Dinnes
Department of Communication
  Sciences and Disorders
College of Health and Human
  Services
Bowling Green State University
Bowling Green, Ohio

Carly Dinnes
Department of Special Education
  and Communication Disorder
Bowling Green State University
Bowling Green, Ohio

Felipe Augusto dos Santos Mendes
School of Physical Therapy
Universidade de Brasília (UnB),
  Campus UnB Ceilândia
and
Master's Programme in
  Rehabilitation Sciences
Universidade de Brasília (UnB)
Brasília, Brazil

Stuart Ekberg
School of Psychology & Counselling
and
Institute of Health & Biomedical
  Innovation
Queensland University of
  Technology
and
Centre for Children's Health
  Research
Brisbane, Australia

Ulrika Ferm
DART Centre for AAC and AT,
  Queen Silvia Children's Hospital
Sahlgrenska University Hospital
Göteborg, Sweden

Belinda Fisher
School of Health & Rehabilitation
  Sciences
University of Queensland
Brisbane, Australia

Mark Halaki
Discipline of Exercise and Sport
  Science
Faculty of Health Sciences
The University of Sydney
Sydney, Australia

Leanne Hassett
Discipline of Physiotherapy, Faculty
  of Health Sciences/Institute for
  Musculoskeletal Health, School
  of Public Health, Faculty of
  Medicine & Health
The University of Sydney
Sydney, Australia

Christopher M. Hayre
Medical Imaging
Institute of Applied Technology
Abu Dhabi, United Arab Emirates
and
University of Suffolk
Suffolk, United Kingdom

Jerry K. Hoepner
Department of Communication
  Sciences and Disorders
University of Wisconsin
Eau Claire, Wisconsin

Kristina Holmgren
Department of Health and
  Rehabilitation
Institute of Neuroscience and
  Physiology, Sahlgrenska
  Academy, University of
  Gothenburg
Göteborg, Sweden

Sandra Houen
School of Early Childhood &
  Inclusive Education
Queensland University of
  Technology
Brisbane, Australia

Karen Hux
Psychology Department
Quality Living, Inc.
Omaha, Nebraska

Bonnie Kaplan
Yale Center for Medical
  Informatics
Yale Bioethics Center Scholar
Yale Information Society Project
  Faculty Affiliated Fellow
Yale Biomedical Ethics Center
  Faculty Affiliate
Solomon Center for Health Law and
  Policy Faculty Affiliate
Yale University
New Haven, Connecticut

Giulio E. Lancioni
Department of Neuroscience and
  Sense Organs
University of Bari
Bari, Italy

S. Lindsay
Bloorview Research Institute
Holland Bloorview Kids
  Rehabilitation Hospital
and
Department of Occupational
  Science & Occupational Therapy
University of Toronto
Toronto, Ontario, Canada

Lili Liu
School of Public Health and Health
  Systems
Faculty of Applied Health
  Sciences
University of Waterloo
Waterloo, Ontario, Canada
and
Department of Occupational
  Therapy
Faculty of Rehabilitation Medicine
University of Alberta
Edmonton, Alberta, Canada

Michelle A. Meade
Department of Physical Medicine
  and Rehabilitation
University of Michigan
Ann Arbor, Michigan

Deborah Minton
Center for Innovation in Transition
  and Employment
Kent State University
Kent, Ohio, United states

Dave J. Muller
University of Suffolk
Suffolk, United Kingdom
and
Disability and Rehabilitation
    Journal, United States

Amanda Nardone
Sargent College of Health and
    Rehabilitation Sciences,
Boston University
Boston, Massachusetts

Silvia Gonçalves Ricci Neri
College of Physical Education
Universidade de Brasília, (UnB)
Brasília, Brazil

Mark F. O'Reilly
Department of Special Education
University of Texas at Austin
Austin, Texas

Marisa Perera
Department of Psychology
University of Miami
Miami, Florida

Emma Power
Speech Pathology
Graduate School of Health
University of Technology Sydney
New South Wales, Australia
and
Speech Pathology
Faculty of Health Sciences
University of Sydney
New South Wales, Australia

Lynn Rampertab
Holland Bloorview Kids
    Rehabilitation Hospital
Toronto, Ontario, Canada

Sofia Ranchordás
University of Groningen
Groningen, The Netherlands
and
Leiden Law School
Leiden University
Leiden, The Netherlands
and
Information Society Project
Yale Law School
New Haven, Connecticut

Adriana Maria Rios Rincon
Department of Occupational
    Therapy
Faculty of Rehabilitation Medicine
University of Alberta
Edmonton, Alberta, Canada

Maziah Mat Rosly
Department of Physiology
Faculty of Medicine
University of Malaya
Kuala Lumpur, Malaysia

Hadi Mat Rosly
Department of Mechatronics
    Engineering
Faculty of Engineering
International Islamic University
    Malaysia
Malaysia

Maziah Mat Rosly
Department of Physiology
Faculty of Medicine
University of Malaya
Kuala Lumpur, Malaysia

Elaine Sampson
West Virginia University
Morgantown, West Virginia

Thomas W. Sather
Department of Communication
Sciences and Disorders
University of Wisconsin
and
Rehabilitation Services
Mayo Health Systems
Eau Claire, Wisconsin

Marcia J. Scherer
Institute for Matching Person and
Technology
Webster, New York

Jeff Sigafoos
School of Education
Victoria University of Wellington
Wellington, New Zealand

Nirbhay N. Singh
Medical College of Georgia
Augusta University
Augusta, Georgia

Callista Stauffer
Center for Innovation in Transition
and Employment
Kent State University
Kent, Ohio, United states

Maryanne Theobald
School of Early Childhood &
Inclusive Education
Queensland University of
Technology
Brisbane, Australia

Maayken van den Berg
College of Medicine and Public
Health/College of Nursing and
Health Sciences
Flinders University
Adelaide, South Australia

Section 1

Introductory Perspective

1

Everyday Technology in Healthcare: An Introduction

Christopher M. Hayre
Institute of Applied Technology
University of Suffolk

Dave J. Muller
University of Suffolk

Marcia J. Scherer
Institute for Matching Person and Technology

CONTENTS

The Value of Everyday Technology in Contemporary Society..........................3
Conceptual Importance of ANT for Health Research...5
Summary 7
References 8

The Value of Everyday Technology in Contemporary Society

In the last decade, the use of what we term 'everyday technology' includes (and is not limited to) smartphones, smartwatches, tablets, computers and gaming consoles and have all rapidly excelled in use worldwide. In 2013, smartphone sales surpassed those of regular cell phones opening up different channels of smartphone applications, social media, photo/video sharing, whilst enhancing virtual interactions of forums and blogs. More recently, we have seen increasing use of smartwatches. Rawassizadeh et al. (2015) identified the approximate growth of smartwatch sales reaching 214 million by 2018 and penetrating health research since 2014, enabling technical function, supported with acceptability and effectiveness in order to enhance the everyday life of individuals. Due to this rapid acceleration, smartwatches are now becoming widely integrated into healthcare systems whereby patient data is remotely synchronised enhancing holistic treatment of patients across an array of clinical contexts. A recent example by Reeder and David (2016) recognised the utility of smartwatches within the intensive care unit. Whilst on the one hand, the authors warn of the possibility for cross-contamination of such devices amongst healthcare professionals, it is also acknowledged that introducing a smartwatch to patients can offer little cross-contamination and thus enable instant data transfer, which can be monitored remotely.

The increasing use of everyday technology within society identifies its multifaceted use, enhancing societal interconnectivity. Moreover, Friedman (2009) suggests that a person working in partnership with technology is generally assumed to be 'better' when compared to an individual unassisted. From a sociocultural perspective the first author reflects on his own sociocultural experiences, following a recent move outside of the United Kingdom, whereby his own smartphone device remained pivotal for him and his family, living and working in a new part of the world. For example, the ability to instantly message and video call family and friends at a time when physically restricted from one another was welcomed. In addition, whilst the smartphone facilitated connectivity with family and friends, it enabled him to keep abreast of news, sustained collaboration with academic peers, helped manage international finances, and possibly more importantly, locate nearby hospitals/clinics, pharmacists, and supermarkets when needed. Reflecting on the use of smartphone device offered virtues that may have led to sociocultural challenges.

This utilisation of smartphones is also evident in other contexts. A study by Kaufmann (2018) examined the use of smartphone use amongst refugees fleeing Syria following civil unrest. The study found that when large numbers of Syrian refugees left their homes, the ability to instantly message family and friends in 'group chats' using WhatsApp enabled a transnational digital community, facilitating the movement of refugees into cities in Central and Western Europe. In this example, smartphones offered many ways to stay in touch and overcome restrictions of physical space, which the study terms 'ordinary co-presence', whereby maintaining a virtual space is achieved for family members across continents (ibid.). In short, the benefits of smartphones have transnational impact, supporting the view that smartphones are simply more than a digital tool – but a device that can impact on an individual's health and well-being. In addition, the work by Kaufmann (2018) offers methodological considerations in light of using everyday technology. For example, due to the researchers inability to meet some individuals in person, the researcher 'joined' the group chat of Syrian refugees using WhatsApp in order to interact and collect data via a digital platform, leading to what the author deemed mobile instant interviewing. Here, then, this demonstrates that everyday technology not only offers an array of empirical opportunities, but importantly novel methodological considerations for researchers who may be restricted. This supports the claim by Horst and Hjorth (2013, p. 94) that smartphones remain an example of 'personalization par excellence' whereby they have the potential to get close to the everyday lives of people.

On the one hand, we have witnessed how smartphones have facilitated everyday lives of individuals, yet, there are also situations where smartphones are seen to hinder social and educational environments. The former has been recognised in sporting spectacles, in particular, basketball and football matches. It has been claimed fans should 'put down their phones and enjoy the sporting spectacle because people can't clap while they're holding their phones' (Hutchins, 2016, p. 421). Similarly, in the Dutch football league, fans have protested, calling for the cessation of fans checking their phones during matches whereby fans should 'support the team and observe the on-field action unfolding' (ibid., p. 425). The latter concerns smartphone use in educational environments, leading to the rise of new legislation. In July 2018, France passed a law affirming that school children will be required to leave their smartphones switched off or at home (RFI, 2018). The ban for 'smart devices' in France has been applied to pupils up to the age of 14–15; however, although schools can still justify the utilisation of smartphones amongst pupils for pedagogical use, extracurricular activities or for disabled pupils, this new legislation has been claimed to 'move France into the 21st century' (ibid., p. 1). The evidence above offers insight into the potential dichotomy associated with smartphone technology, thus whilst central to uncovering its current uses in healthcare, this text also explores wider everyday technologies that can either facilitate or hinder health outcomes.

The general acceptance and value of smartphone devices is thus challenged leading to question a potential paradox. Turkle (2012, p. 280) recognises this paradox from a social perspective whereby there may be a sense of feeling 'alone together' in social interactions whereby smartphone users remain in constant connectedness with their phones, and as a result rarely have each other's full attention when in each other's company (ibid.). This is argued to lead to social interactions becoming 'pausable' as people stop and look down at their mobile screens to check emails, text, social media updates and application notifications (ibid., p. 161). In response, this book advocates for the use of everyday technology and how it can facilitate an array of health outcomes for individuals. Further, it is acknowledged that the use of everyday technology also demonstrates challenges, thus important to strike a balance between what should become a healthy use of everyday technology and not the demise of social interaction.

Conceptual Importance of ANT for Health Research

Information communication technology (ICT) has become increasingly utilised for information and data transfer in the last decade. This has led to a number of countries implementing and continuously updating ICT systems within healthcare organisations in order to manage and enhance patient safety. The use of digitally enabled technologies facilitating exchange of clinical and administrative healthcare is generally accepted, offering value to all actors operating within healthcare environments. Whilst this remains central, this book focuses on the use of ICT that is not necessarily inherent within all healthcare organisations. For example, smartphones, smartwatches, tablets and computer gaming consoles are readily available and already owned by consumers, which offers a unique perspective in how this technology can be utilised by health organisations, without purchasing equipment.

In order to critically examine the role of technology and its role on enhancing health outcomes, the concept of ANT is discussed. ANT focuses on non-human entities and its effects on social lives. For example, an 'actor' within the ANT model is defined as the 'source of an action regardless of its status as a human or non-human' (Cresswell et al., 2010, p. 2). One important feature of ANT is the move away from the idea that technology impacts on humans as an external force, and is replaced with the concept that technology emerged from the social interests of individuals, thus shaping social interactions (Prout, 1996). This leads ANT to be considered as an 'ethno-methodology' as indicated by Latour (2005, p. 72) affirming that:

> ANT is not the empty claim that objects do things, instead of human actors: it simply says that no science of the social can start if the enquiry into who participate in the action is not first discovered.

ANT is typically aligned with its own epistemology and ontology, whereby the world consists of multiple networks, which may include human ideas and concepts, a concept typically aligned to social constructivism whereby the lives of individuals and everyday technology can have multifaceted impact on various individuals (Law, 1992). Further, by critically engaging with the ANT concept it enables the unification of the two overarching concepts inherent within this book – the use of everyday technology and its impact on humans. Theoretically, then, ANT accepts the social connection and equal influence of technology as it now becomes increasingly interconnected into the social lives of individuals. This is evident whereby the majority of individuals now interact with some form of technological device within their daily lives. By reflecting on the first author's experience, we have witnessed how everyday technology is able to connect with family and friends on both practical and emotional levels, thus central to accepting its equal value in contemporary health environments.

The ANT model importantly bridges the rise of everyday technology and human participation demonstrating both social and technological facets. Thus, it could be argued that this book is not only exploring the virtue of everyday technology for health conditions, but also explores the social constructs of multiple realities that remain both complex and fluid. A principal acknowledgement of this text accepts the interconnectivity and necessity of two principal actors: human beings and technology and how this fusion offers opportunities for individuals.

ANT offers an overarching framework of this book that may help interlink technology with pertinent phenomena. In addition, the emergence and development of technology is arguably leading us to become increasingly reliant upon everyday technology, and not simply for social purposes, but for the sustainability of good health. This leads us to acknowledge a paradigm shift in healthcare, whereby the everyday use of technology for organisations can also enable sound outcomes. Further, as technology becomes increasingly accessible and more affordable for consumers, it is likely to play an increasingly pivotal role to users worldwide when it comes to improving individual lives. Thus, by adopting an ANT lens, it can help infer greater understandings of both human and technological change in society, rather than simply considering each as a separate entity. It is therefore anticipated that this book can critically reflect, adapt and welcome innovative technological applications into the health environment and offer discussions outlining both opportunities and challenges.

Summary

This introductory chapter has outlined two key points, which is anticipated to help contextualise the book. First, the authors reflect on the existing effects of what we deem 'everyday technology'. We have identified the sharp rise in consumer ownership of everyday technology and how this now impacts on the social lives of individuals, including that of the author following a recent move overseas. Whilst some evidence highlights social challenges with the use of everyday technology, there is a general acceptance that everyday technology offers practical and emotional virtues, whereby it connects people and aids other facets of our lives. In short, we accept that everyday technology is not only able to enhance social outcomes, but also enhance the outcomes for health conditions, which remains the general focus of this book.

Next, we introduced ANT, a theoretical model that identifies human beings and technology as equal actors. We have argued how this theoretical and ethnomethodological lens can help contextualise the forthcoming work by authors transnationally. Further, as everyday technology continues to develop, it is generally accepted that technology will remain a key actor for practitioners, researchers and patients alike in future years, thus requiring a lens that enables critical appraisal of the use of everyday technology and how it impacts on the health outcomes of individuals.

References

Cresswell, K.M., Worth, A., & Sheikh, A. (2010) Actor-Network Theory and its role in understanding the implementation of information technology developments in healthcare. *BMC Medical Informatics and Decisions Making.* 10(67), pp. 1–11.

Friedman, C.P. (2009) A 'Fundamental Theorem' of biomedical informatics. *Journal of American Medical Informatics Association.* 16(2), p. 169.

Horst, H., & Hjorth, L. (2013) Engaging practices: Doing personalized media. In S. Price, C. Jewitt, & B. Brown (Eds.), *The Sage Handbook of Digital Technology Research* (pp. 87–101). London: SAGE.

Hutchins, B. (2016) We don't need no stinking smartphones!' Live stadium sports events, mediatization, and the non-use of mobile media. *Media, Culture and Society.* 38(3), pp. 420–436.

Kaufmann, K. (2018) Navigating a new life: Syrian refugees and their smartphones in Vienna. *Information, Communication and Society.* 21(6), pp. 882–898.

Latour, B. (2005) *Reassembling the Social: An Introduction to Actor-Network Theory.* Oxford: Oxford University Press.

Law, J. (1992) Notes on the Theory of the Actor-Network: Ordering, strategy and heterogeneity. *Systems Practice.* 5, pp. 379–393.

Prout, A. (1996) Actor-network theory, technology and medical sociology: An illustrative analysis of the metered dose inhaler. *Sociology of Health and Illness.* 18, pp. 198–219.

Rawassizadeh, R., Price, B.A., & Petre, M. (2015) Wearables: Has the age of smart-watches finally arrived? *Communication of the ACM.* 58(1), pp. 45–47.

Reeder, B., & David, A. (2016) Health at hand: A systematic review of smart watch uses for health and wellness. *Journal of Biomedical Informatics.* 63, pp. 269–276.

RFI English Ed. (2018) Society – France outlaw smartphone use in schools. *Paris SyndiGate Media Inc.* [Online] Available at: https://search.proquest.com/docview/2079813733?accountid=17074 (Accessed: January 22nd 2019).

Turkle, S. (2012) *Alone Together: Why we Expect More from Technology and Less from Each Other.* New York: Basic Book.

Section 2

Contemporary Applications in Healthcare

2

Therapy through Play: Advancing the Role of Robotics in Paediatric Rehabilitation

S. Lindsay

Holland Bloorview Kids Rehabilitation Hospital

University of Toronto

L. Rampertab and C.J. Curran

Holland Bloorview Kids Rehabilitation Hospital

CONTENTS

Introduction 12
Objectives 13
Development of an Adapted Group-Based Robotics Programme for
Children with Disabilities 13
    HB FIRST® Robotics Programme 15
Implementation of the HB FIRST® Robotics Programme 17
Adaptations to the Programme 18
    LEGO® Digital Designer 18
    Vocabulary Tools 18
    Visual Schedules 19
    Selection Mats 19
    Digital Instructions for Visual Differences 19
    Communicator 5 Used with Switches 19
Perceived Impacts of the Programme 20
How Everyday Technologies Can Enhance Healthcare Delivery 20
How does Everyday Technology Impact on Practitioners 22
    Fine Motor Skills 22
    Social, Communication and Teamwork Skills 22
    Self-Advocacy, Self-Esteem and Problem-Solving 23
    Career Exploration 24
Impact of Programme on Clinical Staff 25
Future Impact of the Programme 27
Summary 28
References 28

Introduction

Play is a childhood occupation, which is an important aspect of a child's development (Brodin and Lindstrand, 2000) that is recognized by the International Classification of Functioning (World Health Organization, 2007). Play skills help children to initiate and maintain communication skills with peers, develop self-determination, decision-making and problem-solving skills (Case-Smith and O'Brien, 2010; Harkness and Bundy, 2001; Porter et al., 2009; Rios-Rincon et al., 2016). Play can also promote the development of cognition, language and social competence (Nicolopoulou et al., 2009) while enhancing learning and providing a context for intervention strategies for other therapy goals (Morrison et al., 2002).

Exploring how children with disabilities play is important because they engage in free play less often than children without disabilities do, and encounter more barriers in the type and frequency of play activities (Harper et al., 2008; Rios-Rincon et al., 2016; Rubin and Howe, 1985). Such patterns are disconcerting because limited play among children can lead to poor self-esteem and social isolation (Couch et al., 1998; Miller and Reid, 2003). Therefore, having an environment that supports exploration, socialization and learning may help to develop play skills among children with disabilities (Howard et al., 2012). Although play is an important way to motivate children, it is underutilized as a therapeutic intervention (Couch et al., 1998; Majnemer et al., 2008).

A promising play-based intervention is using such mediums as LEGO® MINDSTORM® and WeDo 2.0 that embed technology into playful activity (Lo et al., 2009; Lindsay and Lam, 2018). LEGO® is a familiar toy and is also sufficiently novel when it is incorporated with a robotics component to enhance exploration and development of play (LeGoff and Sherman, 2006). Promoting play skills through the use of robots as a form of therapy has been gaining momentum to increase children's participation (Adams and Cook, 2014). Although research in this area is growing, most robotics programmes are designed for children without disabilities. Few studies to date have explored play within an adapted, group-based, hands-on robotics programme for children with disabilities (Lindsay and Lam, 2018). Having such an approach can help children to learn about science, technology, engineering and math (STEM), an area where people with disabilities are chronically under-represented. By encouraging students to pursue STEM disciplines at an early age through programmes offered outside of the school curriculum can help to build on STEM awareness and potential careers for the future. With the need for more specialized knowledge in the growing fields of information technology, programmes like this become even more important in sparking an interest in STEM.

Objectives

The aim of this chapter is to describe the development and implementation of an adapted group-based robotics programme for children with disabilities, and their experiences within it. Drawing on interviews with staff and children in the programme, this chapter discusses the evolution and development of an adapted group-based robotics programme within a paediatric rehabilitation hospital. Secondly, we explore the perceived impacts of the programme from the perspectives of clinicians and staff implementing the programme and the children engaged in it. Finally, we consider the future impact of the programme, and in particular, how we are building capacity to expand the programme to other sites in the broader community.

Development of an Adapted Group-Based Robotics Programme for Children with Disabilities

We draw on a document review (i.e. meeting minutes, field notes and first-hand experience of the Robotics Co-ordinator and a Director from the rehabilitation hospital delivering the programme) to describe the development and implementation of the HB FIRST® robotics programme. FIRST® (For Inspiration and Recognition of Science and Technology) is a non-profit organization that operates after-school robotics programmes for young people ages 6–18 internationally (FIRST® Robotics Canada, 2015). The mission of FIRST® is to inspire young people to be science and technology leaders, by engaging them in exciting mentor-based programmes that build science, engineering and technology skills, that inspire innovation and that foster well-rounded capacities including self-confidence, communication and leadership.

Holland Bloorview Kids Rehabilitation Hospital provides specialized programmes and clinical care to children with disabilities, which helps them to participate fully in life. Such programmes include cutting-edge research with frontline care to improve the lives of children with disabilities and their families. Within the Centre for Leadership in Participation and Inclusion at Holland Bloorview, a continuum of evidence-informed inpatient, ambulatory and community-integrated services are offered for children and youth with disabilities up to the age of 18 years. Programmes are designed to enhance the quality of life and support optimal transitions across the lifespan for children and youth and their family's specialized services include therapeutic recreation. All individual and group services are specifically tailored to the needs of the individual child and are integrated within larger rehabilitation pathways.

Holland Bloorview Kids Rehabilitation Hospital partnered with FIRST®
Robotics Canada to develop an adapted program (HB FIRST® Robotics) to
provide children with disabilities an opportunity to explore STEM while
also working on therapy goals (Lindsay and Hounsell, 2017). We did this
by adapting a group-based robotics programme that provides experience-
based opportunities with the aim to build self-confidence, independence,
communication, teamwork and STEM skills (Lindsay and Hounsell, 2017).
As an initial step for developing the programme, social scientists lead the
collaborative process, which included clinicians, educators, government and
community groups and families and youth.

The mission of the HB FIRST® robotics programme is to create a program
that teaches building and programming skills using engineering design principles in a social setting that strengthens critical thinking, problem-solving,
teamwork and encourages self-confidence and independence. In developing
the program, we considered the adaptations that were needed to make the
program accessible. It was the first STEM-based programme in the local community that was specifically designed for children with disabilities. A main
challenge was recognizing the varied needs of children that had various types
of disabilities such as autism, cerebral palsy, muscular dystrophy, acquired
brain injury, spinal cord injuries among other developmental conditions. This
meant that each child's specific needs had to be assessed along with an individualized learning strategy to help ensure their success in the programme.

Programme administrators decided that therapeutic recreation specialists
were well suited to deliver programs such as HB FIRST® robotics because
of their underlying principles recognizing leisure, recreation and play as
integral components of quality of life (Carruthers and Hood, 2007). Their
therapy is directed towards functional interventions, leisure, education
and participation opportunities that is designed to restore, remediate and
rehabilitate a person's level of functioning and independence in life activities to promote health and wellness while reducing or eliminating activity
limitations (Carruthers and Hood, 2007). Therapeutic recreation specialists
are trained to show appreciation and respect for individuals and groups,
including recognizing and celebrating diversity in childhood development
(Carruthers and Hood, 2007). They do not equate disability with pathology
and are sensitive to extending the notion of recognizing common worth
through universal programmes (Carruthers and Hood, 2007).

Some of the facilitation strategies that therapeutic recreation specialists
employ are to ensure a fully integrated experience include developmental
recognition, nurturing the talents, skills, capacities and choices of children
(Carruthers and Hood, 2007; Stumbo and Peterson, 1998). In this sense,
utilizing therapeutic recreation specialists to co-facilitate the HB FIRST®
robotics programme helps to ensure group engagement and programmes
that are growth-promoting and challenging, rather than custodial in their
approach (Carruthers and Hood, 2007). Further, within this model of care,
sharing physical and social space offers opportunities for social interactions

and a culture that promotes both friendship and comradery (Carruthers and Hood, 2007). With their specialized training in facilitating group programmes and their expertise in integrating children into an activity, we felt that therapeutic recreation specialists were a natural fit with delivering FIRST® core values (FIRST® Robotics Canada, 2015) into a model of practice where the primary value being one of fun and social opportunity.

HB FIRST® Robotics Programme

The programme involved two separate age groups, juniors, aged 6–8 and intermediates, aged 9–14 (see Table 2.1 for program overview). The junior group involves approximately ten children who work in pairs or groups of three along with a clinical staff member (i.e. therapeutic recreation specialist) and approximately five volunteers who have knowledge of robotics

TABLE 2.1

Overview of HB FIRST® Robotics Programmes

	Junior Ages 6–10 Years*	Intermediate Ages 9–14 Years*
Level 1	This programme is designed to engage and motivate children's interest in learning STEM, which is done through motorized LEGO® models and simple programming. WeDo 2.0 supports a hands-on, 'minds on' learning solution that gives children the confidence to ask questions and to solve real-life problems through testing and evaluating solutions and solving problems	This programme is designed to introduce children to the world of STEM and expose them to discovering robotics, mechanisms and simple machines, programming and use of engineering design practices and mobility of systems of robots. This programme is filled with challenges that allow the children to apply their knowledge
Level 2	This programme focuses on the technologies that people face each day. At every lesson children make a new robot with specific functions. It starts with a problem that children should solve using new knowledge, skills, teamwork and creativity. Embedded in this course are more complex building requirements and programming	This programme is designed for children who have taken level 1 programme. The main objective is to continue to enrich and challenge children's knowledge and skills through a more comprehensive understanding of the mechanical, design, build and programming aspects regarding the MINDSTORMS® in real world challenges

(Continued)

TABLE 2.1 (*Continued*)

Overview of HB FIRST® Robotics Programmes

		Junior Ages 6–10 Years*	Intermediate Ages 9–14 Years*
Girls in STEM		The programme was created to provide a comfortable space for young girls to explore and ignite enthusiasm in STEM and build self-confidence in their ability to achieve success in STEM-based subjects. All of our robotics programmes foster problem-solving and critical thinking. This programme is open to young girls with disabilities aged 6–142	
Size of group		Maximum of ten children per class	
Staffing	Therapeutic recreation	One therapeutic staff (Therapeutic Recreational Specialist or Assistant) per class to oversee children's needs, implement learning strategies and facilitating goals set by children	
	Teaching leads	One per class to teach class curriculum	
	Volunteers		
Timing		2 h per week for 6 weeks	
Kits used		WeDo 2.0 kits + *i*Pads LEGO® Build to express kits	MINDSTORM® EV3
Skills learned and class components		1. **Icebreaker.** Each class begins with an icebreaker activity, which is typically run by therapeutic recreational staff. These interactive and often fun sessions run before the main lesson, and help the children get to know each other and the purpose of the class. The icebreaker is an activity or game that is used to welcome and warm up the conversation among participants in the classroom. 2. **Build to Express activity.** This lasts for 30 min and the methodology is about learning to express themselves while learning to listen to others. Build to express is a teaching process that combines a facilitative order thinking by combining LEGO® model building with open-ended questions.	1. **Icebreaker.** Each class begins with an icebreaker activity. 2. **Small activities.** Each week, small activities help drive home the learning objectives. These build the knowledge of using strong multipurpose structures and programming skills. Children test out each step of this process to better understand the concepts. They are then presented with a challenge for the day. Using the knowledge learned during the lesson, they must apply, test and evaluate their solutions. The class usually ends with a challenge.

(Continued)

TABLE 2.1 (*Continued*)

Overview of HB FIRST® Robotics Programmes

	Junior Ages 6–10 Years*	Intermediate Ages 9–14 Years*
	3. **Projects.** Projects use the WeDo 2.0 and are broken down into three parts. The *Explore* phase allows participants to connect to the task; the *Create* phase allows participants to create a working model of the theme; and the *Share* phase, which allows participants to share their discoveries through documentation and presentations. Projects are divided into three main types: investigative, design a solution or based in reality model.	Main concepts learned include: • Introductions to robotics • Engineering design practices • Creating strong structures • Use of sensors • Developing strategies • Meeting the challenge

* Note: in most cases the age range for the junior group was 6–9 but may have occasionally included children aged 10, based on the clinician's assessment of their abilities.

and/or children with disabilities. Over the course of 6 weeks (2 h each week), children build models using WeDo 2.0 while applying math and science concepts (Lindsay and Hounsell, 2017). Meanwhile, within the intermediate group, there are approximately ten children who work in small groups of two or three. They use LEGO® MINDSTORMS® and learn an introduction to robots, mechanisms and simple machines, programming and design, build and testing a robot in a team environment (Lindsay and Hounsell, 2017).

Implementation of the HB FIRST® Robotics Programme

Given the diverse needs of the children our hospital services, those implementing the programme, were met with many challenges in adapting and implementing the programme. A difficulty in developing the program was to recognize that although the learning objectives were similar to FIRST®, they were not identical. Within FIRST® the desired outcome was accomplished through a universal challenge and it culminates with teams attending local competitions. For the HB FIRST® robotics programme, challenges (i.e. programming and building) were embedded as part of the weekly lesson and the competition happened within a classroom learning environment. This was done primarily because local competitions are loud and noisy, have large number of participants and spectators, are meant to be competitive (and can be somewhat stressful) with closed-door judging sessions and official robot competition round matches. All these components represent potential triggers or stressors for some children, which could hinder their experience of the programme. That, coupled with the length of the day, it was decided that a similar competition could be mimicked within a smaller group setting, over a shorter period of time, allowing for more support for children who required it (Lindsay and Hounsell, 2017).

The programme design needed to include enough breadth and depth to meet the needs of children with a wide range of disabilities, which could include both physical and cognitive differences to make it fully accessible and equitable to all participants. Therefore, we could not apply a one-size fits all approach for this programme. Each child is unique in the way they approach their peers, the staff and the programme. We considered how best to engage them with the programme. Addressing this challenge often required input from interdisciplinary team members to ensure full participation (Lindsay and Hounsell, 2017).

Adaptations to the Programme

The main adaptations that were needed to make this programme accessible included LEGO® digital designer, vocabulary tools for children using augmentative and alternative communication devices, visual schedules for children with autism, selection mats for children who needed help with fine motor skills, digital instructions for children with visual impairments and communicator 5 with switches.

LEGO® Digital Designer

The LEGO® digital designer was created by the LEGO® group as design software. As part of the HB FIRST® robotics programme, this was used by children who did not have the ability through hand-over-hand techniques to build LEGO® models but could manipulate a mouse (Lindsay and Hounsell, 2017). We placed a limited set of LEGO® parts on the building palette to save the child's time looking through an extensive library of bricks to find the pieces in the build instructions. In making this adaptation, each child could continue to build in this virtual environment with their partners building the actual models. Children using this adapted method could test and evaluate the model and compete in the challenge (Lindsay and Hounsell, 2017).

Vocabulary Tools

We observed that children using augmentative and alternative communication devices were at a clear disadvantage during class discussion. As their peers answered questions during the teaching portion of the class, their devices had several static buttons and/or screens of categories that did not contain relevant vocabulary for them to participate in a meaningful discussion. Often times, responses were simple and short. Therefore, we developed a set of vocabulary tools to help children utilize these devices more effectively. Parents or staff could preprogramme relevant scientific vocabulary. Using this adaptive strategy reduced the amount of time it took for a child to type in a response and encouraged them to interact in the discussion in real time.

Visual Schedules

We developed visual schedules (i.e. step-by-step overview of the timing of class events), mostly for the children with autism spectrum disorder. Many children had difficulty coping with transitioning from one activity to another within the classroom (e.g. free play versus structured play). Such transitions often triggered anxiety and sometimes challenging and/or disruptive behaviours. Having these schedules on every desk depicting the sequence of events helped children anticipate the transitions, and reduced anxiety (Lindsay and Hounsell, 2017).

Selection Mats

In the HB FIRST® robotics programme, each child works with a partner to build a model based on a scientific concept. Within this team, each member plays a specific role. The designer was the person who finds the pieces and the engineer puts the pieces together from a set of model instructions. Selection mats were developed by an occupational therapist for the programme to help children with low-fine motor skills (Lindsay and Hounsell, 2017). This mat included six cells. A volunteer working with the designer of the pair would put the correct combination of pieces in one cell and incorrect combinations in the other cells. The child was then able to identify the correct combination and pass them to the engineer in the group (Lindsay and Hounsell, 2017).

Digital Instructions for Visual Differences

Many of the children with visual impairments were not totally absent of vision and were able to read under magnified conditions. Therefore, we produced all the build instructions in digital medium, which allowed images and instructions to be enlarged at the discretion of the child (Lindsay and Hounsell, 2017).

Communicator 5 Used with Switches

This adaptation involved an augmentative and alternative communication method used to help supplement the writing of programming language for children using switch-type devices. For example, it allowed the team to create a limited palette of programming blocks used in both the WeDo 2.0 and MINDSTORM® LabView programs. Such youth could then scan through these palettes and select programming blocks that they used to produce specific functions for the robots. Using this communication method also allowed the team to set up a download feature to send the program to the logic bricks and students could test and evaluate programs in real time. The Communicator 5 program was set up to mimic the programming palettes to include action, flow, sensor and data operation blocks. The program was versatile for multiple switches and easily set up. It could be tailored for single users with custom settings. Indeed, many aspects needed to be considered in adapting and implementing the robotics programme for the diverse needs of children with disabilities. Next, we describe the perceived impact of the programme.

Perceived Impacts of the Programme

For this chapter, we draw on the pilot phase of this project that involved observations, survey and semi-structured interviews with 41 participants (i.e. 18 youth aged 6–13 with various physical or developmental disabilities), 12 parents, 11 staff/volunteers involved with developing/implementing the programme (Lindsay and Hounsell, 2017). The methods of this phase are described in detail elsewhere (Lindsay and Hounsell, 2017).

All youth who participated in the programme were invited to take part in the research component (i.e. survey, observations and interview), for which we received ethical approval from a children's hospital and local university. All eligible participants received an information letter and consent form from researchers. The survey asked about what they liked about the program, what they learned and future aspirations for robotics. Our structured observations involved detailed field notes of youth's interactions and engagement in the programme. In-depth interviews were conducted within 1 week of completing the programme. Questions asked about their experiences in the programme. The qualitative data was analysed thematically (Braun and Clarke, 2006). Informed written consent/assent was obtained from all children and their parents (Lindsay and Hounsell, 2017).

How Everyday Technologies Can Enhance Healthcare Delivery

Youth who participated in the programme, their parents and staff leading remarked on how the robotics as an everyday technology helped enhance the clinical environment. In particular, they noted that the robotics programme created a fun environment and opportunity for children with disabilities to develop some of their therapy goals (e.g., social skills, teamwork, communication skills, fine motor; fostering independence; self-advocacy). For example, one staff involved in delivering the programme said, 'It's also very important to get kids together and to have fun and explore' (key informant 7).

This type of programme brings children together to help them engage in an activity that is adapted to their needs and not otherwise offered in the community. For example, a staff member explained,

> We had a lot of clients and families tell us that they find it really difficult to find things they're interested in and that are inclusive. Then they come here and try to find out what they want, and it just seemed that everybody was just so into the program and that science and technology and engineering; This could be something that they focus on and that could be educational but fun for them. So that was great.
>
> *key informant 9*

A parent of a child in the junior programme commented, 'I think the structure was quite good, working with the partner allowed them to really interact, and it lessened any frustration they might have at being stuck on something because they could sort of talk about it; and the idea of a mentor helping them always gave that resource there to make it sort of easier and get through things. So, I think that the structure was very good. Certainly (JFL-08, male, grade 2) enjoyed it every time, and seemed pretty happy with everything, the way it went'.

A key informant (#4) who was involved with developing the program and also dropped in several times to see the kids in action said, 'the actual robots they built were significant, effective in that the kids that were there were very much engaged in the program, very interested in the teaching and the building part, and working together cooperatively extremely well'. Meanwhile, a clinician involved in delivering the robotics programme shared, 'that helps them continue their learning and also to help build confidence; much of the skills we wanted them to build leadership, friendship, all that stuff' (key informant 6). Other staff noted how the programme enabled an environment to develop social skills. For example, one said that turn-taking and behaving properly in a group 'all of those kinds of things could be goals that are supported in this kind of a programme. Our team had also talked about it afterwards, like using the robotics concepts to support some other therapy goals. So, for example using the robotics because it's fun and it's interesting' (key informant 10, Lindsay and Lam: 267). A parent also mentioned that their son learned a lot now about computers, 'teaching them in a way that is educational and fun, is really good' (JFL-02, male, grade 2).

How does Everyday Technology Impact on Practitioners

Youth, parents and staff noted how children participating in the programme enhanced their fine motor, social, communication and teamwork skills, self-advocacy, self-esteem and problem-solving skills while also engaging in career exploration.

Fine Motor Skills

Some of the children in the programme participated as way to develop their fine motor skills. For example, a parent of a child (male, grade 7) explained, 'we were looking for something to help him with his fine motor skills' (IFL-01parent). Another parent of a child (male, grade 5) said, 'It absolutely helped his fine motor skills and built his confidence and that he can actually build something from the beginning to the end from these little loose pieces to a solid wonderful robot, is quite an accomplishment. So, for me, that's a benchmark to always refer back to like you did that in the group and that was terrific' (IFL-05). Clinicians also noted that they helped some children 'work on fine motor skills and that sort of thing' (key informant 10).

Social, Communication and Teamwork Skills

A parent of a child in the junior programme described how the clinician helped him to develop his communication skills within the robotics programme: 'He needed a little one of his extra support because social communication with his peers, being a new setting, is often weak. So, I think the therapeutic rec therapist helped with that' (parent of JFL-04, male, grade 3).

Some children in the intermediate programme expressed that they wanted to join the programme to develop more friendships. For example, one youth in the intermediate programme said, 'I also kind of wanted to be more social with some of the other kids' (IFL-02, female, grade 7). Another youth commented on the social benefits of participating in the programme. Specifically, they mentioned, 'I liked [him] just being there and learning something different in the environment and interacting with other kids as opposed to being at home and on the computer by myself. The interaction was what I enjoyed' (parent of IFL-01, male, grade 7; Lindsay and Hounsell: 701). Other youth agreed, 'my favorite part of this program was getting to collaborate with others and make friends' (IFL-06, male, grade 5). A boy in the junior programme noted that he 'liked playing with others and celebrating the completion of the project' (JFL2–07, male, grade 3).

For many youth in the programme, particularly those with autism, they wanted to participate in this programme to develop their social and communication skills. Parents and clinicians reported noticing how building robots within this programme helped foster children's communication skills.

For example, a parent describes, 'The clinician made changes on the settings (of the robot) and was intrigued by his partners reactions, that they could do different things to kind of get a different reaction out of each other and things like that' (parent of JFL-04, male, grade 3). A staff member involved in implementing the programme commented, 'it was nice to see how it was benefitting the kids...I think there is an undervalued role for (rehabilitation hospital) in facilitating these social encounters' (key informant 5). Another staff member concurred that 'Definitely the biggest one was making friends and socialization' (key informant 9).

Our findings showed that the robotics programme helped youth to develop their teamwork skills. For example, a female in grade 7 within the intermediate programme mentioned, 'I liked the teamwork...that we were always working in groups and teams, and we all got to pick different ideas to create the best way to do something' (IFL-02). Another female in grade 3 in the junior group described, 'I felt proud that we finished it together' (JFL10, female, grade 3). Meanwhile, parents, who came in to observe the last 10 min of the sessions noted,

> Whenever we would come into the room we'd see that he was actually working harder at things and more patient and the other kids. I could see that he just wanted to jump in there but he held back and made sure that everyone had a chance to get their turn. He said that he enjoyed the interaction with everybody.
>
> *parent of IFL-01, male, grade 7*

Another parent of a child in the junior programme highlighted, 'They created an environment of respect and equal sharing and taking care of one another. I think whether his partner built very slowly or not, it didn't seem to faze him. I think on the days they did build a bit faster, he was just, okay, you build it. I'll take it apart, and now let's rebuild it and you take a turn to build it. So, that was an interesting dynamic to witness' (parent of JFL-07, male, grade 3; Lindsay and Lam, 2018: 268).

Self-Advocacy, Self-Esteem and Problem-Solving

Children, their parents and staff running the program described how engaging in robotics helped them with their self-advocacy, self-esteem and problem-solving skills. For example, a parent of a child in the junior programme told us, 'He is an excellent problem-solver, and he likes to figure out ways to make things work. So, I think the feedback I got from one of the sessions was that he was very good at figuring out how to make things go' (parent of JFL-02, male, grade 2; Lindsay and Lam, 2018: 268). A child in the intermediate group explained, 'it's kind of like a bit of a problem-solving and there's opportunity there for others kids too' (IFL-02, female, grade 7). To illustrate, a child said,

> What they were teaching I thought was really good and just showing the kids' stuff like how to build a robot and what you need to get it to going and doing all the fun little races. That way the kids could really see their robot in action and feel like they've accomplished something.
>
> *IFL-01, male, grade 7*

Children, parents and staff in the programme reported noticing changes in self-esteem over the course of the programme. For example, a parent of a child mentioned, 'I think it did wonders for his self-esteem first of all because at the end of the program when they got those medals he was so proud. He wore that medal all week at school' (parent of JFL-05, male, grade 2). A staff member similarly shared, 'It definitely gives them a new shine, like they're glowing with achievement; this accomplishment that they were able to do every single week' (key informant 1).

Another parent of a youth in the intermediate group explained how the program helped him to realize his abilities and potential. To illustrate, they said,

> It was a fantastic experience to be part of something that was more at his cognitive level and to be able to participate in it using his, power chair and access these things with his power chair as opposed to relying on someone to run it for him. So, it was a great experience for us and for him because it's very difficult to find things that he can do on his own. This was something that was interesting for him and that he was able to successfully run on his own.
>
> *parent of IFL-06, male, grade 5; Lindsay and Hounsell (2017): p. 701*

Career Exploration

Many youth involved and their parents described how their involvement in the robotics programme helped them to explore their career interests. For example,
  a parent explained,

> He likes a lot of computer stuff and I thought this might be something that he'd be interested in. He did enjoy it so it did work out...because he is mentioning about getting into game design and stuff. So, I think robotics would be also good. So, I'm looking to see what else is out there so he can continue learning and hopefully he'll want to continue later on in his life.
>
> *parent of IFL-01, male, grade 7*

Another parent described a similar experience, 'it was a wonderful opportunity. He doesn't get exposure to that at all. I wasn't sure what his interest would be so it'd be nice to see if that would spark an interest in him' (parent of IFL-05, male, grade 6). Meanwhile, a youth described, 'I decided to take part in it because I didn't know a lot about robotics…it might be a cool experience, plus there are some high schools nearby who offer robotics programmes. So, I thought maybe looking down the road I could see if that was something I was interested in' (IFL-02, female, grade 7).

Other younger participants in the junior level programme also described what they learned. A parent shared,

> It is something that he really enjoyed and learned a lot and got a lot out of it.
> Actually, from some of the things he learned in class he went to school and then he was telling the teachers all of the things he had learned the day before and the teacher was like, that program sounds incredible.
>
> *JFL-05, male, grade 2*

Another parent told us about their child's experience: 'He always had the interest but I think it really encouraged him that he could do it. And that he was excellent at it. I think it's brought forth that interest even more, which is terrific. I think that even at this young age he's found that niche. Which some people search for a very long time. He's definitely interested and that's something we need to move forward with for sure' (parent of JFL-05 male, grade 2).

A parent of a child in the junior programme mentioned, 'The best thing that happened as a result of his involvement in the program is that it led to more exploration of robotics' (parent of JFL-07, male, grade 3). Further, a staff member involved in running the program explained how it created an opportunity to explore their career interests:

> It's pushing the clients that I see into the fields of science, computers and technology and taking the fear out of those. I saw value in those clients on the computer and programming…They can be independent and they can build and create something and see the value in that for play, but also for possible learning.
>
> *key informant 7*

Impact of Programme on Clinical Staff

The staff who were involved in developing and/or implementing the robotics programme commented on their perceived impact. For example, one staff member described how working with children with disabilities helped her to realize their abilities. She explained,

> I saw all of these kids working so hard and being able to achieve so much, but at the same time they had their potentials pushed to the

limit and they just kept aspiring to do more with it...this just opened my eyes to a new gateway of opportunities and that the kids definitely are capable of learning and being able to do more...they seemed more independent and the parents have been able to give them that independence because they've been able to do all these projects themselves and we're just giving them these tools.

key informant 1

Other staff reported noticing the abilities of the children during the course of this programme. For example, 'I think it exceeded expectations for what the kids would be able to accomplish in six weeks...One of the things that was the most helpful along the way in the programme was talking directly with the parents and hearing their insights of what they liked, hearing their enthusiasm...It was really rewarding' (key informant 6).

Another staff shared a similar experience: 'It's been really fun to see with all the kids and their growth from the first week to like now, just being able to see them implement everything we've taught them into a new structure, without us telling them anything; they're just doing it on their own. It's been life-changing' (key informant 2). An additional staff member recalled the impact that the programme had on them:

We had a blast. Sometimes you teach students and you never know whether they're getting the concepts or not, and when they went to challenge day in both classes, I think we were pleasantly surprised to see kids using the concepts that they had learned in previous classes. It was just so rewarding to see that they were getting the concepts, and they were using some of the principles that were taught. It was great to see them be competitive, and have fun, and sort of be strategic with one another and come up with strategies and we saw that in both the junior room and in the senior room, which was totally amazing to see that.

key informant 3

One key informant who was involved in developing and adapting the programme to address the needs of youth with disabilities said, 'When you got there you just didn't want to leave because you saw it having such a profound effect on the kids...staff that were able to customize whatever that particular child needed to make sure that they had a rewarding experience, and that's really important' (key informant 4).

A staff member involved in delivering the programme shared, 'You go in and let's build some LEGO®. You're as empowered as you are by the kids because everything you're doing is for the kids. Even some small role that I had in helping this programme come together. It's really cool that I could be a part of it' (key informant 6). Overall, one staff summarizes it best: 'I think the biggest success was the enjoyment that the participants had' (key informant 10).

Future Impact of the Programme

Given the importance of recreation and leisure participation to children with disabilities and their families, staff at Holland Bloorview Kids Rehabilitation Hospital set out to develop a model providing a vision of services that would guide programme planning and development outside of the hospital walls. This model was designed to articulate the key principles and strategies needed to support community-focused therapeutic recreation and life skills services, along with community development and the generation of sustainable community services. The model (King et al., 2013) supports a change in thinking from a traditional individually focused deficit model of intervention to a community level strength- and resource-based approach (Bazyk et al., 2015).

Holland Bloorview Kids Rehabilitation Hospital's ecological model of community focused programming provides a solid framework that serves to drive the methodology of strategic partnership building and is responsive to the needs of children and youth with disabilities across the full spectrum of community services. Using a four-part ecological model of community-focused recreation service and life skills services is based on philosophical principles that lie at the heart of client/family-centred care, therapeutic recreation (King et al., 2013), community development and health promotion. The model offers services required to support community members and community organizations to become their own agents of change in the quest to promote the participation of children and youth with disabilities in recreation and leisure activities and community life. The model also provides a vision where community members take responsibility and have capacity to bring about changes they desire, supported by consultation and training services from Holland Bloorview as required.

The idea of broadening our horizons to offer robotics programmes outside of the hospital and in local communities stemmed from our strategic plan, where a key priority is partnering to drive the integration of care and services. Building strategic partnerships with community partners and families will help to enhance integrated robotics programming in the community.

Through developing partners across the province (e.g. other children's treatment centres), we set out to identify gaps in service provision and potential sites where the robotics programme could be implemented. Holland Bloorview Kids Rehabilitation Hospital, where this programme was first adapted and implemented, has now linked with several other children's treatment centres to help get them started in setting up a similar adapted robotics program. We developed a toolkit (e.g. involving tips on budgeting and grant excerpts, curriculum information, programme logistics and equipment management, volunteer recruitment and training and adaptive tools) that can be shared with other hospitals and children's treatment centres. We have been training other centres on how to operationalize robotics programmes and co-develop sustainable strategies to ensure its longevity.

Summary

This chapter described the development and implementation of an adapted group-based robotics programme for children with disabilities and their experiences within it along with the perceived impacts of the programme from staff perspectives. Our findings showed that the children enjoyed the programme and clinical staff made several adaptations and overcame many challenges to enhance the inclusion and participation of children with various types of disabilities. Our findings show how a familiar toy such as LEGO® can be combined with robotics to enhance children's rehabilitation therapy. The programme is now being adopted in several other children's treatment centres.

References

Adams, K. & Cook, A. 2014. Programing and controlling robots using scanning on a speech generating communication device: A case study. *Technology and Disability*, 25, 49–59.

Bazyk, S., Demirjian, L., Laguardia, T., Thompson-Repas, K., Conway, C. & Michaud, P. 2015. Building capacity of occupational therapy practitioners to address the mental health needs of children and youth: A mixed-methods study of knowledge translation. *American Journal of Occupational Therapy*, 69, DOI: 10.5014/ajot.2015.019182.

Braun, V. & Clarke, V. 2006. Using thematic analysis in psychology. *Qualitative Research in Psychology*, 3, 77–101.

Brodin, J. & Lindstrand, P. 2000. Reflections on children with disabilities and computer play. *European Rehabilitation*, 3, 153–158.

Carruthers, C. & Hood, C. 2007. Building a life of meaning through therapeutic recreation: The leisure and well-being model. *Therapeutic Recreation Journal*, 41, 276–297.

Case-Smith, J. & O'Brien, J. 2010. *Occupational Therapy for Children*, Maryland Heights, MO, Mosby Elsevier.

Couch, K., Deitz, J. & Kanny, E. 1998. The role of play in paediatric occupational therapy. *American Journal of Occupational Therapy*, 52, 111–117.

First® Robotics Canada. 2015. FIRST robotics Canada 2015 annual report. www.firstroboticscanada.org/main/wp-content/uploads/ 2015-Year-End-Report.pdf.

Harkness, L. & Bundy, A. 2001. The test of playfulness and children with physical disabilities. *Occupational Therapy Research Journal*, 21, 73–89.

Harper, C., Symon, J. & Frea, W. 2008. Recess is time-in: Using peers to improve social skills of children with autism. *Journal of Autism and Developmental Disorders*, 38, 815–826.

Howard, A., Park, C. & Remy, S. 2012. Using haptic auditory intervention tools to engage students with visual impairments in robot programming activities. *IEEE Transactions in Learning Technology*, 5, 87–95.

King, K., Curran, C. & McPherson, A. 2013. A four-part ecological model of community-focused therapeutic recreation and life skills services for children and youth with disabilities. *Child: Care, Health and Development*, 39, 325–336.

Legoff, D. & Sherman, M. 2006. Long-term outcome of social skills intervention based on interactive LEGO play. *Autism*, 4, 317–329.

Lindsay, S. & Hounsell, K. 2017. Adapting a robotics program to enhance participation and interest in STEM among children with disabilities. *Disability and Rehabilitation: Assistive Technology*, 12, 694–794.

Lindsay, S. & Lam, A. 2018. Exploring types of play in an adapted robotics program for children with disabilities. *Disability and Rehabilitation: Assistive Technology*, 13, 263–270.

Lo, J., Chi, P. & Wang, H. 2009. Pervasive computing in play-based occupational therapy for children. *Pervasive Computing*, 8, 66–73.

Majnemer, A., Shovel, M. & Law, M. 2008. Participation and enjoyment of leisure activities in school-aged children with cerebral palsy. *Developmental Medicine and Child Neurology*, 50, 751–758.

Miller, S. & Reid, D. 2003. Doing play: Competency, control and expression. *Cyberpsychology Behaviour*, 6, 623–632.

Morrison, R., Sainato, D. & Benchaaban, D. 2002. Increasing play skills of children with autism using activity schedules and corresponding training. *Journal of Early Intervention*, 25, 58–72.

Nicolopoulou, A., De, S. & Ilgaz, H. 2009. Using the transformative power of play to educate hearts and minds: From Vgotsky to Vivian Paley and beyond. *Mind Culture and Activity*, 17, 42–58.

Porter, M., Hernandez-Reif, M. & Jessee, P. 2009. Play therapy: A review. *Early Child Development and Care*, 179, 1025–1040.

Rios-Rincon, A., Adams, K. & Magill-Evans, J. 2016. Playfulness in children with limited motor abilities when using a robot. *Physical and Occupational Therapy in Pediatrics*, 36, 232–246.

Rubin, K. & Howe, N. 1985. Toys and play behaviour: An overview. *Top Early Child Special Education*, 5(3), 1–9.

Stumbo, N. & Peterson, C. 1998. The leisure ability model. *Therapeutic Recreation Journal*, 32, 82–96.

World Health Organization. 2007. International classification and functioning, disability and health: children and youth version: ICF-CY. https://apps.who.int/iris/handle/10665/43737.

3

Alzheimer's and mHealth: Regulatory, Privacy and Ethical Considerations

Bonnie Kaplan
Yale University

Sofia Ranchordás
University of Groningen

CONTENTS

Introduction 32
mHealth 33
   Expected Benefits 33
   mHealth for Alzheimer's 35
U.S. Regulatory Environment 36
   Regulatory Agencies 37
      Safety and Efficacy – The FDA 37
   Privacy and Security Regulation – Health Insurance Portability and
   Accountability Act, the FCC and the FTC 38
Privacy and Security Regulatory Challenges 39
   Data Collection 39
   Involvement of Multiple Actors 40
   Device Vulnerability 40
   Transmission and Storage 40
   'Sensor Fusion' and Re-Identification 41
   mHealth Privacy Policies 41
Burdens on mHealth Users 42
Consent 43
Discussion 44
Conclusions 45
Acknowledgements 45
References 46

Introduction

About 50 million people worldwide have dementia, and with someone developing dementia every 30 s (Alzheimer's Disease International 2018), that number is projected to reach 75–82 million by 2030 (Greenblatt 2017, Alzheimer's Disease International). It is a major cause of disability, with overwhelming physical, psychological, social and economic effects not only on people with the disease, but also on their caregivers, families, friends and society at large. Dementia is an untreatable 'syndrome in which there is deterioration in memory, thinking, behaviour and the ability to perform everyday activities' (Greenblatt 2017).

In 2015, dementia's total global societal cost was estimated at US$ 818 billion, equivalent to 1.1% of global gross domestic product (GDP), and expected to rise above US$ trillion. About 20% of that was for direct medical care costs; while 40% of each was for direct social sector and informal care costs, making dementia equivalent to the eighteenth largest economy in the world (Alzheimer's Disease International, Greenblatt 2017). It is no surprise that the World Health Organization recognises dementia as a public health priority and that The Lancet Commission on Dementia Care declared it 'the greatest global challenge for health and social care in the 21st century' (Greenblatt 2017, Livingston et al. 2017).

Alzheimer's contributes to 60%–70% of dementia cases (Greenblatt 2017). Although most people with dementia live in low-income countries, in the United States, 5.7 million people are estimated to have Alzheimer's, or one in ten people over the age of 65, with annual direct costs in 2018 estimated at US$ 227 billion. Families bear 70% of the lifetime costs of unpaid care, long-term care, and out-of-pocket expenses. As the sixth leading cause of death in the United States, and the fifth leading cause of death among those age 65 and older, Alzheimer's is the only top ten cause of death in the United States that cannot be prevented, cured or even slowed. The disease disproportionately affects African-Americans and Hispanics, who are 1.5–2 times as likely to be affected as older whites and women, who account for about two-thirds of those affected (Alzheimer's Association 2018).

This chapter focusses on mobile Health (mHealth) smartphone applications (apps) and wearables for Alzheimer's patients. It provides an overview of mHealth, the applicable U.S. regulatory framework and related ethical issues. While these new technologies can empower and improve the quality of life of many patients and caregivers, there is much unsupported optimism and few evidence-based mHealth services (Byambasuren et al. 2018, Bondaronek et al. 2018, Marcolino et al. 2018, Tomlinson et al. 2013). As The Lancet Commission on Dementia Care notes (Livingston et al. 2017):

> ... evidence on the effectiveness for most devices is not available. Caution is therefore needed to protect people with dementia from overselling of ineffective and potentially unsafe devices. Technology is not a replacement for human contact.

We describe common uses, promises and benefits of mHealth in Alzheimer's care as examples that especially highlight significant considerations common to other areas of mHealth, as well as other health information technologies. Alzheimer's apps are especially poignant because they target fears about becoming demented.

We next examine the U.S. regulatory environment, not only because it is a giant technological market with worldwide influence, but also because regulatory and ethical issues in the United States exemplify considerations that are significant elsewhere. The European Union (EU)'s regulatory environment is becoming increasingly relevant to all technology companies through changes in data protection regulation, EU court decisions and fines for monopoly and privacy violations. At the time of this writing, not only is the regulatory status in the EU in flux, the regulatory environment in the United States also is changing. Though it is too early to assess long-term effects, the trend seems to be that the EU is moving towards stricter regulation while the United States is loosening regulation.

We explain why regulatory, privacy and security concerns might be more apparent in the case of mHealth apps developed for Alzheimer's disease patients and their caregivers, especially considering concerns about privacy, user burdens and consent in light of cognitive impairment. Most people are unaware of these issues. They also are unaware of potential privacy breaches and security implications of apps and devices. Health privacy issues are particularly exacerbated because users with Alzheimer's, dementia or other mental diseases might be unable to give informed consent to the tracking and data collection that are often part of these apps (Howe 2012). We discuss these ethical issues as well as regulatory ones.

---

mHealth

Expected Benefits

mHealth encompasses 'any medical and public health practice supported by mobile devices, such as mobile phones, patient monitoring devices, personal digital assistants and other wireless devices' (European Commission 2014). This includes wearable and implantable technologies integrated with a mobile device or sensors, such as smart soles, watches, bracelets, pendants and the well-known Fitbit.

By early 2018, over 318,000 mHealth apps were available for download, up from more than 100,000 health apps reported in 2015 (Byambasuren et al. 2018, Xu and Liu 2015). mHealth applications support a broad array of healthcare services by providing customised diagnosis, disease management and monitoring and lifestyle or well-being advice. They are expected to make the doctor–patient relationship more cooperative, help patients save money, revolutionise physical examinations, improve mental states, give patients more control over their medical decisions and disease management, assume some of clinicians' jobs and responsibilities, improve outcomes and access to healthcare services, decentralise and democratise medicine, reduce healthcare spending and 'level the playing field in patients' favor … Ultimately chang[ing] the future of healthcare forever' (Byambasuren et al. 2018, YML Media Labs 2018). mHealth applications are praised for promoting health by providing real-time feedback to users, motivating users to change unhealthy lifestyle habits and facilitating the use of medical devices to monitor health conditions (World Health Organization 2011). mHealth also helps patients overcome the stigma of seeking some healthcare services, such as mental healthcare (Gard 2012, Lopez and Patten 2013, Price et al. 2014). mHealth, like the broader category of eHealth, is promoted as improving services and access to healthcare providers (including specialty services) through consultation, communication with patients and intervention (McCubbin 2006); reducing disparities in healthcare accessibility; decreasing travel time for both patient and clinician and empowering patients. These expected benefits also could lead to changes in infrastructure that would provide seamless and continuous care available on a more equitable basis by allowing inter-organisational cooperation and the ready flow of information between patients and providers, wherever located (Kaplan and Litewka 2008).

mHealth is appealing to clinicians who see the possibility to better connect to and understand individual patients and for patients to create communities (Masters 2015). Researchers promote the combination of mobile apps, health platforms, tele-imaging, teleconsultation, wearable technology and Internet of Things (IoT) as helping shape personalised and precision medicine initiatives with mobile technology.

The U.S. Congress, agencies and insurance companies also have been 'sympathetic' to mHealth products (Cortez 2014). The World Health Organization too has supported mHealth apps that offer the promise of expanded and more affordable access to healthcare, particularly in developing countries (van Heerda et al. 2012). The European Commission also acknowledged the potential of mHealth to play a part in transforming healthcare and increasing its quality and efficiency (European Commission 2014).

mHealth has the potential for patient empowerment, disease prevention, monitoring and pre-disease screening and assessment, efficient and effective treatment and generating and collecting public health and medical research data. However, there are concerns surrounding privacy, security, consent, cost-effectiveness and other legal and ethical issues (Kaplan and Litewka 2008). There is little evidence of mHealth's effectiveness or safety (ABC News 2018, Byambasuren et al. 2018, Yasini et al. 2016). Additionally, although by 2012, more than 88% of adults in the United States owned mobile phones, and 31% used them to access health information, ethnic minority groups in the United States are more likely to own mobile and smartphones and use them for health information access (Atienza et al. 2015). These same ethnic minorities have a higher incidence of Alzheimer's (Alzheimer's Association 2018); these issues will have a disproportionate impact on vulnerable populations.

mHealth for Alzheimer's

Technology companies and application developers see a potential market in developing tools to address dementia prevention and care. The Lancet Commission on Dementia Care identified technological innovations that may be useful in dementia care by monitoring behaviour, environment and physiological signs with various devices and wearable sensors, cognitive and memory aids, online support, companionship and information (Livingston et al. 2017).

Assisted living centres and dementia units use Alexa, Amazon Echo's voice-activated smart home assistant to help seniors access news, connect with others, remind them to take their medicines or dress for the weather, alert others if they fall and take on other duties of caregivers, despite potential privacy violations (Newman 2018). Apple's Mind Share, smart home assistants Amazon Echo and Google Nest and digital platforms like Neurotrack and Quest Diagnostic's CogniSense are used to track cognitive performance and measure physiological changes in the hopes of identifying connections between lifestyle, behaviour and medical condition (Leescher 2017, van Wagenen 2018). Researchers and others are using Fitbit or Garmin's Vivosmart activity tracker to collect data that could lead to identifying disease markers.

Products like Global Positioning System (GPS) tracking devices that can be worn or just carried in a pocket or purse empower patients and caregivers by helping track patients and informing caregivers of patients' whereabouts and mitigating the risk of wandering. The Alzheimer's Association Comfort Zone Check-In, for example, offers 'comprehensive web-based location management service. Families can remotely monitor a person with Alzheimer's by receiving automated alerts throught [*sic*] the day and night when a person has travelled beyond a preset zone' (Alzheimer's Association 2018). Alznav, another application, allows users to locate family members, order a taxi and find their way home. It automatically notifies family members and caregivers if the user has left a pre-established secure area (Fraunhofer Portugal). However, tracking apps could be compromised by an Alzheimer's patient's tendency to lose or forget a smartphone's location. Consequently, wearable technologies such as GPS SmartSoles (GPS SMARTSOLE) can be more effective for patients with dementia. Without the conspicuousness of a bracelet or pendant designed to detect falls and track individuals' locations, these tracking devices can be used by people with a variety of cognitive disorders, including traumatic brain injury, autism and Alzheimer's disease (Jackman 2014).

Other apps offer memory training services, assistance with performing basic tasks and activities of daily living, scheduling of treatment alerts and medication reminders, sharing information with doctors and caregivers or providing promising tools and games for cognitive improvement or access to speech pathologists who help with aphasia (Garvin 2017, Leescher 2017, Mukherjee 2013, Wicklund 2016, 2017a,b). One such aid, Backup Memory, enables users to upload photographs, videos and textual information about their friends and family in the hope that these reminders might slow down the disease's progression (Samsung Newsroom 2015).

mHealth offers promise for Alzheimer's patients and support for patients and their caregivers, very often, for free (Metcalf 2014). However, as we often hear: 'when something online is free, you're not the customer, you're the product' (Hoofnagle and Whittington 2014). In addition to the many potential benefits, there also are potential pitfalls, including regulatory issues, privacy, consent and burden on users.

U.S. Regulatory Environment

Recent news coverage has brought more attention to how private data, including data related to health, is collected, analysed and sold: Facebook giving data access to device makers or scanning postings to respond to what may be suicidal thoughts, fitness apps revealing users' locations, health insurers teaming up with data brokers and Google with Fitbit, and apps to monitor users' phone habits for mood or memory changes or signs of stress (Allen 2018, Allison 2018, Dance et al. 2018, Health Data Management 2018, Singer 2018, Tan 2018, Whittaker 2018). These reports illustrate that, despite efforts to provide heightened protection to private health information, the problem of surveillance in general is applicable to mHealth apps and wearable devices that collect data about the users and sometimes their caregivers. People nonetheless often are unaware of the privacy issues, as app developers typically fail to provide transparent information on potential data collection, mining and third-party disclosure (Sunyaev et al. 2015).

Despite the advantages of mobile applications for healthcare, there are important legal and ethical concerns in addition to privacy (Kaplan and Litewka 2008, Nouri et al. 2018, Yasini et al. 2016). One is the need for more clarity concerning product safety and liability. Potential inaccurate use by patients and physicians using transmitted information for diagnosis raises questions of doctor's liability if a patient is injured by diagnosis based on faulty or inaccurate information from monitoring devices (Yang and Silverman 2014). Lack of demonstrated safety and efficacy, as discussed below, is another issue.

Problems are compounded when crossing state or national boundaries. mHealth apps must comply with an array of international and sectorial regulations and frameworks (Mars and Scott 2010). Users carry their phones with them when travelling, so mHealth apps may need to comply with local legislation and different countries' regimes (Avancha et al. 2012). As for many other new technologies, business models require tailoring to local language, regulations and market characteristics.

Regulatory Agencies

U.S. mHealth regulation is a highly fragmented, complex patchwork of federal statutes, state legislation and multiple agencies' regulations (Yang and Silverman 2014, Helm and Georgatos 2014). At the federal level, mHealth services are at the intersection of broadband, technology and health, so subject to the jurisdiction of multiple agencies, including the Food and Drug Administration (FDA)'s regulation of medical devices, the Federal Trade Commission (FTC)'s regulation of unfair and deceptive practices and the Federal Communication Commission (FCC)'s oversight of communications. In addition, mHealth apps often involve cross-jurisdictional medical services (e.g. a patient in Phoenix, AZ being diagnosed by a physician in Boston, MA), raising clinical practice licensure and malpractice concerns, which are primarily regulated by states where relevant laws differ.

Safety and Efficacy – The FDA

Among its many duties, the FDA is the primary agency regulating safety and efficacy of medical devices. However, it generally does not regulate mHealth safety and efficacy. Many mHealth apps are not developed by physicians or programmers with medical training, and few have been subject to the rigorous testing required for medical devices or pharmaceuticals (Bondaronek et al. 2018, Byambasuren et al. 2018, Marcolino et al. 2018). This lack of testing is partly because the FDA's oversight of devices depends on whether an app is intended to perform a medical device function, i.e. when it is employed for the diagnosis of a disease or other condition, or its cure, mitigation, treatment or prevention (Kramer et al. 2012, United States Government 2016, 2017). FDA jurisdiction therefore excludes apps that 'help patients (i.e., users) self-manage their disease or conditions without providing specific treatment or treatment suggestions; provide patients with simple tools to organize and track their health information; help patients document, show, or communicate potential medical conditions to health care providers'; applications for administrative and financial purposes, lifestyle and wellness programmes (e.g. calorie counting and nutrition apps), some portions of electronic health records and care coordination applications (United States Government, Department of Health and Human Services, Food and Drug Administration 2015).

Device regulation is in flux as, at the time of this writing, the FDA is developing new guidance and taking public commentary related to medical devices. Partly this is in response to Section 3060 of the 21st Century Cures Act of 2016, which removed certain software functionalities from the definition of device. These include software functions 'for maintaining or encouraging a healthy lifestyle….such as weight management, physical fitness, relaxation or stress management, mental acuity, self-esteem, sleep management, or sexual function' (United States Government 2017). The FDA consequently cannot regulate such software as a device.

Additionally, the FDA also began developing a new approach to regulation which, instead of focusing on the devices themselves, pre-certifies, for streamlined pre-market review, companies 'for the quality of their software design, testing, clinical practices, real-world performance monitoring, and other appropriate capabilities' (United States Government 2018). Industry and professional organisations are urging the FDA to clarify these new directions, concerned that the criteria for whether specific software is a device are ambiguous and warning of 'lingering confusion among developers and clinicians trying to determine whether specific decision support software is, or is not, considered a device' (American Medical Informatics Association 2018), while industry representatives contend that the FDA has no authority to remove software as a medical device from the standard 510(k) pre-market submission process (Lim 2018). Regardless of the outcome of these developments, it is clear that many mHealth apps have not been and will not be regulated or tested for safety or efficacy.

Privacy and Security Regulation – Health Insurance Portability and Accountability Act, the FCC and the FTC

The United States differs from the omnibus EU approach to device and privacy regulation. Instead, privacy is governed by a complex patchwork of rules at the federal and state level. For example, because mHealth services involve communications networks, the FCC is partially responsible for their regulation, which includes the data privacy provision of the Communications Act (United States Government, Federal Trade Commission 2015).

The Health Insurance Portability and Accountability Act (HIPAA), which governs privacy and security of clinical data, applies only to mHealth platforms managed by a 'covered entity' (for example, doctors, nurses, hospitals and other healthcare professionals and organisations) (Helm and Georgatos 2014). Neither commercial nor research apps are covered by HIPAA. Further, HIPAA protects only identifiable 'health information', i.e. only clinical data, so does not include data gathered by many commercial mHealth apps. Health research data is regulated by the Common Rule, which also does not apply to commercial mHealth apps (Rothstein 2005). Further limitations of health data privacy protections are discussed elsewhere (Kaplan 2014, 2015).

Consequently, consumer protection laws and FTC enforcement have been the primary means for enforcing privacy protections for mobile apps (United States Government 2011). The FTC is charged with preventing unfair or deceptive practices and ensuring compliance with contracts, including privacy agreements and security safeguards. It sanctions unsubstantiated claims about products and requires companies to abide by their user agreements, including enforcing vendors' privacy policies, or violating the

Children's Online Privacy Protection Act (COPPA) by collecting personal information from children without their parents' consent (United States Government 2013). Additionally, with heightened concern over cybersecurity, including Congressional and security agencies' investigations of election meddling and Facebook privacy violations, The House Energy and Commerce Committee and also the health industry began seeking financial support and guidance, including clarifying 'whether FDA guidance on post-market cybersecurity is binding' (Ravindranath 2018).

Privacy and Security Regulatory Challenges

mHealth raises privacy and security concerns. In the United States and EU alike, privacy laws have not yet fully accounted for aspects of mHealth. It is likely that app developers may not be covered by laws regulating personal health information (Avancha et al. 2012, Evans 2011, Hall and McGraw 2014, Luxton et al. 2011, Yang and Silverman 2014). Existing laws are considered open, outdated and based on obsolete technology (European Commission 2015, Martínez-Pérez et al. 2015). Technical or engineering control standards often fill the regulatory gaps, while legal and health informatics research tends to focus on methods for securing systems or techniques, such as authentication and encryption, rather than address the cross-border and privacy and security legal issues inherent to mHealth (Martínez-Pérez et al. 2015, Williams and Maeder 2015).

mHealth apps and wearable technology collect, process and transmit sensitive health information and general data about patients and their caretakers. This data can be aggregated, reused and mined, making privacy and security concerns more salient than ever (Kaplan 2014, 2015). Related legal and ethical concerns are highlighted below.

Data Collection

Smartphones, tablets and wearables connected to other devices allow for the continuous collection of a broad range of data over extended periods and locations, and send it wirelessly to a mobile device (usually a smartphone) for storage and analysis. These technologies also register information from their users or people in the surrounding area. This data may be widely distributed to third parties, often for advertising purposes (Kotz 2011). Tracking location, social interactions and lifestyle data violates an expectation of privacy, but most users are neither fully aware of what data is collected nor how it is used and reused (Shklovski et al. 2014).

In addition, these apps leave these users' private health information and other personal details vulnerable to exploitation by the app developer and third-party advertisers (Motti and Caine 2015). Often data is collected without distinguishing between different contexts (e.g., a wandering patient with memory loss versus a private meeting between patient and friend). However, consumer attitudes about privacy and security are highly contextualised (Nissenbaum 2010). It matters what kind of information and how sensitive or personal it is perceived to be; where, when, who is accessing or seeing the information and why it is being accessed (Atienza et al. 2015, Motti and Caine 2015, Prasad et al. 2011). Elderly people, for example, value their independence but accept devices, such as in-home monitoring or wearable identification, if the devices help them maintain independence (Virkki and Raumomen 2013). They may be willing to share data with physicians, who have a duty of keeping the information confidential, but fear depressing or alarming their families or impairing their sense of independence if they share data with family members (Prasad et al. 2011, Boise et al. 2013).

Involvement of Multiple Actors

Safeguarding privacy is especially challenging because mHealth involves multiple people and a variety of apps, contributing to a diversity of practices and expectations. In addition to patients, clinicians, caregivers and family members, mHealth apps may involve call centres, telecommunications, data storage service providers and patient-monitoring companies. They use information they collect for wellness advice, diagnosis, treatment and follow-up. Further, mobile devices typically have hidden data stores and logs that others might obtain (Nagaty 2015). Patient-users may not understand that all these entities have access to the information. In addition, information about people other than the patient, such as others whom the person visits or who are in photographs, can become available through these apps.

Device Vulnerability

Smartphones are vulnerable to many security threats, including malware and other software that can damage or alter health information. mHealth apps might be hacked or send unencrypted information. Unencrypted online communication and third-party hosting and storage services make it possible to intercept or tamper with information, especially if the device is stolen or lost. Users of mHealth apps who are less aware of these risks might expose themselves to threats by sharing passwords and phones or by being less cautious about secure Internet connections (Zubaydi et al. 2015).

Transmission and Storage

Electronic platforms themselves are vulnerable to third-party attacks (Zubaydi et al. 2015). The huge volume of data an mHealth app generates necessitates cloud data storage. Cloud computing allows for cost savings, storage management, platform strength, resource availability, backup and recovery and decreased IT maintenance, but also means consumers disclose, often without being aware of it, private health information to the cloud provider (Gilmer 2013, Hon et al. 2012, Nagaty 2015, Schwartz 2013).

'Sensor Fusion' and Re-Identification

mHealth sensors can contribute to so-called 'sensor fusion', that is, combining sensor data from different sources to allow complex inferences to be drawn from collected data, such as inferring someone's mental state from how that person walks or holds the phone (Hall and Llinas 1997, Peppet 2014). Unique individual features, such as gait, included in the data may be difficult to anonymise or de-identify per HIPAA requirements, if even covered by HIPAA (Schwartz and Solove 2011).

mHealth Privacy Policies

Patients and research subjects are required to sign authorisation (for HIPAA) or consent (for research) forms or accept click-through commercial agreements that make data about them available to many different parties. App privacy policies are long, confusing and tucked away in complex fine print Terms of Use agreements (Steele 2015). Few users understand the implications of what is covered, what might happen to data once it is released or how it may be combined with other data in ways that could threaten their privacy (Berg 2014). Policies may not address data ownership or specify what data the app or wearable collect (Peppet 2014). Others beyond the immediate user also may have their privacy compromised or information about them, such as location or photo identification, shared without their permission or knowledge (Such and Criado 2018).

Privacy policies are often drafted for 'superusers', that is, highly tech-savvy individuals who read every single word and understand the app's default options (Tere and Polonetsky 2013). In addition, privacy features require sophisticated users who are aware of user-level privacy controls; encryption and authentication methods; available antitheft mechanisms; where data is stored and how it is secured or existing hardware, software, storage and network vulnerabilities. This information, even if provided, is not always read or understood.

Permission for data release and acceptance of app user agreements is obtained when people are more vulnerable or have an immediate need or wish to purchase an app (Bolchini et al. 2004). Users may simply accept vendor agreements when they acquire an app without reading or understanding what the privacy policy is – assuming there is a privacy policy. A 2013 study of the 600 most commonly used apps revealed that less than one-third had privacy policies and that about two-thirds of policies did not specifically address the application. Furthermore, the privacy policies were lengthy and written at college-level reading grade (Sunyaev et al. 2015). Unsurprisingly, users often do not read these policies and simply accept them, so they have no adequate and accessible notice or choice regarding disclosing personal information (Hughes and Goldstein 2015). mHealth apps' privacy policies are generally difficult to understand for an average user, let alone an Alzheimer's patient with cognitive limitations.

Burdens for privacy and security protection appear to be placed on users, who are expected to educate themselves on security features and to take appropriate precautions (European Commission 2014, Premarathne et al. 2015).

Burdens on mHealth Users

mHealth assumes competent and willing users, even though this is not always the case in mental health (Kramer et al. 2013). mHealth devices also treat users as subject to surveillance and persuasion, and assume that responsible users will act in accordance with the need for constant measurement and follow a device's advice and strictures (Lupton 2012). They further assume that devices are not shared, lost or stolen. Burdening individuals with expectations that they be informed and thoughtful about protecting privacy and security may be threatening rather than empowering. Placing responsibility for privacy and security on potential users, rather than on manufacturers or developers, is a tall order for any user (Hall and McGraw 2014), let alone those with dementia.

Although not all dementia patients are elderly, considering the elderly's special vulnerabilities is a useful way to identify significant issues. App design may preclude users with limited technical skills, such as the elderly or people who lack dexterity or visual acuity (Blaschke et al. 2009). Font size is not only an issue for reading agreements, but also for reading and responding to displays; most mobile apps necessarily use small fonts. Usability problems that cause confusion may contribute to inadvertently providing or releasing information that compromises someone's privacy. Even though most of the few usability studies have focussed on dementia apps (3 of the 22 reviewed) (Zapata et al. 2015), more research is needed to address display size, colour and organisation; pulse control or typography and other aspects of usability for the elderly, impaired or cognitively challenged.

Although consumers generally trade off privacy concerns and potential benefits (Atienza et al. 2015), their concerns are legitimate. A number of health app providers have already shared patients' information with other companies (European Commission 2014). Moreover, these privacy and security risks stem not only from the unauthorised sharing of data but also due to the physical risks which might arise if this data is intercepted, hacked and tampered with. Privacy and security concerns are exacerbated for patients with cognitive limitations (Kramer et al. 2013).

Consent

Consumers tend to ignore complicated and often unintelligible privacy policies. This lack of transparency undermines informed consent as patients have little idea of what is protected or what information about them involves health data (Kaplan 2016). They consent to the collection and dissemination of personal information without being fully informed (Nehf 2005).

For data, informed consent refers to the widely recognised right of a patient to know what information is being held, how it is being used and the right to correct and control it (Kaplan 2015). Patients' consent is required to use identifiable data for research and authorisation for its use for clinical purposes – but only for data covered by the Common Rule or HIPAA, neither of which generally covers commercial mHealth apps. Few patients understand the click-through agreements they sign and their data may be made available in ways they do not expect (Haynes 2007). Even fewer will consider implications of de-identification and the potential for re-identification. Consent therefore is not particularly 'informed' (Kaplan 2015).

Consent is more of an issue for users with dementia than it is for the mentally competent. They may not be given much choice from their families or medical insurance companies about using mHealth applications and wearing tracking devices, even when they are able to make such decisions (Kaplan and Litewka 2008). In addition, Alzheimer's patients may feel dehumanised by mHealth apps because they interfere with their personal autonomy and assume their consent to 24/7 surveillance (Jin 2013). Competence underlies ideals of patient empowerment, consent and mHealth. Alzheimer's patients' competence may vary over time and circumstance. To complicate matters, it is worth asking to what extent should prior decisions, made when the patient was competent, control their later destinies, when their preferences and circumstances may be different (Brodoff 2010), or whether Alzheimer's apps should incorporate 'rolling informed consent' (Novitzky et al. 2015, Howe 2012).

It is also likely that Alzheimer's patients, like most elderly, have co-morbidities that predate their diagnosis. What earlier data should be released, possibly despite prior lack of consent, if it may be relevant to later treatment? What memories should be encapsulated for later presentation that may comfort or serve as life-enhancing reminders to an Alzheimer's patient, even if that information previously was kept private? 'Privacy self-management', or the ability of consumers to decide on cost and benefits of privacy may not be an option for Alzheimer's patients (Solove 2013). These patients are not only uninformed, they may be unable to understand the terms of use of most apps.

Relying on informed consent in the case of mHealth is a weak privacy protection because most individuals do not understand either the privacy policies, if they even exist and are read, or the trade-offs. With little, if any, transparency about further data uses, data is distributed in numerous unexpected ways. Users usually have little choice but to sign off or click on a user agreement (Hall and McGraw 2014, Kaplan 2014, 2015, Rothstein and Talbot 2007). In addition, personality changes and memory loss in the case of mental health patients raise the disturbing question of just who is consenting when personality changes, when memory fails, and when behaviour is different from what it used to be.

Even if the patient is the only user, mHealth applications can involve the transmission of data related to other people who have not given consent. This is especially true of location tracking, where microphones, cameras or other sensors can pick up caregivers, family members, friends and others in the location. These people also may appear in photographs and other memory aids (Hall and McGraw 2014, Kumar et al. 2013).

Discussion

In addition to the general health privacy and security considerations analysed in this chapter, mHealth for treating and monitoring Alzheimer's disease faces two interrelated major regulatory challenges: the inadequacy of existing privacy legislation and the uncertainty of future legislation or device regulation, both in general and also to account for the specific vulnerabilities of Alzheimer's patients. But more can be done beyond addressing regulatory challenges.

Privacy considerations would be easier if transparency was improved and policy complexity reduced. People should know and understand what kinds of protections and potential data use accompany using an app or sharing health information. They should be able to consent via an easily understandable policy and be informed as to what privacy expectations and recourses they may have through HIPAA or other regulation. It would be simpler, if various government regulations and policies were harmonised and transparent rather than confusing and fragmented. Efforts could be better targeted if more were known about the current state of public knowledge and expectations, so misconceptions could be addressed better.

Regulatory shortcomings need addressing as well. These include inconsistencies of governance of different kinds and sources of data, lack of clarity about data ownership, dangers of data aggregation and secondary use, insufficiency of de-identification, weak sanctions and little means of recourse for violations and how and which apps are vetted. Moreover, regulatory requirements should not be treated as a ceiling, so that compliance is not seen simply as checking boxes or satisfying the letter of the rules, but as a floor on which to build ethical and practical approaches.

Consumer and patient education also would help, as would clearer policies, media reporting and advising by healthcare professionals. These professionals should be better informed so they can make wiser recommendations to their patients and others who consult them and be cognisant of potential vulnerabilities involved in mHealth apps, especially for more vulnerable patients.

Developers and vendors should not unduly burden potential customers and should not take advantage of their fears concerning their well-being or their understandable hopes regarding how helpful the technologies may be. Apps, as well as policies, could be better designed to make privacy options more readily apparent, screens more readable and defaults more in line with user expectations. Best practices could be identified and disseminated by bringing together industry, communities of practice, research from multiple disciplines, patients and other consumers. Incentive structures could be explored that would help encourage innovative and ethical practice.

The vast potential for patient-generated data to provide valuable resources for improving healthcare, public health and research also needs protecting. As in other areas of healthcare, careful consideration is needed to achieve the promise of advances possible through access to the volumes of data being produced, while also protecting patients. Lastly, more public discussion and deliberation could help provide more thoughtful policy and practice.

Conclusions

mHealth can be tremendously helpful and valuable. It can enable services that otherwise would not be readily available, support patients and caregivers, improve lives and health and be a rich resource for research. The challenge is to enable these benefits while protecting patients and others. We focussed this chapter primarily on privacy and related issues in mHealth, using apps for Alzheimer's as a telling way to examine the regulatory and healthcare environment. The mHealth sector is developing free from most regulatory constraints. It offers few protections for privacy and security of personal health information, data collection, safety or cost-effectiveness. (Whittaker 2012, ABC News 2018). While the situation for mHealth needs addressing in general, apps for Alzheimer's disease and other mental health conditions might require more legal attention than others because these patients often cannot give informed consent to data collection and processing, but still have the right to privacy.

Acknowledgements

We wish to thank Shlomit Yanitsky-Ravid for encouraging this work and for her and Laura Langone's editorial suggestions.

References

ABC News (2018) There are 250,000 fitness and health apps—but little evidence they work, [online], available: www.abc.net.au/news/2018-05-17/mhealth-apps-wellness-and-fitness-apps-not-always-proven-to-work/9758720 [Accessed July 24, 2018].

Allen, M. (2018) Health insurers are vacuuming up details about you—and it could raise your rates, ProPublica, July 17, 2018,

Allison, C. (2018) Fitbit and Google team up on health, with doctors set to receive patient data, [online], available: www.wareable.com/fitbit/fitbit-google-cloud-data-health-6035 [Accessed July 20, 2018].

Alzheimer's Association (2018) 2018 Disease facts and figures, [online], available: www.alz.org/alzheimers-dementia/facts-figures [Accessed July 17, 2018].

Alzheimer's Disease International (2018) Dementia statistics, [online], available: www.alz.co.uk/research/statistics [Accessed July 17, 2018].

American Medical Informatics Association (2018) AMIA urges more work on FDA's decision support guidance, [online], available: www.amia.org/news-and-publications/press-release/amia-urges-more-work-fda%E2%80%99s-decision-support-guidance [Accessed July 24, 2018].

Atienza, A. A., Zarcadoolas, C., Vaughon, W., Hughes, P., Patel, V., Chou, W.-Y. S. and Pritts, J. (2015) Consumer attitudes and perceptions on mHealth privacy and security: Findings from a mixed-methods study, *Journal of Health Communication*, 20, 673–679.

Avancha, S., Baxi, A. and Kotz, D. (2012) Privacy in mobile technology for personal healthcare, *ACM Computing Surveys*, 45(1), Article 3, 1–54.

Berg, J. W. (2014) The E-health revolution and the necessary evolution of informed consent, *Indiana Health Law Review*, 11(2), 589–608.

Blaschke, C. M., Freddolino, P. P. and Mullen, E. E. (2009) Ageing and technology: A review of the research literature, *British Journal of Social Work*, 39(4), 641–656.

Boise, L., Wild, K., Mattek, N., Ruhl, M., Dodge, H. H. and Kaye, J. (2013) Willingness of older adults to share data and privacy concerns after exposure to unobtrusive in-home monitoring, *Gerontechnology*, 11(3), 428–435.

Bolchini, D., He, Q., Antón, A. I. and Stufflebeam, W. (2004) "I need it now': Improving web usability by contextualizing privacy policies," In Koch, N., Fraternali, P. and Wirsing, M., eds., *Web Engineering: 4th International Conference ICWE 2004*, Munich, Germany, July 26–30, Springer, 31–44.

Bondaronek, P., Alkhaldi, G., Slee, A., Hamilton, F. L. and Murray, E. (2018) Quality of publicly available physical activity apps: Review and content analysis, *JMIR mHealth Uhealth*, 6(3), e53, [online], available: https://mhealth.jmir.org/2018/3/e53/ [Accessed March 21, 2018].

Brodoff, L. E. (2010) Planning for Alzheimer's disease with mental health advance directives, *The Elder Law Journal*, 17, 238–308.

Byambasuren, O., Sanders, S., Beller, E. and Glasziou, P. (2018) Prescribable mHealth apps identified from an overview of systematic reviews, *npj Digital Medicine*, 1, 1–12, [online], available: www.nature.com/articles/s41746-018-0021-9.pdf [Accessed June 22, 2018].

Cortez, N. (2014) The mobile health revolution, *UC Davis Law Review*, 47, 1173–1230.

Dance, G. J. X., Confessore, N. and Laforgia, M. (2018) Facebook gave device makers deep access to data on users and friends, *The New York Times*, June 3, 2018.

European Commission (2014) Green Paper on mobile health (mHealth), [online], available: https://ec.europa.eu/digital-single-market/en/news/green-paper-mobile-health-mhealth [Accessed August 14, 2018].

European Commission (2015) Summary report on the public consultation on the green paper on mobile health, [online], available: https://ec.europa.eu/digital-single-market/en/news/summary-report-public-consultation-green-paper-mobile-health [Accessed August 14, 2018].

Evans, B. J. (2011) Much ado about data ownership, *Harvard Journal of Law and Technology*, 25(1), 69–130.

Fraunhofer Portugal. AlzNav, [online], available: http://alznav.projects.fraunhofer.pt/ [Accessed September 23, 2018].

Gard, A. (2012) Bridging the disparities gap with mobile technology, [online], available: http://clinicians.org/bridging-the-disparities-gap-with-mobile-technology-2/ [Accessed September 20, 2018].

Garvin, K. (2017) Can brain games and exercise prevent dementia? We don't know yet, [online], available: https://labblog.uofmhealth.org/rounds/can-brain-games-and-exercise-prevent-dementia-we-dont-know-yet [Accessed July 17, 2018].

Gilmer, E. (2013) Privacy and security of patient data in the cloud: Cloud providers' and consumers' responsibilities under US law, [online], available: www.ibm.com/developerworks/cloud/library/cl-hipaa/ [Accessed September 20, 2018].

GPS SMARTSOLE. [online], available: www.gpssmartsole.com/ [Accessed June 19, 2016].

Greenblatt, C. (2017) Dementia, [online], available: www.who.int/news-room/fact-sheets/detail/dementia [Accessed July 17, 2018].

Hall, D. L. and Llinas, J. (1997) An introduction to multisensor data fusion, *In Proceedings of the IEEE International Symposium*, January 1997, 6–23, [online] available: https://ieeexplore.ieee.org/document/554205 [Accessed June 12, 2019].

Hall, J. L. and McGraw, D. (2014) For telehealth to succeed, privacy and security risks must be identified and addressed, *Health Affairs*, 33(2), 216–221.

Haynes, A. W. (2007) Online privacy policies: Contracting away control over personal information? *Penn State Law Review*, 111(3), 586–624.

Health Data Management. (2018) Google continues work to use machines for health analytics, [online], available: www.healthdatamanagement.com/articles/google-continues-work-to-use-machines-for-health-analytics [Accessed July 20, 2018].

Helm, A. M. and Georgatos, D. (2014) "Privacy and mHealth: How mobile health 'apps' fit into a privacy framework not limited to HIPAA," *Syracuse Law Review*, 64(1), 131–179.

Hon, W. K., Millard, C. and Walden, I. (2012) "Who is responsible for 'personal data' in cloud computing?—the cloud of unknowing, part 2," *International Data Privacy Law*, 2(1), 3–18.

Hoofnagle, C. J. and Whittington, J. (2014) Free: Accounting for the costs of the Internet's most popular price, *UCLA Law Review*, 61, 606–670.

Howe, E. (2012) Informed consent, participation in research, and the Alzheimer's patient, *Innovations in Clinical Neuroscience*, 9(5–6), 47–51.

Hughes, P. P. and Goldstein, M. (2015) Privacy, security, and regulatory considerations as related to behavioral health information technology, In Marsch, L.,

Lord, S. and Dallery, J., eds., *Behavioral Healthcare and Technology: Using Science-Based Innovation to Transform Practice*, Oxford: Oxford University Press, 224–238.

Jackman, T. (2014) George Mason professor champions shoes with GPS tracking for Alzheimer's patients, *Washington Post*, February 14, 2014.

Jin, S. (2013) Private use of electronic tracking devices on individuals with dementia: Balancing possible ethical and legal issues with potential safety benefits, *Annals of Health Law: Advance Directive*, 22, 14–41, [online], available: www.luc.edu/law/academics/journals-publications/annalsofhealthlaw/advancedirective-archive/issue_10.html, [Accessed June 12, 2019].

Kaplan, B. (2014) Health data privacy, *Institute for Social and Policy Studies Working Paper* 14-028, [online], available: https://ssrn.com/abstract=2510429, unpublished [Accessed October 18, 2018].

Kaplan, B. (2015) Selling health data: De-identification, privacy, and speech, *Cambridge Quarterly of Healthcare Ethics*, 24(3), 256–271.

Kaplan, B. (2016) How should health data be used? Privacy, secondary use, and big data sales, *Cambridge Quarterly of Healthcare Ethics*, 25(2), 312–329.

Kaplan, B. and Litewka, S. (2008) Ethical challenges of telemedicine and telehealth, *Cambridge Quarterly of Healthcare Ethics*, 17(4), 401–416.

Kotz, D. (2011) A threat taxonomy for mHealth privacy, *In Proceedings of the Workshop on Networked Healthcare Technology (nethealth), IEEE Computer Society Press*, Bangalore, India, January 6–8.

Kramer, D. B., Xu, S. and Kesselheim, A. S. (2012) Regulation of medical devices in the United States and European Union, *New England Journal of Medicine*, 366, 848–855.

Kramer, G., Mishkind, M. D., Luxton, D. C. and Shore, J. H. (2013) Managing risk and protecting privacy in telemental health: An overview of legal, regulatory, and risk-management, In Cover, F., Myers, K. and Turvey, C., eds., *Telemental Health: Clinical, Technical, and Administrative Foundations for Evidence-Based Practice*, Waltham, MA: Elsevier, 83–107.

Kumar, S., Nilsen, W. J., Abernethy, A., Atienza, A., Patrick, K., Pavel, M., Riley, W. T., Shar, A., Spring, B., Spruijt-Metz, D., Hedeker, D., Honavar, V., Kravitz, R., Lefebvre, R. C., Mohr, D. C., Murphy, S. A., Quinn, C., Shusterman, V. and Swendeman, D. (2013) Mobile health technology evaluation: The mHealth evidence workshop, *American Journal of Preventive Medicine*, 45(2), 228–236.

Leescher, D. (2017) Digital health technologies for Alzheimer's disease, [online], available: https://davidleescher.wordpress.com/2017/01/30/digital-health-technologies-for-alzheimers-disease/ [Accessed July 17, 2018].

Lim, D. (2018) Industry seeks clarity on latest FDA pre-cert working model, [online], available: www.healthcaredive.com/news/industry-seeks-clarity-on-latest-fda-pre-cert-working-model/528180/ [Accessed July 24, 2018].

Livingston, G., Sommerlad, A., Orgeta, V., Costafreda, S. G., Huntley, J., Ames, D., Ballard, C., Banerjee, S., Burns, A., Cohen-Mansfield, J., Cooper, C., Fox, N., Gitlin, L. N., Howard, R., Kales, H. C., Larson, E. B., Ritchie, K., Rockwood, K., Sampson, E. L., Samus, Q., Schneider, L. S., Selbæk, G., Teri, L. and Mukadam, N. (2017) Dementia prevention, intervention, and care, *Lancet*, 390(10113), 2673–2734.

Lopez, M. H. Gonzalez-Barrera, A. and Patten, E. (2013) Closing the digital divide: Latinos and technology adoption, [online], available: www.pewhispanic.org/2013/03/07/closing-the-digital-divide-latinos-and-technology-adoption/ [Accessed September 20, 2018].

Lupton, D. (2012) M-health and health promotion: The digital cyborg and surveillance society, *Social Theory and Health*, 10, 229–244.

Luxton, D. D., McCann, R. A., Bush, N. E., Mishkind, M. C. and Reger, G. M. (2011) mHealth for mental health: Integrating smartphone technology in behavioral healthcare, *Professional Psychology: Research and Practice*, 42(6), 505–512.

Marcolino, M. S., Oliveira, J. A. Q., D'Agostino, M., Ribeiro, A. L., Alkmim, M. B. M. and Novillo-Ortiz, D. (2018) The impact of mHealth interventions: Systematic review of systematic reviews, *JMIR mHealth and uHealth*, 6(1), e23, [online], available: http://mhealth.jmir.org/2018/1/e23/ [Accessed September 23, 2018].

Mars, M. and Scott, R. E. (2010) Global e-health policy: A work in progress, *Health Affairs*, 29(2), 237–243.

Martínez-Pérez, B., de la Torre-Díez, I. and López-Coronado, M. (2015) Privacy and security in mobile health apps: A review and recommendations, *Journal of Medical Systems*, 39, 181–188.

Masters, C. (2015) Role of Mobile Health (mHealth) in precision medicine, [online], available: http://blog.centerforinnovation.mayo.edu/2015/09/23/role-of-mobile-health-mhealth-in-precision-medicine/ [Accessed September 20, 2018].

McCubbin, C. N. (2006) Legal and ethico-legal issues in e-healthcare research projects in the UK, *Social Science and Medicine*, 62(11), 2768–2773.

Metcalf, D. (2014) Next generation solutions in mHealth, In Krohn, R. and Metcalf, D., eds., *mHealth Innovation: Best Practices from the Mobile Frontier*, Chicago, IL: HIMSS Publishing, 297–304.

Motti, V. G. and Caine, K. (2015) Users' privacy concerns about wearables: Impact of form factor, sensors and type of data collected. In Brenner, M., Christin, N., Johnson, B. and Rohloff, K., eds., *Financial Cryptography and Data Security: FC 2015 International Workshop*, San Juan, Puerto Rico, January 30, Springer, 231–244.

Mukherjee, S. (2013) How smartphones are revolutionizing home care for Alzheimer's and Autism patients, [online], available: https://thinkprogress.org/how-smartphones-are-revolutionizing-home-care-for-alzheimers-and-autism-patients-341c87c46c87/ [Accessed July 17, 2018].

Nagaty, K. A. (2015) A secured hybrid cloud architecture for mHealth care, In Adibi, S., ed. *Mobile Health: A Technology Road Map*, Cham: Springer, 541–588.

Nehf, J. P. (2005) Shopping for privacy online: Consumer decisions: Matching strategies and the emerging market for information privacy, *University of Illinois Journal of Law, Technology, and Policy*, 2005(1), 1–54.

Newman, L. H. (2018) Don't freak out about that Amazon Alexa eavesdropping situation, *Wired*, May 24, 2018.

Nissenbaum, H. (2010) *Privacy in Context: Technology, Policy, and the Integrity of Social Life, Stanford Law Books*, Stanford, CA: Stanford University Press.

Nouri, R., Kalhori, S. R. N., Ghazisaeedi, M., Marchand, G. and Yasini, M. (2018) Criteria for assessing the quality of mHealth apps: A systematic review, *Journal of the American Medical Informatics Association*, 25(8), 1089–1098.

Novitzky, P., Smeaton, A. F., Chen, C., Irving, K., Jacquemard, T., O'Brolcháin, F., O'Mathúna, D. N. and Gordijn, B. (2015) A review of contemporary work on the ethics of Ambient Assisted Living Technologies for people with dementia, *Science and Engineering Ethics*, 21, 707–765.

Peppet, S. R. (2014) Regulating the Internet of Things: First steps toward managing discrimination, privacy, security, and consent, *Texas Law Review*, 83, 85–176.

Prasad, A., Sorber, J., Stablein, T., Anthony, D. and Kotz, D. (2011) Exposing privacy concerns in mHealth, *In Proceedings of the 2nd USENIX Conference on Health Security and Privacy*, San Francisco, CA, Berkeley, CA: USENIX Association, 1–2.

Premarathne, U. S., Han, F., Liu, H. and Khalil, I. (2015) Impact of privacy issues on user behavioural acceptance of personalized mHealth services, In Adibi, S., ed. *Mobile Health: A Technology Road Map*, Cham: Springer, 1089–1109.

Price, M., Yuen, E. K., Goetter, E. M., Herbert, J. D., Forman, E. M., Acierno, R. and Ruggiero, K. J. (2014) mHealth: A mechanism to deliver more accessible, more effective mental health care, *Clinical Psychology and Psychotherapy*, 21(5), 427–436.

Ravindranath, M. (2018) Health industry asks government for help on cybersecurity, *Politico* [online], available: www.politico.com/newsletters/morning-ehealth/2018/06/29/health-industry-asks-government-for-help-on-cybersecurity-268015 [Accessed July 24, 2018].

Rothstein, M. A. (2005) Research privacy under HIPAA and the Common Rule, *Journal of Law, Medicine and Ethics*, 33(1), 154–159.

Rothstein, M. A. and Talbot, M. (2007) Compelled authorizations for disclosure of health records: Magnitude and implications, *American Journal of Bioethics*, 7(3), 38–45.

Samsung Newsroom (2015) Samsung volunteers in Tunisia develop app for Alzheimer's patients, [online], available: https://news.samsung.com/global/samsung-volunteers-in-tunisia-develop-app-for-alzheimers-patients [Accessed August 15, 2018].

Schwartz, P. M. (2013) Information privacy in the cloud, *University of Pennsylvania Law Review*, 16, 1623–1662.

Schwartz, P. M. and Solove, D. J. (2011) PII problem: Privacy and a new concept of personally identifiable information, *New York University Law Review*, 86(6), 1814–1894.

Shklovski, I., Mainwaring, S. D., Skuladottir, H. H. and Borgthorsson, H. (2014) Leakiness and creepiness in app space: Perceptions of privacy and mobile app use, *In Proceedings of the 32nd annual ACM conference on Human factors in computing systems*, April 26–May 1, 2347–2356. New York: ACM..

Singer, N. (2018) How companies scour our digital lives for clues to our health, *The New York Times*, February 25, 2018.

Solove, D. J. (2013) Introduction: Privacy self-management and the consent dilemma, *Harvard Law Review*, 126, 1880–1903.

Steele, A. (2015) An emergency room in your living room: Privacy concerns as health information moves outside context, *Virginia Journal of Law and Technology*, 19(2), 389–454.

Such, J. M. and Criado, N. (2018) Multiparty privacy in social media, *Communications of the ACM*, 81(8), 74–81.

Sunyaev, A., Dehling, T., Taylor, P. L. and Mandl, K. D. (2015) Availability and quality of mobile health app privacy policies, *Journal of the American Medical Informatics Association*, 22, e28–e33.

Tan, R. (2018) Fitness app Polar revealed not only where U.S. military personnel worked, but where they lived, *The Washington Post*, July 18, 2018.

Tere, O. and Polonetsky, J. (2013) A theory of creepy: Technology, privacy and shifting social norms, *Yale Journal of Law and Technology*, 16(1), 59–102.

Tomlinson, M., Rotheram-Borus, M. J., Swartz, L. and Tsai, A. C. (2013) Scaling up mHealth: Where is the evidence? *PLOS Medicine*, 10(2), e1001382, [online], available: https://doi.org/10.1371/journal.pmed.1001382 [Accessed September 20, 2018].

United States Government, Department of Health and Human Services, Food and
Drug Administration (2015) Mobile medical applications: Guidance for industry and food and administration staff, [online], available: www.fda.gov/
media/80958/ [Accessed July 1, 2019].

United States Government, Federal Trade Commission (2011) "'Acne cure' mobile app
marketers will drop baseless claims under FTC settlements," [online], available: www.ftc.gov/news-events/press-releases/2011/09/acne-cure-mobile-app-
marketers-will-drop-baseless-claims-under [Accessed March 17, 2016].

United States Government, Federal Trade Commission (2013) Path social
networking app settles FTC charges it deceived consumers and improperly collected personal information from users' mobile address books, [online], available:
www.ftc.gov/news-events/press-releases/2013/02/path-social-networking-
app-settles-ftc-charges-it-deceived [Accessed September 23, 2018].

United States Government, Federal Trade Commission (2015) Protecting and promoting the open Internet, FCC-15-24, [online], available: www.federalregister.gov/
documents/2016/12/21/2016-30766/protecting-and-promoting-the-open-internet
[Accessed September 23, 2018].

United States Government, Federal Trade Commission (2016) Mobile health apps
interactive tool, [online], available: www.ftc.gov/tips-advice/business-center/
guidance/mobile-health-apps-interactive-tool [Accessed September 23, 2018].

United States Government, Food and Drug Administration (2017) Changes to existing
medical software policies resulting from Section 3060 of the 21st Century Cures
Act: Draft guidance for industry and Food and Drug Administration staff,
[online], available: www.fda.gov/downloads/medicaldevices/deviceregulation-
andguidance/guidancedocuments/UCM587819.pdf [Accessed July 24, 2018].

United States Government, Food and Drug Administration (2018) Developing a
Software Pre certification Program: A working model, [online], available:
www.fda.gov/downloads/medicaldevices/digitalhealth/digitalhealthprecert-
program/UCM611103.pdf [Accessed July 24, 2018].

van Heerda, A., Tomlinson, M. and Swartz, L. (2012) Point of care in your pocket: A
research agenda for the field of mHealth, *Bulletin of the World Health Organization*,
90, 393–394.

van Wagenen, J. (2018) Wearables and health IT boost Alzheimer's research, *HealthTech
Magazine*, [online], available: https://healthtechmagazine.net/article/2017/06/
wearables-and-health-it-boost-alzheimers-research [Accessed July 17, 2018].

Virkki, J. and Raumomen, P. (2013) Perpectives for wearable electronics in healthcare
and childcare, *E-Health Telecommunication Systems and Networks*, 2, 58–63.

Whittaker, R. (2012) Issues in mHealth: Findings from key informant interviews,
JMIR, 14(5), e129, [online], available: https://www.jmir.org/2012/5/e129/
[Accessed September 23, 2018].

Whittaker, Z. (2018) Fitness app Polar exposed locations of spies and military personnel,
ZDNet, [online], available: www.zdnet.com/article/fitness-app-polar-exposed-
locations-of-spies-and-military-personnel/ [Accessed July 18, 2018].

Wicklund, E. (2016) Study: Telehealth helps dementia patients recover 'lost' words,
[online], available: https://mhealthintelligence.com/news/study-telehealth-
helps-dementia-patients-recover-lost-words [Accessed July 17, 2018].

Wicklund, E. (2017a) Global project to develop mHealth games for clinical treatment,
[online], available: https://mhealthintelligence.com/news/global-project-to-
develop-mhealth-games-for-clinical-treatment [Accessed July 17, 2018].

Wicklund, E. (2017b) Mobile health app helps seniors reduce their risk for Dementia, [online], available: https://mhealthintelligence.com/news/mobile-health-app-helps-seniors-reduce-their-risk-for-dementia [Accessed July 17, 2018].

Williams, P. and Maeder, A. J. (2015) Security and privacy issues for mobile health, In Adibi, S., ed. *Mobile Health*, Cham: Springer 1067–1088.

World Health Organization (2011) mHealth: New horizons for health through mobile technologies, *Global Observatory for eHealth Series*, 3, [online], available: www.who.int/goe/publications/goe_mhealth_web.pdf [Accessed September 20, 2018].

Xu, W. and Liu, Y. (2015) mHealth apps: A repository and database of mobile health apps, *JMIR mHealth and uHealth*, 3(1), e28, [online], available: http://mhealth.jmir.org/2015/1/e28/ [Accessed September 23, 2018].

Yang, Y. T. and Silverman, R. D. (2014) Mobile health applications: The patchwork of legal and liability issues suggests strategies to improve oversight, *Health Affairs*, 33(2), 222–227.

Yasini, M., Beranger, J., Desmaraism, P., Perez, L. and Marchand, G. (2016) mHealth quality: A process to seal the qualified mobile health apps, In Hoerbst, A., Hackl, W. O., de Keizer, N., Prokosch, H. U., Hercigonja-Szekeres, M. and de Lusignan, S., eds., *Exploring Complexity in Health: An Interdisciplinary Systems Approach - Proceedings of MIE2016, Munich, Germany, August 28–September 2, European Federation for Medical Informatics (EFMI) and IOS Press*, 205–209.

YML Media Labs (2018) The future of healthcare: How mobile medical apps give control back to us, [online], available: https://ymedialabs.com/future-of-healthcare [Accessed July 24, 2018].

Zapata, B. C., Fernández-Alemán, J. L., Idri, A. and Toval, A. (2015) Empirical studies on usability of mHealth apps: A systematic literature review, *Journal of Medical Systems*, 39, 1–19.

Zubaydi, F., Salah, A., Alou, F. and Sagahyroon, A. (2015) Security of mobile health (mHealth) systems. *In 15th IEEE International Conference on Bioinformatics and Bioengineering (BIBE)*, Belgrade, Serbia, November 2–4, IEEE.

4

Exergaming for Health and Fitness Application

Maziah Mat Rosly

University of Malaya

Hadi Mat Rosly

International Islamic University Malaysia

Mark Halaki

The University of Sydney

CONTENTS

Introduction: A Serious Game, Exergaming...53
The Technology and Mechanics of Exergaming...55
Exergaming in Exercise, Sports and Rehabilitation Settings.........................56
Promoting Exergaming for Active Living...58
Challenges and Recommended Future Directions for Exergaming in
Health...61
Considerations and Conclusion..64
References...65

Introduction: A Serious Game, Exergaming

Games are an interactive activity designed for diversion and entertainment purposes. Current gaming platforms come in tabletop and electronic formats, where each format was developed based on an entertaining game scenario or 'progress'. Tabletop games may come in board (Monopoly®), card (Uno®), blocks (Jenga®) or in-table (foosball) types. Electronic games utilise platforms such as video projectors or virtual reality environments, and are termed video games. An electronic game's mechanics generally include aspects related to progress, badges (achievements) and levels that are collectively abbreviated as PBL. However, the structural parts of electronic games constitute three elements of 'input', 'compute' and 'output' that form a dynamic paradigm or interaction cycle (Djaouti et al., 2008). Inputs are signals from a joystick, a control module, pressure sensors, cameras, etc. that provide a command. The rules of the digital games are programmed with algorithms in the 'compute' part and are used to evaluate the input and produce the output. Computing these algorithms may constitute artificial intelligence, as it creates a dynamic gaming interactivity. The 'output' is a response to the move and could be in a form of a countermovement, an interaction or other. Video games have been utilised in education, health, engineering, military, politics and business to bring together user-centred experiences that add pedagogical values, including fun and competition. Video games used in such fields for purposes other than entertainment are collectively termed 'serious games'.

Serious games are defined as any piece of software designed to connect a serious purpose to the gaming structure (Djaouti et al., 2011) in order to capture the attention of a more global audience, encourage creativity and innovation. 'Exergaming' is a motion video game designed to integrate active bodily movements for in-game control. This genre of video gaming comes under the titular serious games, due to its use in health promotion, which sometimes borrow elements of gamification. The application of game thinking or elements in a traditionally non-gaming context is termed 'gamification' (Landers, 2014; Rutledge et al., 2018). It is a design technique applied to facilitate the learning experience and improve engagement of a particular activity's goal, and has distinctly different design and implementation concepts than serious games. Gamification differs from a serious game in that gamifying is usually applied to an existing learning activity or curriculum to facilitate achievement of the activity or curriculum's goals. An example of this includes gamifying lecture quizzes using mobile applications, such as kahoot (http://kahoot.it), or rating student presentations by use of mentimeters (www.menti.com).

Exergaming began as an active video game designed to fulfil objectives specific to a serious game's objective, which is to promote active bodily movements instead of the traditional sedentary gaming. The introduction of exergaming for commercial game console platforms was popularised by the Nintendo® Company in 2006 with the introduction of the Wii system (Miyachi et al., 2010). Other major game console producers, such as Sony PlayStation, Microsoft Xbox and XaviX systems, followed suit with their own versions of movement-controlled gaming interfaces (Tanaka et al., 2012). Interfaces used for in-game exergaming control can range from having motion tracking sensors (Sony Eye Camera and Move controllers, Nintendo Wii®, Xbox Kinect), foot-operated pads (Dance Dance Revolution by Konami®), arm ergometry (GameCycle® or GameBike®) or musical instruments (Guitar Hero©). These exercise systems integrated into video gaming were originally designed with the goal of providing a fun and motivating exercise platform (Fitzgerald et al., 2004; Guo et al., 2006). However, as research progressed into the area of exergaming, collective studies revealed potential in providing equal opportunities to sports participation among children, elderly group, individuals with physical disabilities or health issues and marginalised women.

The Technology and Mechanics of Exergaming

The combination of video gaming and active body movements for in-game control seen in exergaming produced a physical exertion level that can be considered as 'exercise activities'. User interactivity typically featured in sports-like motion games such as tennis, boxing and kayaking are featured in three dimensional rotation (Tanaka et al., 2012; Burns et al., 2012; Fitzgerald et al., 2004; Gaffurini et al., 2013; O'Connor et al., 2002; Warburton et al., 2009; Mat Rosly et al., 2017a) that is planned, structured and repetitive. It uses various types of game controllers as dynamic interfaces, including, but not limited to motion tracking sensors, such as accelerometers, gyroscopes and cameras, foot-operated pressure pads or force platforms, arm crank/bicycle ergometers and musical instruments. These exergames were conceptualised with the goal of improving physical activity levels among sedentary gamers by creating a need to actively move while playing video games. Exergaming, essentially, requires specific rules for gameplay, where a certain level of skill and mastery are achieved overtime. When this field of exercise is played competitively as an individual or in cooperative or team play, the term exergaming can be classified as a sports competition.

Some exergames have incorporated virtual reality to immerse the user in the exergame and promote their engagement. A virtual reality experience requires four key elements: a virtual world, immersion, sensory feedback (responding to user input) and interactivity (Sherman and Craig, 2018). However, aspects of exergaming could incorporate virtual reality environments such as semi-immersive (head-mounted sets) or fully immersive displays. A typical fully immersive virtual reality setup takes the form of a cube-like space, in which images are displayed by a series of projectors located on the floors and walls. It can also include additional equipment to enhance the experience by providing speakers, wall-mounted tracking sensors and olfactory devices (smell diffusers). In essence, virtual reality is better understood as an artificial environment that is constructed with a concept that included interactive graphics, force-feedback, sound, smell or taste recognition. The type of virtual reality environment appropriate for exergaming is entirely dependent on the budget allocated to producing the game and the goals to accomplish stakeholders' needs.

The use of head-mounted sets to provide the virtual reality environment has the common side effects of dizziness or discomfort. Therefore, most exergames do not utilise any head-mounted displays or any other special visual apparatus in order to feel immersed within the virtual exergaming environment. Instead, projector screens, television or monitors are used to display the output produced while exergaming. The predicted side effects of dizziness or discomfort is prevented, as well as the elimination of a source of encumbrance that might hinder the motor response of participants while exergaming. Although newer head-mounted displays produced in the form of stereoscopic glasses are considerably less cumbersome than previous models, current available reports of their use in rehabilitation or exercise present limited findings (Borrego et al., 2018). Future work should consider potential improvements on the exergaming system by utilising the fully immersive virtual reality displays, as it may improve the exergaming experience further. However, total engagement via fully immersive virtual reality enhancements may not be as budget friendly, can be tedious to set up and would not be easily portable.

Exergaming in Exercise, Sports and Rehabilitation Settings

Exercise is known to be a subset of leisure time physical activity that is planned, structured and repetitive for the purpose of conditioning any part of the body (Caspersen et al., 1985). Physical activities that are dose-response sufficient to enable improvements in fitness and reduce risk of cardiometabolic diseases are recommended by current guidelines (Haskell et al., 2007). These activities, if known to be of adequate intensity are collectively understood as 'dose-potent' (Mat Rosly et al., 2017a,b), a term coined to mean a moderate-vigorous aerobic exercise intensity, performed within bouts of 10 min (Garber et al., 2011). However, this measure of 'dose-potency' omitted the amount of time and frequency spent on the exercise over a week that enables an estimate of physical activity level. In addition, any form of competitive exercise, played according to specific rules, is called sports. This general term for sports embraces the exercise umbrella and relates to a specific profession, which requires practice to attain a level of expertise.

Movement control from users who are actively participating within an exergaming environment, promotes engagement during exercise. Studies conducted on exergaming feasibility include various targeted populations, such as obese or overweight children, elderly, individuals with physical disabilities or other health conditions, and marginalised women who are in confinement, showed promising outcomes. Exergames utilizing balance boards have been used to train the elderly population in fall preventions, as well as improving their cognitive skills. Sports-type exergaming, such as Move Boxing or GameCycling, has also been steadily introduced as an alternative to traditional methods of exercise among individuals with physical disabilities. Unlike custom exergaming systems, however, most commercially available exergames were not initially designed for attaining specific rehabilitation goals in mind. Alternatively, exergaming has several advantages over conventional exercise equipment. This can include being more affordable, readily available in the market, significantly more enjoyable, easier to set up, motivating to participate in and dose-potent feasible, even in a sitting position (Mat Rosly et al., 2017a,c).

Exergames are now increasingly introduced as an exercise training intervention in many research studies. The intensities used in most studies were self-imposed by the participants themselves and were heavily subjected to their level of enjoyment (Mat Rosly et al., 2017a–c; Malone et al., 2016). Conventional types of exercise equipment (e.g. arm cranking, treadmill) have allowed titration of moderate-vigorous exercise intensity within any desired training zone, by easily controlling the workload and speed. Titrating the exergame's intensity, within specific training zones can be difficult to achieve due to the dynamic response and player interaction. This is related to specifications involved in the 'compute' algorithms within the exergaming programme, which may not tally well with the 'input' mechanism or produced efficiently through players' 'output'. Additionally, exergaming training are heavily influenced by any progress with different levels, where for instance, the system's artificial intelligence, if included, may capture the opponents play style and react differently over the proceeding rounds. It is theoretically possible to maintain an expected training zone while exergaming by altering the player input mechanics, speed, difficulty level and adding resistance weights during gameplay, but further research would be needed to validate this. Exergames could incorporate parameters such as heart rate, perceived exertion and metabolic energy expended to achieve this.

Earlier in the millennia, conventional video games were first integrated into an arm ergometer or wheelchairs for propulsion and control, demonstrating better enjoyment than the traditional arm cranking, whilst also being intensity adequate (O'Connor et al., 2002; Widman et al., 2006). Further research into this area concluded that exergaming with higher intensity correlated with higher perceived enjoyment (Malone et al., 2016) and adherence (Widman et al., 2006). However, there are limited numbers of cohort studies that report on exergaming outcomes compared to traditional forms of exercise, since most were cross-sectional observations. Studies on exergaming for individuals with physical disabilities have concentrated on commercially available video game consoles such as Nintendo Wii (Gaffurini et al., 2013), PlayStation Move (Mat Rosly et al., 2017a,c), Xbox Kinect (Malone et al., 2016) and the XaviX (Burns et al., 2012) systems. The issue with this approach is that exergames commercially available were designed for the able-bodied population and are rarely suitable for individuals with mental disorders, intellectual or physical disabilities. Additionally, the different mechanical specifications of each exergaming exercise platforms noted different levels of exertion and enjoyment. Most notably, PlayStation Move controllers have higher specifications that include accelerometers, gyroscopes and geomagnetic sensors that are suitable for three-dimensional motion detection. This includes full-arm axial rotation detection, even in a sitting position where it improves user motion detection and enhances the exergaming experience.

Modifications and adaptations to these exergames may be necessary to allow players with neurological or physical disabilities partake in sports exergaming interventions (Hernandez et al., 2012). Console hardware that support exergames based on traditional exercise equipment (i.e. GameCycle or GameBike) has been shown to sufficiently produce intensities adequate to improve cardiometabolic health (Warburton et al., 2009; Widman et al., 2006). Ideally, achieving dose-potent exergaming intensity can be done by tailoring the gameplay to fit type of players' disability category, functional range of movement and position (sitting, standing or body-weight supported) (Mat Rosly et al., 2017a; Malone et al., 2016). The flexibility and dynamic integration of the exergaming's software and hardware could be adapted as a vigorous intensity type of sport even for individuals with a low range of ambulation status and disability, such as those with tetraplegia. An example of this would be the Move Kayaking (Mat Rosly et al., 2017a), where adaptations involved different 'input' mechanisms, by changing the gameplay settings from DualShock® controller based to Move controller position recognition, requiring active arm axial movements. Alternatively, lower extremity-based exergames in the form of floor pads, seen in dance video games have also been adapted for upper extremity tabletop exergaming (Rowland and Rimmer, 2012).

Promoting Exergaming for Active Living

Exergaming has been used to improve health among children (Sheehan and Katz, 2013), busy college students (Graves et al., 2010), females with several socio-environmental constraints (Roopchand-Martin et al., 2015; Staiano and Calvert, 2011), post-partum mothers confined to their homes (Tripette et al., 2014; Elliott-Sale et al., 2014) and individuals with physical disabilities (Mat Rosly et al., 2017b) or mental disorders (Barnes and Prescott, 2018). Over the last decade, the use of exergaming have reported increasing advantageous results in alleviating symptoms related to a series of mental health issues such as anxiety (Barnes and Prescott, 2018), depression (Reger et al., 2012) and attention-deficit hyperactivity disorders (Benzing et al., 2018). Studies have shown that exergames prove more beneficial among children, adolescents and females as opposed to the adult males (Sheehan and Katz, 2013; Tripette et al., 2014; Roopchand-Martin et al., 2015; Staiano and Calvert, 2011; Graves et al., 2010). Exergaming has the ability to tackle some of the barriers reported for dose-potent activities and offer an alternative to traditional or conventional exercise types. The concept of exergaming allows users from rural areas or those who are confined to their homes to partake in sports and exercise within the comfort of their own homes.

Home-based exergaming programmes deployed among obese and overweight school-going children showed promising results in adherence, improving health metabolic as well as social gameplay (Staiano et al., 2018). However, the adherence rate to these home-based programmes among children may not be long lasting as their interest span can be easily swayed by other interests. The technology behind exergaming training platforms should, therefore, include rapid update cycles, in terms of new software or hardware, in order to capture adherence and motivation among children. More recently, exergaming as a physical education programme has been implemented in schools, in an effort to reduce the growing trends of sedentary lifestyle and obesity (Chen and Sun, 2017). An online exergaming competition can also make the exercise experience more engaging for children, especially when cooperative or competitive play environments are introduced (Kooiman et al., 2016). This exergaming programme showed better adherence rate, since it is conducted within extracurricular activities designed within a more disciplined school schedule. Future efforts should also implement such programmes among schools catering for children with physical or intellectual disabilities as part of their education portfolio.

Motherhood can be challenging for post-partum women to partake in regular exercise, as their confinement period requires demanding time and attention to fulfil the needs of a growing infant. This challenge is also exacerbated by concerns of leaking and incontinence following labour among new mothers. Exercising at home may provide limited options for rapid and continued sports participation for these mothers. Therefore, the introduction of exergaming among post-partum women within the comfort of their homes is an interesting approach to promote active lifestyle during confinement. In developing countries or countries with cultural or religious restrictions for females, this exergaming training platform may prove beneficial for their weekly dose of exercise. In essence, it would also be possible to use exergaming as a tool to interact/cooperate online, for social or competitive exergaming, especially for these pockets of special women with limited freedom of expression (Marker and Staiano, 2015). However, restricted network connectivity may prove challenging to overcome when using online exergaming features. Gradually, the promotion of cheaper alternative telecommunications, as technology improves, can provide expansion of Internet viable areas, feasible for exergaming.

In the elderly population, exergaming is a viable therapeutic tool that promotes dynamic improvements in their cognitive and cardiometabolic parameters. Older populations are prone to risks of fall, depressive symptoms and cognitive impairments, which reduce their quality of life as they age. The combined elements of active bodily movements, higher activity enjoyment, focus and engagement provided within exergaming alleviates anxiety, fear and depression among the elderly. Dance types of exergaming, for instance, have been indicated to decrease depressive symptoms in fallers and increase balance dynamics among older community-dwelling population (Rodrigues et al., 2018). In addition, skills accumulated during exergaming can be transferred to real-life abilities by training the sensorimotor and cognitive re-functioning (Harris et al., 2015). Although physical activity recommendations among the older population is lower than the recommendations for the younger population, dose-potent exercise is still an important component in any type of intervention, and exergaming should not be an exception. The readiness to change their behavioural attitude during this period is difficult, but exergaming intervention showed some measure of effectiveness, when deployed in a community-based programme (Sowle et al., 2017). As such, identifying methods to improve physical activity among this population proves very challenging.

Barriers related to exercise participation among individuals with physical disabilities were apparent within four categorical frameworks categorised as physical limitations, personal characteristics, socio-environmental factors and current available economic policies. The socio-demographic setting may heavily impact the weight of the perceived barriers in different categories, where this can range within developed or developing countries. Developed nations like the United States noted significant differences in exercise barriers among those with low-household income, compared to the higher-income group (Hwang et al., 2016). Interestingly, these barriers were not apparently different in a Malaysian study sample (Mat Rosly et al., 2018), which represented a developing country's socioeconomic demography. However, most studies conducted globally echoed the issue of sedentary lifestyle among individuals with physical limitations, with only 50% of their study sample reported being physically active (Anneken et al., 2010; Martin Ginis et al., 2010). These findings denote that the ability to finance continued active lifestyles will influence perceived barriers but did not necessarily affect the likelihood of exercise participation.

Physical limitations can include a number of aspects such as prevalence of wheelchair use, presence of pain while exercising and the need for assistance. One of the defining predictor of participation in intensity adequate aerobic exercise was factors related to wheelchair use (Mat Rosly et al., 2018; Anneken et al., 2010; Jaarsma et al., 2014). This also associates strongly with socio-environmental aspects of being a wheelchair user, as the ability to finance transportation costs and fitness facility fees were known issues that these individuals face. These issues were exacerbated by the fact that not having exercise equipment at home can even reduce the odds of them exercising (Cowan et al., 2013). Additionally, participating in wheelchair sports exercise most often required skills or body functions that are challenging for many individuals with physical disabilities. Home-based exergaming programmes can focus on delivering television or online-based training assistance, where individuals can partake in exergaming activities within the comforts of their own homes. Further work could look into the feasibility of home-exergaming for such individuals prior to deployment and advocate for policies to change the nature of physical training content delivery.

The perception of pain during exercise was commonly reported by individuals experiencing disabilities related to traumatic injuries (Mat Rosly et al., 2017c, 2018). However, pain resulting from any traumatic injury to the neural nervous systems is known to be non-nociceptive, exacerbated by its chronic neuropathic nature (Varoto and Cliquet, 2015). Neuropathic pain is difficult to manage clinically, with pharmacological interventions only providing temporary symptomatic relief. Exergaming environments have documented evidence of pain distraction whilst exercising (Mat Rosly et al., 2017c; Pekyavas and Ergun, 2017). This may be attributed to the pathway mechanics of pain stimulation, which could be overlapped by the visual and auditory feedback during exergaming (Jerdan et al., 2018). However, there is not enough evidence to support reduction of chronic pain through non-pharmacological interventions in these individuals, and further work is needed to support this claim (Boldt et al., 2014). An important key strength for deploying exergaming as a feasible exercise modality is the perceived enjoyment supporting its use, as reported by several studies among those with neurological disabilities (Malone et al., 2016; Widman et al., 2006; Mat Rosly et al., 2017c). Higher enjoyment scores were reported to improve motivation and maintain adherence rates to exercise (Pekyavas and Ergun, 2017; Widman et al., 2006), which may help in alleviating ongoing perception of pain.

Self-motivation, high level of exercise interest and the physically active identity are some of the essence of personal characteristics affecting exercise adherence, despite the ongoing physical and socio-environmental limitations. These barriers related to personal characteristics were more widely reported among the high-income individuals (Cowan et al., 2012; Mat Rosly et al., 2018), whilst socioeconomic and environmental barriers were associated with the low-income group. Essentially, exergaming programmes can be prescribed in a mix-and-match fashion to cater for the selected needs of community-dwelling individuals with disabilities. This is because exergaming programmes have the potential to elicit positive changes despite the ongoing debate among health professionals on the side effects of prolonged use, such as addiction to video games or increased social anxiety. Strategic methods of exercising through exergaming can address barriers considered as 'blind-spots', likely to be of no interest, too lazy to exercise, being afraid to leave home or not worth the time, that were reported by individuals with physical disabilities. It is known that motivation is a strong driver to exercise participation, and this is particularly apparent among the wheelchair-active population (Crawford et al., 2008; Kehn and Kroll, 2009).

Challenges and Recommended Future Directions for Exergaming in Health

Exergames were pioneered in the 20th century, by their first generation of active video gaming, where a number of previous studies have demonstrated the therapeutic effectiveness of exergames targeted at individuals with Parkinson's disease, cerebral palsy, stroke or spinal cord injury (Cooper et al., 1995; Fitzgerald et al., 2004; O'Connor et al., 2002; Rowland and Rimmer, 2012). These exergaming systems can be extremely expensive, with costs ranging from USD 10,000 to 50,000 (Guo et al., 2006; Cooper et al., 1995) that are most often only deployed at a rehabilitation facility and must be custom ordered. In contrast, commercially available exergame systems (such as the Xbox Kinect, Nintendo Wii or PlayStation Move) are produced to be relatively more affordable (~USD300) and easily available for the consumer market. In general, exergaming systems are believed to be a less expensive alternative to regular exercise equipment. This is due to its varied interactivity, owing to the wide availability of off-the-shelf exergames that have been heavily commercialised, well received and well-funded by their respective parent companies. It made exergaming more conducive for home-based physical training compared to conventional exercises or other intervention programmes. No studies have investigated the cost efficacy of exergaming intervention versus traditional training. However, promoting increased physical activities and consequently their health in general, can benefit from lesser reliance on assisted care and fewer hospitalisations (Miller and Herbert, 2016).

The introduction of virtual reality-enhanced simulation can improve the exergaming experience as previous studies demonstrated higher-quality gameplay were associated with higher exercise intensity and perceived enjoyment (Malone et al., 2016; Mat Rosly et al., 2017b). Regular sports activities easily and readily available for the common able-bodied population, such as real-life kayaking, hard-core boxing and sword duelling would not be feasible for those with physical disabilities. Other directions of exergaming can include providing platforms for athletes to train and enhance their skills when factors such as weather, space or ability become an issue. Exergaming platforms now have the ability to provide an alternative form of sports competition that is vigorous in intensity, useful for various populations with limitations and is enhanced via a digital network environment (Mat Rosly et al., 2017a; MacIntosh et al., 2017). Exergaming can, therefore, be introduced as a moderate-vigorous intensity aerobic exercise training programme, with the capability to provide higher enjoyment for individuals with physical disabilities (Mat Rosly et al., 2017c). Participants actively involved in physical activity utilising exergaming have the potential to improve specific aspects of skill acquisition and executive functions (Benzing et al., 2018).

Current research into exergaming has now extended into other areas of intervention, further broadening the scale of exergaming uses. These approaches can include cognitive behavioural therapies for mental health concerns covering anxiety, depression as well as post-traumatic stress disorders. The initial stages of gaming research reported that casual video games alone have shown significant reductions in anxiety (Fish et al., 2014) and depressive (Russoniello et al., 2013) symptoms. Mobile health applications that have been gamified, through use of interactive activities, adding challenge modules and rewarding points provide potential solution to improve and facilitate cognitive behavioural therapies (Pramana et al., 2018). This gamification process can improve user engagement, retention and engagement, reinforcing compliance in treatment delivery. However, research in this field appears to be extremely limited, as early findings have only suggested that therapeutic video games have potential in helping individuals with anxiety reduce their symptoms to clinically measurable outcomes. It has not been shown to be superior to pharmaceutical interventions or cognitive behavioural therapies. There are no reported active exergaming pre-post trials comparing its efficacy against traditional management interventions to support this yet.

Challenges arise when researchers attempt to develop and design an exergame specifically to suit the needs of individuals with physical disabilities, especially for those with impaired upper-limb functions (tetraplegia/ hemiplegia). Their different injury types, motor power, hand grip or range of function most often require personalised modifications to suit different gameplays. For instance, the paddle case in Move Kayaking (Mat Rosly et al., 2017a) for individuals with tetraplegia must be adjustable in length, preferably longer, in order to allow a more simplified kayaking movement feasible for any paralysis occurring in various muscles related to upper-limb axial rotation (Trevithick et al., 2007). To accommodate for weak handgrips seen in impaired upper-limb functions, the Move controller's handles may benefit from using specialised gripping gloves such as the Active Hands (The Active Hands Company, Rumbush, United Kingdom). The exergame's haptic sensors, known as the camera detecting movements, must be adjusted in height to suit wheelchair-bound players. The width should be calibrated to follow the arm-to-arm length parameters, since this allows in-depth three-dimensional motion capture analysis and avoid uncaptured user input. In particular, the PlayStation Move's eye camera and wand controllers are able to produce high-definition depth resolution that provides the fastest 'output' mechanics in exergaming. This is important, since poor recognition of arm axial rotation movement due to low-depth resolution and prolonged latency period can cause frustration in players. However, the use of the Move controllers may be difficult for users with weak handgrips, but could be easily accommodated for with the aforementioned grip gloves.

In order to promote integrated exergaming developments geared for specific targeted population, an interdisciplinary collaboration effort should be optimised by combining expertise from different disciplines. The multidisciplinary input is important in tailoring different types of exergaming for each need of the individual. The range of motion, flexibility and functional mobility can differ heavily between different types of disability. Cognitive impairments seen in the elderly can also affect their ability to evaluate timing, balancing or motor coordination. However, several issues during the development process may hamper effective communication that complicates exergame development coordination. This can include use of different terminologies by different disciplines, parallel developments taking place at different locations, allocating funding, human and technological resources. Ideally, there should be an exergaming trainer, who should be skilled and knowledgeable enough to deliver the training content and module. This way, the programme can utilise the full potential of the given exergaming console system used. Researchers could focus more on adapting current available exergames for targeted specific population, as it is more cost-efficient. This can enhance the feasibility and efficacy of exergaming as a form of sport or exercise whilst providing robust guidelines needed for exergaming education in health. The most challenging future work would be to develop an exergaming training platform that fully combines both upper- and lower-limb movement mechanisms. This may provide better cardiometabolic and respiratory improvements, when compared to isolated upper- or lower-body exergaming.

   With the current advancements of technology in the video game industry, using commercially available exergaming training platforms can prove challenging as explicit features and specifications of certain consoles may limit wide-use application. Older console models, such as Xbox Kinect, XaviX or Nintendo Wii, being no longer produced in the market or region locked and the newer models, such as Xbox One nor Nintendo Switch, not being backwards compatible, further limits the clinical rehabilitation impact and adoption of these off-the-shelf games to existing users. Recently, gaming disorders have now been officially recognised by the World Health Organization as an addiction illness, as defined in the eleventh Revision of the International Classification of Diseases (ICD-11) released by the World Health Organisation in 2018. It is important to be informed that sedentary games and active exergaming are distinctly different, with the latter directed more towards improving physical lifestyle and well-being. Additionally, a higher duration of hours spent on exergaming, do not imply bordering features of exercise addiction, as it is most often a result of a different underlying disorder, and dose-potent physical training is promoted for a healthier lifestyle. There are many described advantages to exergaming, an active form of serious games genre that have so far, not been reported to warrant addiction yet. However, long-term implications to prolonged participation in moderate-vigorous aerobic exergaming, can lead to overuse injuries, but this is largely seen in all other sports as well.

Considerations and Conclusion

Exergames, a combination of active bodily movements and video gaming, are a genre of serious games designed to achieve health outcomes through a series of processes called gamification. Collective studies revealed better immersion, motivation and enjoyment perceived during exergaming rather than conventional exercise programmes. Achievements obtained during exergaming, in the gaming environment, provide a sense of progressive development for participants to adhere in continuous exercise. It has been demonstrated to yield broad positive outcomes, given the high appeal of gaming in general. These can include improving exercise participation, transferable skill acquisition and motivating engagement. Exergames are especially appealing to special groups of population, as well as different age categories, owing to their intrinsic motivation (fun) enhancing aspects. Pockets of groups have been identified to benefit from exergaming: children, who generally play extensive amounts of games and thereby may be prone to exergaming; elderly, who benefit from continued active engagement; individuals with disabilities, who can perform these exergaming activities even in wheelchairs; and finally, marginalised women, whom may have been disadvantaged from experiencing equality for sports participation due to expected cultural norms. These targeted populations face large disparities, and inequality still persists in access to exercise and sports services. Organisations and communities have made significant strides towards lifting marginalised populations out of social deprivation related to exercise. There is a growing need to address sedentary lifestyles, and available exergaming training platforms can promote comprehensive opportunities for them.

References

Anneken, V., Hanssen-Doose, A., Hirschfeld, S., Scheuer, T. & Thietje, R. 2010. Influence of physical exercise on quality of life in individuals with spinal cord injury. *Spinal Cord*, 48, 393–399.

Barnes, S. & Prescott, J. 2018. Empirical evidence for the outcomes of therapeutic video games for adolescents with anxiety disorders: Systematic review. *JMIR Serious Games*, 6, e3.

Benzing, V., Chang, Y. K. & Schmidt, M. 2018. Acute physical activity enhances executive functions in children with ADHD. *Scientific Reports*, 8, 12382.

Boldt, I., Eriks-Hoogland, I., Brinkhof, M. W., de Bie, R., Joggi, D. & von Elm, E. 2014. Non-pharmacological interventions for chronic pain in people with spinal cord injury. *The Cochrane Library*, 28, CD009177.

Borrego, A., Latorre, J., Alcañiz, M. & Llorens, R. 2018. Comparison of Oculus Rift and HTC Vive: Feasibility for virtual reality-based exploration, navigation, exergaming, and rehabilitation. *Games for Health*, 7, 151–156.

Burns, P., Kressler, J. & Nash, M. 2012. Physiological responses to exergaming after spinal cord injury. *Topics in Spinal Cord Injury Rehabilitation*, 18, 331–339.

Caspersen, C. J., Powell, K. E. & Christenson, G. M. 1985. Physical activity, exercise, and physical fitness: Definitions and distinctions for health-related research. *Public Health Reports*, 100, 126–131.

Chen, H. & Sun, H. 2017. Effects of active videogame and sports, play, and active recreation for kids physical education on children's health-related fitness and enjoyment. *Games for Health*, 6, 312–318.

Cooper, R. A., Vosse, A., Robertson, R. N. & Boninger, M. L. 1995. An interactive computer system for training wheelchair users. *Biomedical Engineering: Applications, Basis and Communications*, 7, 52–60.

Cowan, R. E., Nash, M. S. & Anderson-Erisman, K. 2012. Perceived exercise barriers and odds of exercise participation among persons with SCI living in high-income households. *Topics in Spinal Cord Injury Rehabilitation*, 18, 126–127.

Cowan, R. E., Nash, M. S. & Anderson, K. D. 2013. Exercise participation barrier prevalence and association with exercise participation status in individuals with spinal cord injury. *Spinal Cord*, 51, 27–32.

Crawford, A., Hollingsworth, H. H., Morgan, K. & Gray, D. B. 2008. People with mobility impairments: Physical activity and quality of participation. *Disability and Health*, 1, 7–13.

Djaouti, D., Alvarez, J. & Jessel, J. P. 2011. Classifying serious games: The G/P/S model. In Patrick Felicia (ed.), *Handbook of Research on Improving Learning and Motivation through Educational Games: Multidisciplinary Approaches*, IGI Global, Vol. 2, pp. 118–136.

Djaouti, D., Alvarez, J., Jessel, J. P., Methel, G. & Molinier, P. 2008. A gameplay definition through videogame classification. *International Journal of Computer Games Technology*, 4, 1–7.

Elliott-Sale, K., Hannah, R., Bussell, C., Parsons, A., Woodrow Jones, P. & Sale, C. 2014. A pilot study evaluating the effects of a 12 week exergaming programme on body mass, size and composition in postpartum females. *International Journal of Multidisciplinary and Current Research*, 2, 131–138.

Fish, M. T., Russoniello, C. V. & O'Brien, K. 2014. The efficacy of prescribed casual videogame play in reducing symptoms of anxiety: A randomized controlled study. *Games for Health*, 3, 291–295.

Fitzgerald, S. G., Cooper, R. A., Thorman, T., Cooper, R., Guo, S. & Boninger, M. L. 2004. The GAME (Cycle) exercise system: Comparison with standard ergometry. *The Journal of Spinal Cord Medicine*, 27, 453–459.

Gaffurini, P., Bissolotti, L., Calza, S., Calabretto, C., Orizio, C. & Gobbo, M. 2013. Energy metabolism during activity-promoting video games practice in subjects with spinal cord injury: Evidences for health promotion. *European Journal of Physical and Rehabilitation Medicine*, 49, 23–29.

Garber, C. E., Blissmer, B., Deschenes, M. R., Franklin, B. A., Lamonte, M. J., Lee, I. M., Nieman, D. C., Swain, D. P. & American College of Sports Medicine. 2011. American College of Sports Medicine position stand. Quantity and quality of exercise for developing and maintaining cardiorespiratory, musculoskeletal, and neuromotor fitness in apparently healthy adults: Guidance for prescribing exercise. *Medicine and Science in Sports and Exercise*, 43, 1334–1359.

Graves, L. E., Ridgers, N. D., Williams, K., Stratton, G., Atkinson, G. & Cable, N. T. 2010. The physiological cost and enjoyment of Wii Fit in adolescents, young adults, and older adults. *Journal of Physical Activity and Health*, 7, 393–401.

Guo, S., Grindle, G. G., Authier, E. L., Cooper, R. A., Fitzgerald, S. G., Kelleher, A. & Cooper, R. 2006. Development and qualitative assessment of the GAME cycle exercise system. *IEEE Transactions on Neural Systems and Rehabilitation Engineering*, 14, 83–90.

Harris, D. M., Rantalainen, T., Muthalib, M., Johnson, L. & Teo, W. P. 2015. Exergaming as a viable therapeutic tool to improve static and dynamic balance among older adults and people with Idiopathic Parkinson's disease: A systematic review and meta-analysis. *Frontiers in Aging Neuroscience*, 7, 167.

Haskell, W. L., Lee, I. M., Pate, R. R., Powell, K. E., Blair, S. N., Franklin, B. A., Macera, C. A., Heath, G. W., Thompson, P. D. & Bauman, A. 2007. Physical activity and public health: Updated recommendation for adults from the American College of Sports Medicine and the American Heart Association. *Medicine and Science in Sports and Exercise*, 39, 1423–1434.

Hernandez, H., Graham, T. C., Fehlings, D., Switzer, L., Ye, Z., Bellay, Q., Ameer Hamza, M., Savery, C. & Stach, T. 2012. Design of an exergaming station for children with cerebral palsy. *Proceedings of the 2012 ACM Annual Conference on Human Factors in Computing Systems*, Austin, Texas, USA. 2619.

Hwang, E. J., Groves, M. D., Sanchez, J. N., Hudson, C. E., Jao, R. G. & Kroll, M. E. 2016. Barriers to leisure-time physical activities in individuals with spinal cord injury. *Occupational Therapy in Health Care*, 30, 215–230.

Jaarsma, E. A., Dijkstra, P. U., Geertzen, J. H. & Dekker, R. 2014. Barriers to and facilitators of sports participation for people with physical disabilities: A systematic review. *Scandinavian Journal of Medicine and Science in Sports*, 24, 871–881.

Jerdan, S. W., Grindle, M., van Woerden, H. C. & Kamel Boulos, M. N. 2018. Head-mounted virtual reality and mental health: Critical review of current research. *JMIR Serious Games*, 6, e14.

Kehn, M. & Kroll, T. 2009. Staying physically active after spinal cord injury: A qualitative exploration of barriers and facilitators to exercise participation. *BMC Public Health*, 9, 168.

Kooiman, B. J., Sheehan, D. P., Wesolek, M. & Reategui, E. 2016. Exergaming for physical activity in online physical education. *International Journal of Distance Education Technologies*, 14, 1–6.

Landers, R. N. 2014. Developing a theory of gamified learning: Linking serious games and gamification of learning. *Simulation and Gaming*, 45, 752–768.

Macintosh, A., Switzer, L., Hwang, S., Schneider, A. L. J., Clarke, D., Graham, T. C. N. & Fehlings, D. L. 2017. Ability-based balancing using the gross motor function measure in exergaming for youth with cerebral palsy. *Games for Health*, 6, 1–7.

Malone, L. A., Rowland, J. L., Rogers, R., Mehta, T., Padalabalanarayanan, S., Thirumalai, M. & Rimmer, J. H. 2016. Active videogaming in youth with physical disability: Gameplay and enjoyment. *Games for Health*, 5, 333–341.

Marker, A. M. & Staiano, A. E. 2015. Better together: Outcomes of cooperation versus competition in social exergaming. *Games for Health*, 4, 25–30.

Martin Ginis, K., Latimer, A. E., Arbour-Nicitopoulos, K. P., Buchholz, A. C., Bray, S. R., Craven, B. C., Hayes, K. C., Hicks, A. L., McColl, M. A., Potter, P. J., Smith, K. & Wolfe, D. L. 2010. Leisure time physical activity in a population-based sample of people with spinal cord injury part I: Demographic and injury-related correlates. *Archives of Physical Medicine and Rehabilitation*, 91, 722–728.

Mat Rosly, M., Halaki, M., Hasnan, N., Mat Rosly, H., Davis, G. M. & Husain, R. 2018. Leisure time physical activity participation in individuals with spinal cord injury in Malaysia: Barriers to exercise. *Spinal Cord*, 56, 806–818.

Mat Rosly, M., Halaki, M., Mat Rosly, H., Cuesta, V., Hasnan, N., Davis, G. M. & Husain, R. 2017a. Exergaming for individuals with spinal cord injury: A pilot study. *Games for Health*, 6, 279–289.

Mat Rosly, M., Mat Rosly, H., Davis, G. M., Husain, R. & Hasnan, H. 2017b. Exergaming for individuals with neurological disability: A systematic review. *Disability and Rehabilitation*, 39, 727–735.

Mat Rosly, M., Mat Rosly, H., Hasnan, N., Davis, G. M. & Husain, R. 2017c. Exergaming boxing versus heavy bag boxing: Are these equipotent for individuals with spinal cord injury? *European Journal of Physical and Rehabilitation Medicine*, 53, 527–534.

Miller, L. E. & Herbert, W. G. 2016. Health and economic benefits of physical activity for patients with spinal cord injury. *ClinicoEconomics and Outcomes Research*, 8, 551–558.

Miyachi, M., Yamamoto, K., Ohkawara, K. & Tanaka, S. 2010. METs in adults while playing active video games: A metabolic chamber study. *Medicine and Science in Sports and Exercise*, 42, 1149–1153.

O'Connor, T. J., Fitzgerald, S. G., Cooper, R. A., Thorman, T. A. & Boninger, M. L. 2002. Kinetic and physiological analysis of the GAME(Wheels) system. *Journal of Rehabilitation Research and Development*, 39, 627–634.

Pekyavas, N. O. & Ergun, N. 2017. Comparison of virtual reality exergaming and home exercise programs in patients with subacromial impingement syndrome and scapular dyskinesis: Short term effect. *Acta Orthopaedica et Traumatologica Turcica*, 51, 238–242.

Pramana, G., Parmanto, B., Lomas, J., Lindhiem, O., Kendall, P. C. & Silk, J. 2018. Using mobile health gamification to facilitate cognitive behavioral therapy skills practice in child anxiety treatment: Open clinical trial. *JMIR Serious Games*, 6, e9.

Reger, G. M., Holloway, K. M., Edwards, J. & Edwards-Stewart, A. 2012. Importance of patient culture and exergaming design for clinical populations: A case series on exercise adherence in soldiers with depression. *Games for Health*, 1, 312–318.

Rodrigues, E. V., Gallo, L. H., Guimarães, A. T. B., Melo Filho, J., Luna, B. C. & Gomes, A. R. S. 2018. Effects of dance exergaming on depressive symptoms, fear of falling, and musculoskeletal function in fallers and nonfallers community-dwelling older women. *Rejuvenation Research*, 21(6), 518–526.

Roopchand-Martin, S., Nelson, G., Gordon, C. & Sing, S. Y. 2015. A pilot study using the XBOX Kinect for exercise conditioning in sedentary female university students. *Technology and Health Care*, 23, 275–283.

Rowland, J. L. & Rimmer, J. H. 2012. Feasibility of using active video gaming as a means for increasing energy expenditure in three nonambulatory young adults with disabilities. *PMR*, 4, 569–573.

Russoniello, C. V., Fish, M. & O'Brien, K. 2013. The efficacy of casual videogame play in reducing clinical depression: A randomized controlled study. *Games for Health*, 2, 341–346.

Rutledge, C., Walsh, C. M., Swinger, N., Auerbach, M., Castro, D., Dewan, M., Khattab, M., Rake, A., Harwayne-Gidansky, I., Raymond, T. T., Maa, T., Chang, T. P. & Quality Cardiopulmonary Resuscitation (QCPR) Leaderboard Investigators of the International Network for Simulation-Based Pediatric Innovation, R., and Education (INSPIRE). 2018. Gamification in action: Theoretical and practical considerations for medical educators. *Academic Medicine*, 93, 1014–1020.

Sheehan, D. P. & Katz, L. 2013. The effects of a daily, 6-week exergaming curriculum on balance in fourth grade children. *Journal of Sport and Health Science*, 2, 131–137.

Sherman, W. R. & Craig, A. B. 2018. *Understanding Virtual Reality: Interface, Application, and Design*. Morgan Kaufmann: San Francisco, 6.

Sowle, A. J., Francis, S. L., Margrett, J. A., Shelley, M. C. & Franke, W. D. 2017. A community-based exergaming physical activity program improves readiness-to-change and self-efficacy among rural-residing older adults. *Journal of Aging and Physical Activity*, 25, 432–437.

Staiano, A. E., Beyl, R. A., Guan, W., Hendrick, C. A., Hsia, D. S. & Newton, R. L. J. 2018. Home-based exergaming among children with overweight and obesity: A randomized clinical trial. *Pediatric Obesity*, 13(11), 724–733.

Staiano, A. E. & Calvert, S. L. 2011. Wii tennis play for low-income African American adolescents' energy expenditure. *Cyberpsychology*, 5, 4.

Tanaka, K., Parker, J. R., Baradoy, G., Sheehan, D., Holash, J. R. & Katz, L. 2012. A comparison of exergaming interfaces for use in rehabilitation programs and research. *Journal of the Canadian Game Studies Association*, 6, 69–81.

Trevithick, B. A., Ginn, K. A., Halaki, M. & Balnave, R. 2007. Shoulder muscle recruitment patterns during a kayak stroke performed on a paddling ergometer. *Journal of Electromyography and Kinesiology*, 17, 74–79.

Tripette, J., Murakami, H., Gando, Y., Kawakami, R., Sasaki, A., Hanawa, S., Hirosako, A. & Miyachi, M. 2014. Home-based active video games to promote weight loss during the postpartum period. *Medicine and Science in Sports and Exercise*, 46, 472–478.

Varoto, R. & Cliquet, A. 2015. Experiencing functional electrical stimulation roots on education, and clinical developments in paraplegia and tetraplegia with technological innovation. *Artificial Organs*, 39, E187–E201.

Warburton, D. E., Sarkany, D., Johnson, M., Rhodes, R. E., Whitford, W., Esch, B. T., Scott, J. M., Wong, S. C. & Bredin, S. S. 2009. Metabolic requirements of interactive video game cycling. *Medicine and Science in Sports and Exercise*, 41, 920–926.

Widman, L. M., McDonald, C. M. & Abresch, R. T. 2006. Effectiveness of an upper extremity exercise device integrated with computer gaming for aerobic training in adolescents with spinal cord dysfunction. *The Journal of Spinal Cord Medicine*, 29, 363–370.

5

Technology Solutions and Programs to Promote Leisure and Communication Activities with People with Intellectual and other Disabilities

Giulio E. Lancioni
University of Bari

Nirbhay N. Singh
Augusta University

Mark F. O'Reilly
University of Texas

Jeff Sigafoos
Victoria University of Wellington

CONTENTS

Introduction 72
Assistive Technology for Leisure Activities 73
  Programs to Help People Access Brief Stimulation Events 73
  Programs to Help People Control a Television Device 74
  Programs to Help People Choose among Stimuli 74
Assistive Technology for Communication 75
  Programs to Help People Make Verbal Requests 75
  Programs to Help People Make Telephone Calls or Use Text Messages 77
Assistive Technology for Leisure and Communication 78
  Programs with the First Technology Arrangement 79
  Programs with the Second Technology Arrangement 80
  Programs with the Third Technology Arrangement 81
Discussion 82
References 84

Introduction

People with intellectual and other disabilities (e.g. motor and sensory impairments) may have serious problems in independently managing leisure activities and communication and thus largely rely on the support of others (Badia et al., 2013; Lancioni et al., 2017b; Sutherland et al., 2014; Taylor & Hodapp, 2012). Indeed, many of these people may fail to independently access simple everyday activities, such as listening to music and watching television or videos, due to the fact that they cannot (properly) use regular equipment and computer systems available to access those activities (Dahan-Oliel et al., 2012; Lancioni et al., 2017a,b). The same people may not possess speech abilities to successfully communicate or simply interact with relevant partners in their immediate environment (i.e. caregivers and staff) and/or may be unable to independently establish an interaction with distant partners due to their inability to use telephone devices and equivalent means to get in touch with those partners (Hatakeyama et al., 2015; Lancioni et al., 2014b; McMillan & Renzaglia, 2014; van der Meer et al., 2012).

There is ample consensus on the view that the aforementioned situation is deleterious and efforts need to be made to address the problems and curb their negative implications (Foley & Ferri, 2012; Lancioni & Singh, 2014c). One intervention approach to tackle the problems and facilitate progress within the aforementioned areas relies on the use of assistive technology (Federici & Scherer, 2012; Meder & Wegner, 2015; Mihailidis et al., 2016; Stasolla et al., 2015). With the expression 'Assistive Technology' one generally refers to any type of device or tool that can help the user reach objectives that he or she could never attain independently (i.e. without the support of such an instrument/device). For example, a person with intellectual disability and extensive motor impairment could never be expected to manage independent access to preferred stimuli and choose among them. Yet, assistive technology could make the objective attainable. The person could be automatically presented with brief samples of a variety of stimuli and provided with a microswitch (i.e. a sensor that is connected to the device presenting the stimuli and can be activated with minimal responses). With the use of such technology, the person would be allowed to access the stimuli he or she prefers by activating the microswitch in relation to the corresponding samples (Lancioni et al., 2012, 2013b). Similarly, a person with intellectual disability and severe memory problems would not be expected to remember the time of the day when specific activities are due and would hardly manage to remember the steps that the activity includes. Assistive technology solutions could enable that person to mitigate the impact of his or her problems by (1) reminding him or her of the activities at the appropriate time and (2) providing verbal or pictorial instructions for the single steps of the activities in the correct sequence (Gillespie et al., 2012; Lancioni et al., 2016c).

This chapter is an effort to explore a variety of assistive technology solutions evaluated over the years to help persons with intellectual and other disabilities (e.g. intellectual and motor or sensory disabilities) deal with leisure and/or communication activities independently. More specifically, the chapter is focused on (1) technology solutions devised to help people engage in leisure activities, (2) technology solutions devised to help people engage in communication activities and (3) technology solutions devised to help people engage in both leisure and communication activities. For each of these groups of technology solutions, a number of studies are summarized as illustrative examples of the technology employed and of the intervention programs carried out with the support of such technology.

Assistive Technology for Leisure Activities

Programs to Help People Access Brief Stimulation Events

These types of programs require that the participant (1) possesses small responses (e.g. hand, head or lip movements) that can be detected by microswitches/sensors and (2) has clear preferences for environmental stimuli. It also requires that the microswitch used for the participant is connected to a computer or other electronic device, which is set up to regulate the delivery of stimuli contingent on the participant's target responses (Mechling, 2006; Roche et al., 2015; Shih et al., 2011; Tam et al., 2011). For example, Lancioni et al. (2001) carried out a study aimed at enabling two children with intellectual and extensive motor disabilities to access brief periods of preferred stimulation by emitting simple vocalization responses. The responses were monitored through a microswitch consisting of a sound-detecting device connected to a throat microphone, which was not affected by any form of environmental sound. The microphone was kept at the children's larynx by means of a neckband. During the baseline, the microswitch served only to record the vocalization responses (i.e. their frequency during the sessions). During the intervention, the microswitch served to record the responses and also to trigger an electronic device that delivered brief periods of preferred stimulation contingent on the emission of those responses. Both children showed a clear increase in response frequency during the intervention, thus indicating that they enjoyed the stimulation and were actively engaged to increase its availability.

Shih et al. (2009) assessed whether an adolescent and an adult with profound intellectual disabilities and extensive motor impairment would learn to use thumb poke responses to control preferred environmental stimulation. The microswitch used for the participants was an adapted computer mouse and their response consisted of poking with their thumb the mouse's scroll wheel. The responses were transmitted wirelessly to a mini computer, which was connected to (and arranged to regulate) a television set. The television set was inactive during the baseline phases and presented brief music events and videos contingent on the participants' response during the intervention and post-intervention phases. Data showed that both participants increased their response levels during the intervention and post-intervention periods, indicating their ability to pursue stimulation events independently and their consistent interest for the stimulation.

Programs to Help People Control a Television Device

Watching television can be considered a very common leisure activity. Persons with intellectual disability and/or severe motor impairment may not be able to switch 'on' and 'off' the television set or may be unable to move from one channel to another when they are no longer interested in what they are watching. An early study aimed at circumventing this problem (Lancioni et al., 2007) assessed a microswitch-aided program with a young man who (1) presented with severe spastic tetraparesis with no functional movement of arms, hands, legs and trunk and (2) had very limited and difficult-to-understand speech. The technology included two types of microswitches linked to the television's remote control via a prearranged electronic device. The first microswitch (i.e. a pressure sensor) was linked to the participant's face and served to choose the on/off, the channels, or the volume functions. Once the function was selected, the man could operate any choice through the second type of microswitches (optic sensors), which were at the corner of his mouth and could be activated with tongue movements. The positive results obtained with the man and the favourable social validation of the program provided by teacher trainees interviewed about it, motivated new efforts to upgrade the program.

One of those efforts led to set up a computer-aided television system (Lancioni et al., 2014a). The system included a microswitch, a portable computer and a commercial software package (USB TDT AVerTV Volar Green HD A835-ECO plus mini antenna). This package allowed the participants to watch television through a portable computer by activating a microswitch. Microswitch activations served to move forward through the channels available as well as to switch the television on and off. The package was successfully tested with two participants with advanced amyotrophic lateral sclerosis who could activate a mouth microswitch through mild biting pressure and a sound-detecting microswitch with throat microphone through brief sound emissions, respectively.

Programs to Help People Choose among Stimuli

A technology-aided program to allow people to access a variety of environmental stimuli and choose among them may rely on (1) a computer system prearranged to present samples of the stimuli available and respond to the participant's choices and (2) a microswitch device with which to choose the stimuli most wanted. In essence, samples would be presented in succession with brief intervals between one another. Activating the microswitch in overlap or immediately after a sample would trigger the computer and allow the participant to access the corresponding stimulus for a preset period of time (e.g. 20–25 s). Abstaining from microswitch activation would signify lack of choice and thus enable the computer to progress through the presentation of samples until a choice occurs. The program also allows an individual to ask for the repetition of a specific stimulus event. The individual can make such request by activating the microswitch as soon as a stimulus event ends. In that case, the computer would not proceed with new sample presentations but would extend the stimulus event that was just ended. This type of program was reported in several studies (Lancioni et al., 2011b, 2012, 2013b, 2016a). For example, Lancioni et al. (2011b) applied the program with two adults with intellectual, motor and sensory disabilities. Sixteen stimuli were available at each session. Twelve of them were deemed preferred by the participants (i.e. pieces of songs or familiar voices/stories) while four were considered non-preferred (i.e. distorted sounds). This set up allowed to ascertain that the participants (1) were purposeful in their choice behaviour, that is, they chose stimuli deemed preferred and avoided the others and (2) had clear preferences for some of the stimuli. In fact, some of the stimuli were chosen more frequently and more extensively. Additionally, the participants showed mood improvement during the program sessions.

A different program arrangement, relying on the same computer and microswitch technology mentioned above, was reported by Lancioni et al. (2016a). Their study involved two adults affected by moderate intellectual disabilities and visual and motor impairment. At the beginning of each intervention session, the computer presented visually and verbally three music options, one at a time in sequence. When the participant chose one of the options (i.e. by activating the microswitch within 4 s from the presentation of such option), the computer proceeded to present four choice alternatives concerning that option. For example, if the participant had chosen the 'Female singers' option, the computer presented four female singers (i.e. one at a time). The participant could now choose one of the singers. Following this choice, the computer proceeded to present five songs of that singer. At this point, the participant was allowed to choose one of the songs and listen to it. At the end of the song or as soon as it was interrupted by the participant (i.e. via microswitch activation), the computer started a new sequence. Data showed that both participants were successful in using the technology and managed to choose and access preferred songs independently.

Assistive Technology for Communication

Programs to Help People Make Verbal Requests

Using verbal utterances as communication means is certainly an advantage compared to using signs and pictorial representations (Sigafoos et al., 2009; van der Meer et al., 2012, 2017). Indeed, verbal utterances are immediately understood by anybody inside and outside of the education/rehabilitation or care context in which the person spends time. The type of technology available to help non-verbal people express themselves verbally is the speech-generating device (SGD). A variety of SGDs exist and the ways in which they are used can also vary across contexts and people (Kagohara et al., 2013; Lorah et al., 2015; Mullennix & Stern, 2010; van der Meer et al., 2017). For example, Schepis and Reid (1995) used an SGD for an adult who was reported to be in the profound range of intellectual disability and presented with extensive motor impairment. The SGD was set up to make four verbal requests concerning four preferred items. The participant could activate any request by touching the corresponding picture on the SGD's panel. Initially, the participant was introduced to the device and helped to use it. Then, the participant was provided with the device for specific parts of the day. Data showed that the participant used the device to make a number of requests, and as a consequence the amount of interaction between staff and participant increased.

Lancioni et al. (2016b) evaluated a specific SGD for three adults whose disabilities also included blindness or minimal residual vision. The device's front panel was divided into 15 mini sections each of which contained an optic sensor. Each optic sensor was covered by a small object or tag with Braille referring to a specific activity that was deemed to be of interest for the participant. Removing an object or tag (freeing the optic sensor underneath) led (1) the device to verbalize the request for the activity that was represented by that object or tag and (2) a caregiver or staff person to approach the participant and help him to carry out the activity requested. The device was available for lengthy periods of time during the day and the participants used it effectively with the consequence that they made several requests and engaged in a variety of activities. The participants also expressed preference for the sessions with the SGD compared to other activities of the day and staff expressed a favourable opinion about the device's usability and impact.

Ricci et al. (2017) assessed an SGD that involved the use of mini objects or cardboard chips with pictures (as representations of preferred activities) and a smartphone with five participants with intellectual disabilities combined with motor impairment, deafness or blindness. The mini objects were used for the participants affected by blindness, and the pictures were used for the participants with functional vision. The smartphone was fixed at the participants' chest while the mini objects and pictures were attached to a plastic pad, which was at the participants' waist. The mini objects and pictures were supplied with special frequency code labels that made them recognizable for the smartphone fitted with a near-field communication module. Placing a mini object or a picture in contact with the smartphone led this to recognize the activity the picture or object represented and utter (through a dedicated software previously installed) a verbal request for that activity. The request was easily heard and promptly satisfied within the context. All participants learned to use the SGD. Following the intervention period, the participants were reported to make between 5 and 12 requests per 20-min session and to show preferences among activities. Staff interviewed about the device provided fairly positive ratings of it.

Programs to Help People Make Telephone Calls or Use Text Messages

Persons with intellectual and motor or visual disabilities may find great difficulties in interacting (i.e. via telephone calls or text messages) with significant people not present in their immediate environment, because they cannot use telephone devices independently (Al-Mouth & Al-Khalifa, 2015; Hreha & Snowdon, 2011; Lancioni et al., 2014b). Yet, making telephone calls or exchanging messages could be quite relevant for the persons' social and affective contact and thus should be pursued as a rehabilitation target. A way to enable those persons to manage the calls or the messages independent of staff assistance would involve the use of technology. For example, Lancioni et al. (2011a) reported the use of a computer-aided telephone system linked to a microswitch to enable a man who presented with degenerative retinopathy, ataxia and mild intellectual disability and a woman with blindness and motor impairment functioning at the borderline level to make telephone calls. The initial microswitch activation led the prearranged computer to ask the participant which one of the specific groups presented (e.g. family, male friends or female friends) he or she wanted to call. The participant's microswitch activation in relation to a group led the computer to list the names available within that group, one at a time. Microswitch activation in relation to one of those names led the computer to place a call to that person. At the end of the conversation with that person (or in case of no reply), the participant activated the microswitch to disconnect the telephone line and make the telephone available for a new call. The sequence for the new call was as described above. Using the aforementioned technology, the participants were able to make a variety of calls and to reach mean conversation times of about 9 min within 20-min sessions.

Lancioni et al. (2014b) reported two single-case studies aimed at promoting independent performance of telephone calls with the use of two different technology solutions. In the first study, they included a woman with moderate intellectual disability and visual and motor impairments, who was provided with a technology package similar to that described in the study previously reviewed. As soon as the woman activated the microswitch, the computer started to present the names of the persons available for a call. Twelve names/persons were available. After the presentation of each name, a computer statement reminded the woman that she had to activate the microswitch if she wanted to call that person. The computer was set to start a new call sequence (following the same conditions described above) after 15–25 s had elapsed from the end of the previous call or in relation to the woman's microswitch activation. Data showed that during the intervention phases and the post-intervention check (with the technology), the woman managed a mean of about six calls per 10-min session, with about four of those calls being answered.

The second study involved a man who was considered to have a mild to moderate intellectual disability, presented with blindness and possessed clear, easily discriminable speech. He was provided with a Galaxy S3 smart-phone with the S-voice module. The names and telephone numbers of the 14 persons available for the man's telephone calls had been recorded in the device's database. Specifically, the man had been guided to record those names in the device. Before the first telephone call of each session, the man was required to provide an access word (i.e. a greeting word) to activate the device. Thereafter, he was to use the word 'Call', followed by the name of the person with whom he wanted to get in touch to start a telephone call. He had to use the word 'Stop' to end a call when it was completed or if there was no answer from the person called. Data showed that the man was highly successful in performing his telephone calls independently throughout the intervention phases and the post-intervention check.

Lancioni et al. (2010) set up a program of text messaging for two adults who presented with mild intellectual disability, extensive motor impairment, visual impairment or blindness and minimal (difficult-to-decode) speech due to acquired brain injury. The technology included a prearranged computer, a global system for mobile communication and two microswitches (i.e. an optic sensor and a pressure device for the two participants, respectively). The computer was set up to present information/instructions, respond to the micro-switches, send out messages and verbalize incoming messages. The first microswitch activation led the computer to present the names of individuals to whom messages could be sent. New microswitch activation in relation to one of the individuals led the computer to present a list of message topics (e.g. concerning health, work, love and greetings) for that individual. Microswitch activation in relation to one of the topics led to the presentation of the mes-sages available within that topic. Microswitch activation in relation to a spe-cific message led the computer to send that message out to the individual previously selected. An incoming message was signalled to the participant who could get it read by activating the microswitch. Both participants learned to independently send out their messages and to have incoming messages read to them.

Assistive Technology for Leisure and Communication

The technology solutions and intervention programs reviewed above were aimed at supporting either leisure or communication. Yet, many people with intellectual and other disabilities could benefit from the opportu-nity to engage in both leisure and communication activities. Indeed, they could freely shift from one type of activity to the other with increased benefit in terms of quality of engagement, social image and personal satisfaction (Lancioni et al., 2013a). Based on this notion, three main technology arrangements were developed to allow the participants to access both types of activities independently. The first and most basic arrangement included the presence of two or three microswitches/sensors. One or two of those microswitches were linked to stimulation sources. The other microswitch was linked to an SGD that served to call for the attention of the caregiver or staff (Lancioni et al., 2013a). The second arrangement relied on the use of a computer device set-up to present the leisure and communication options and a microswitch that the participant could use to select (via the computer) any of those options (Lancioni et al., 2016a). The third arrangement relied on the use of one or two smartphones (Lancioni et al., 2018).

Programs with the First Technology Arrangement

One of the studies relying on the first technology arrangement involved 11 participants whose ages varied between childhood and adolescence (Lancioni et al., 2009). Their intellectual disability was estimated to be in the severe to profound range. Ten of them also presented with visual impairment that varied from severe disability level or minimal residual vision to total blindness. Two small responses were selected for each participant (e.g. hand pushing, vocalization and head movements). One served for accessing stimulation while the other served for activating the SGD. The microswitches included, among others, pressure sensors, throat microphones, tilt instruments and optic sensors. The SGDs involved microswitches (such as those mentioned above) connected to a vocal output apparatus. Microswitches and SGDs were linked to an electronic device that regulated the delivery of brief periods of preferred stimulation and the activation of a vocal utterance, respectively. The vocal utterance consisted of one of several phrases asking for the attention of the caregiver or staff member. The response to this request (during the intervention phases) included (1) expressions of joy and excitement (that could also be accompanied by events such as hand clapping and foot stamping) and (2) combinations of those expressions with physical contact, such as caressing and embracing. The participants were first taught to use the microswitch then they were taught to use the SGD. Eventually, they were provided with both the microswitch and the SGD simultaneously. Data showed that all participants managed to use the microswitch and SGD, thus accessing preferred stimulation and calling for (and receiving) social contact and attention.

Lancioni et al. (2008a,b) carried out studies, which differed from the one reviewed above in that an extra microswitch was available. That is, the five participants included in the studies, who were affected by severe/profound intellectual, motor and visual disabilities, were provided with a combination of two microswitches and an SGD. Data showed that all participants learned to operate the microswitches and the SGD achieving high levels of leisure and communication engagement throughout the sessions.

Programs with the Second Technology Arrangement

Lancioni et al. (2016a) reported a study in which leisure and communication options were available for two adults, who presented with moderate intellectual disability combined with motor and visual impairments. The technology involved a prearranged computer with screen and sound amplifier, a mobile communication modem and a microswitch. Sessions started with the computer presenting, verbally and through images, three options, that is, 'music', 'videos' and 'telephone'. The options were illuminated in sequence (one at a time) for a few seconds. Following the participant's selection of one option (i.e. through the activation of the microswitch while the option was illuminated), the computer shifted to a second page containing the choice alternatives related to the option just selected. Specifically, if the participant had selected 'music', the computer would present the titles of six to eight songs. Selection of a song (i.e. through the microswitch) led the computer to play that song. The same process was enacted in case the participant selected the 'videos'. If the participant selected the 'telephone' option, the computer presented the names of six to eight people available for telephone calls. Selection of one of these people led the computer to set up a telephone call with him or her. At the end of the call or in case the number of the persons called were engaged, the computer reset starting to show the three options again. Both participants learned to use the technology successfully and operated several choices within the 10-min sessions available. Choices of songs and videos were more frequent than choices of telephone calls. Yet, the levels of calls remained consistent throughout the study.

Lancioni et al. (2017b) carried out a study with nine participants (adults) affected by mild/moderate or moderate intellectual disability as well as motor and visual or auditory impairments. Their study was an extension of the one reported above. In practice, each participant was presented with three or four options among which he or she could choose. The options could include combinations such as (1) songs, sport videos, slide shows and telephone calls; (2) songs, comedy videos and text messages; and (3) comedy videos, sport videos, text messages and telephone calls. Only one of the nine participants did not have a communication option due to her severe hearing impairment and inability to read. The technology worked as described in the previous study. If a participant chose the text messages option, the computer presented the names and/or photos of the individuals available for messaging. Once the participant had selected the individual to whom the message was to be sent, the computer presented the messages available for that individual verbally (except in one case in which they were presented in written form). Essentially, different sets of messages were prearranged for each of the people available for messaging and the participant was to choose the message to send out through the microswitch. Incoming messages were automatically read or printed by the computer. All participants were successful in using the technology and showed high levels of engagement. While one of the participants could only engage in leisure activities (see above), the other eight participants managed to engage in both leisure and communication activities. Leisure engagement was, however, predominant.

Programs with the Third Technology Arrangement

Recently, efforts have been made to develop alternatives to the technology arrangements of the second type. Those alternatives were to be somewhat simpler than the previous arrangements and based on common/normalizing technology devices. In practice, the new, third technology arrangement was aimed at replacing the computer systems, microswitch and mobile communication mode with one or two smartphones. One of the studies carried out in this area (Lancioni et al., 2017a) included five participants who were affected by blindness or severe visual impairment and had a level of functioning compatible with mild intellectual disability. All participants were capable of producing clear verbal utterances. The technology set-up for these participants involved a Samsung Galaxy A3 with standard functions such as the S-Voice, Internet connection, contacts unit and media player. The contacts unit was used to store the names and telephone numbers of the people identified as communication partners for the participants. The media player was used to store a large number of MP3 files concerning leisure options (e.g. singers/songs, comedians, games, sport and food recipes). At the beginning of the study, the participants went through a voice recognition procedure to ensure that the smartphone would subsequently discriminate their verbal utterances and respond to them. During the sessions, the participants were to start with an entry word and then proceeded to utter their requests. Requests for the leisure activities could involve the name of the activity option (e.g. the name of a comedian) and the name of the specific piece within that option (e.g. a comic sketch's title). Requests for placing a telephone call or sending a message required that the participants utter the word 'call' or 'message' and the name of the partner to call or reach via message. All participants learned to use the smartphone successfully and were actively engaged in leisure and communication activities for most of the session time.

Lancioni et al. (2018) adapted the aforementioned smartphone-based program to the condition of five participants who presented with moderate intellectual disability, visual and/or motor impairments and poor speech skills, and thus could not use verbal utterances to make requests. To circumvent the speech problem, the adapted version of the program was to allow the participants to use mini objects or pictures for their requests. The objects and pictures, which represented the leisure and communication activities (1) were fitted with frequency code labels and (2) were used in combination with two Samsung Galaxy A3 smartphones. The first smartphone was equipped with near-field communication and music player functions, and audio files with operational words and leisure and communication requests. It also included a special application allowing it to verbalize the audio files in connection with the code labels of objects and pictures. The second smartphone matched the one described in the previous study (Lancioni et al., 2017a). To make a request, the participants were to place a mini object or picture with coded label on the back of the first smartphone. This smartphone read the label and verbalized the request of the corresponding activity. The verbalization activated the S-Voice of the second smartphone, which then presented the leisure activity or placed a phone call, depending on the type of request carried out. The results of this study with the adapted technology were very similar to those reported in the previous study in which the participants used verbal utterances to make their requests.

Discussion

The technology solutions and technology-based programs reviewed can be taken to indicate that there are intervention options available for a variety of individuals with intellectual and other disabilities. Indeed, research evidence is encouraging as to the possibility of supporting individuals with different types and different levels of disabilities and helping them reach leisure and communication goals that would be unachievable without technology. Notwithstanding the research evidence, the adoption and daily use of those programs and technology solutions may not be a foregone conclusion. Similarly, a successful outcome of those programs and solutions may not be necessarily guaranteed.

Adoption and use of technology solutions within daily contexts are much more likely and realistic when the following criteria are met: (1) the technology is easily available and affordable in terms of costs, (2) the setting up of the technology is manageable within the contexts and (3) staff personnel are adequately prepared to use the technology and convinced of its beneficial effects (Borgestig et al., 2017; Federici & Scherer, 2012; Kuo et al., 2013; Pérez-Cruzado & Cuestas-Vargas, 2017). With regard to the first criterion, one might argue that the technology components (e.g. computers, interfaces, microswitches and smartphones) examined in this chapter are relatively affordable in terms of cost and, with a few exceptions, are commercially available and thus can be directly purchased.

Regarding the second criterion (i.e., setting up the technology), two sets of requirements must be clear. First, the technology components needed for different programs are to be assembled and/or are to be fitted with basic software or commercial applications. For example, a microswitch needs to be interfaced with a computer or other electronic device. Similarly, computers, special SGDs and smartphones or tablets require some form of standard (commercially available) application or dedicated software to perform the functions required within the program. Secondly, the aforementioned devices as well as SGDs need to be fitted with a variety of stimulus events, verbal cues/instructions, visual images or mini objects representing the stimuli (choice options and activities). In light of the above, one can argue that satisfying the second criterion requires a certain level of expertise and definite time investment, which might not always be available in daily contexts.

With regard to the third criterion, the most important point to underline is that staff needs to be prepared about the technology solutions being introduced and the ways in which such technology should be used. Effective staff preparation that may require direct demonstration and supervision is critical for staff to manage the technology adequately. Adequate management of the technology may be one of the two basic conditions for staff to accept it as part of their daily intervention protocol. The other condition would be the experience of positive intervention results in concomitance with the use of the technology solutions.

Achievement of positive intervention results require that (1) the technology solutions applied match the characteristics of the participants and respond to their abilities and needs or interests and (2) the intervention conditions are adequately set up. With regard to the match between technology and user, one can follow some of the guidelines proposed within the 'The Matching Person and Technology Model' (Corradi et al., 2002) and look for the technology arrangement that makes the participant more comfortable. The issue of participant comfortableness may have different meanings across different participants (Scherer et al., 2011). For example, for participants at the low spectrum who are exposed to microswitch-aided programs aimed at promoting stimulation control, comfortableness may primarily concern the easiness of the response required to activate the microswitch (e.g. hand movement, mouth opening and eyelid closure). For participants included in technology-aided programs aimed at supporting stimulus choice, comfortableness may concern both the easiness of the response required for activating the microswitch and the suitability of the intervals separating the stimulus samples during their presentation. For participants included in smartphone-based programs, comfortableness would mainly concern the easiness of the response required to operate choices (i.e. the verbal utterances or the use of mini objects).

A number of intervention conditions implemented during the technology-based program can influence the progress and final outcome of the program. For example, the use of effective prompting strategies may be critical to facilitate the participant's responding, and let him or her discover the impact of it, at the beginning of the program. Similarly, prompt fading may be important to avoid any interruption or slowdown of responding (Pierce & Cheney, 2008). The relevance of the stimuli or activities provided during the sessions (e.g. contingent on microswitch activations available for choice) may determine the participants' level of motivation and consequently their level of initiative and the strength of their response performance (Lancioni et al., 2013a). The use of session lengths matching the participants' optimal engagement time (e.g. in terms of physical resilience or stimulation and activity interest) would certainly have a positive impact on the program outcome.

In conclusion, this chapter has examined a number of studies as illustrative examples of the research literature concerning technology-aided intervention solutions to help people with intellectual and other disabilities engage in leisure, communication or both leisure and communication activities. Within each activity area (i.e. leisure, communication, and leisure and communication combined), different types of technology solutions and technology-aided programs were described. Those technology solutions and programs can help serve people with different needs and abilities and provide them with an opportunity to increase their positive engagement in an independent manner with possible benefits for their general condition, their mood as well as their social image and quality of life (Brown et al., 2013).

References

Al-Mouth, N., & Al-Khalifa, H. S. (2015). The accessibility and usage of smartphones by Arab-speaking visually impaired people. *International Journal of Pervasive Computing and Communications*, 11, 418–435.

Badia, M., Orgaz, M. B., Verdugo, M. A., & Ullán, A. M. (2013). Patterns and determinants of leisure participation of youth and adults with developmental disabilities. *Journal of Intellectual Disability Research*, 57, 319–332.

Borgestig, M., Sandqvist, J., Ahlsten, G., Falkmer, T., & Hemmingsson, H. (2017). Gaze-based assistive technology in daily activities in children with severe physical impairments: An intervention study. *Developmental Nurorehabilitation*, 20, 129–141.

Brown, I., Hatton, C., & Emerson, E. (2013). Quality of life indicators for individuals with intellectual disabilities: Extending current practice. *Intellectual and Developmental Disabilities*, 51, 316–332.

Corradi, E., Scherer, M. J., & Lo Presti, A. (2002). Measuring the assistive technology match. In: S. Federici & M. J. Scherer (Eds.), *Assistive Technology Assessment Handbook* (pp. 49–65). London: CRC Press.

Dahan-Oliel, N., Shikako-Thomas, K., & Majnemer, A. (2012). Quality of life and leisure participation in children with neurodevelopmental disabilities: A thematic analysis of the literature. *Quality of Life Research*, 21, 427–439.

Federici, S., & Scherer, M. J. (Eds.). (2012). *Assistive Technology Assessment Handbook*. London: CRC Press.

Foley, A., & Ferri, B. A. (2012). Technology for people, not disabilities: Ensuring access and inclusion. *Journal of Research in Special Education Needs*, 12, 192–200.

Gillespie, A., Best, C., & O'Neill, B. (2012). Cognitive function and assistive technology for cognition: A systematic review. *Journal of the International Neuropsychological Society*, 18, 1–19.

Hatakeyama, T., Watanabe, T., Takahashi, K., Doi, K., & Fukuda, A. (2015). Development of communication assistive technology for persons with deaf-blindness and physical limitation. *Studies in Health Technology and Informatics*, 217, 974–979.

Hreha, K., & Snowdon, L. (2011). We all can call: Enhancing accessible cell phone usage for clients with spinal cord injury. *Assistive Technology*, 23, 76–80.

Kagohara, D. M., van der Meer, L., Ramdoss, S., O'Reilly, M. F., Lancioni, G. E., Davis, T. N., Rispoli, M., Lang, R., Marschik, P. B., Sutherland, D., Green, V. A., & Sigafoos, J. (2013). Using iPods and iPads in teaching programs for individuals with developmental disabilities: A systematic review. *Research in Developmental Disabilities*, 34, 146–156.

Kuo, K. M., Liu, C. F., & Ma, C. C. (2013). An investigation of the effect of nurses' technology readiness on the acceptance of mobile electronic medical record systems. *BMC Medical Informatics and Decision Making*, 13, 88. doi: 10.1186/1472-6947/13/88.

Lancioni, G. E., O'Reilly, M., Oliva, D., & Coppa, M. M. (2001). A microswitch for vocalization responses to foster environmental control in children with multiple disabilities. *Journal of Intellectual Disability Research*, 45, 271–275.

Lancioni, G. E., O'Reilly, M., Singh, N., Sigafoos, J., Chiapparino, C., Stasolla, F., Bosco, A., de Pace, C., & Oliva, D. (2007). Enabling a young man with minimal motor behavior to manage independently his leisure television engagement. *Perceptual and Motor Skills*, 105, 47–54.

Lancioni, G. E., O'Reilly, M., Singh, N., Sigafoos, J., Oliva, D., & Severini, L. (2008a). Enabling two persons with multiple disabilities to access environmental stimuli and ask for social contact through microswitches and a VOCA. *Research in Developmental Disabilities*, 29, 21–28.

Lancioni, G. E., O'Reilly, M., Singh, N., Sigafoos, J., Oliva, D., & Severini, L. (2008b). Three persons with multiple disabilities accessing environmental stimuli and asking for social contact through microswitch and VOCA technology. *Journal of Intellectual Disability Research*, 52, 327–336.

Lancioni, G. E., O'Reilly, M., Singh, N., Sigafoos, J., Didden, R., Oliva, D., Campodonico, F., de Pace, C., Chiapparino, C., & Groeneweg, J. (2009). Persons with multiple disabilities accessing stimulation and requesting social contact via microswitch and VOCA devices: New research evaluation and social validation. *Research in Developmental Disabilities*, 30, 1084–1094.

Lancioni, G. E., Singh, N., O'Reilly, M., Sigafoos, J., Signorino, M., Oliva, D., Alberti, G., Carrella, L., & de Tommaso, M. (2010). A special messaging technology for two persons with acquired brain injury and multiple disabilities. *Brain Injury*, 24, 1236–1243.

Lancioni, G. E., O'Reilly, M., Singh, N., Sigafoos, J., Oliva, D., Alberti, G., & Lang, R. (2011a). Two adults with multiple disabilities use a computer-aided telephone system to make phone calls independently. *Research in Developmental Disabilities*, 32, 2330–2335.

Lancioni, G. E., Singh, N., O'Reilly, M., Sigafoos, J., Alberti, G., Oliva, D., & Buono, S. (2011b). A technology-aided stimulus choice program for two adults with multiple disabilities: Choice responses and mood. *Research in Developmental Disabilities*, 32, 2602–2607.

Lancioni, G. E., Singh, N. N., O'Reilly, M. F., Green, V., Oliva, D., Buonocunto, F., Sacco, V., Biancardi, E. M., & Di Nuovo, S. (2012). Technology-based programs to support forms of leisure engagement and communication for persons with multiple disabilities: Two single-case studies. *Developmental Neurorehabilitation*, 15, 209–218.

Lancioni, G. E., Sigafoos, J., O'Reilly, M., Singh, N. (2013a). *Assistive Technology: Interventions for Individuals with Severe/Profound and Multiple Disabilities*. New York: Springer.

Lancioni, G. E., Singh, N., O'Reilly, M., Sigafoos, J., Oliva, D., & D'Amico, F. (2013b). Technology-aided programs to enable persons with multiple disabilities to choose among environmental stimuli using a smile or a tongue response. *Research in Developmental Disabilities*, 34, 4232–4238.

Lancioni, G. E., Ferlisi, G., Zullo, V., Settembre, M. F., Singh, N., O'Reilly, M., & Sigafoos, J. (2014a). Two men with advanced amyotrophic lateral schlerosis operate a computer-aided television system through mouth or throat micro-switches. *Perceptual and Motor Skills*, 118, 883–889.

Lancioni, G. E., Singh, N., O'Reilly, M., Sigafoos, J., Boccasini, A., La Martire, M. L., & Lang, R. (2014b). Case studies of technology for adults with multiple disabilities to make telephone calls independently. *Perceptual and Motor Skills*, 119, 320–331.

Lancioni, G. E., & Singh, N. N. (Eds.). (2014c). *Assistive Technologies for People with Diverse Abilities*. New York: Springer.

Lancioni, G. E., O'Reilly, M., Singh, N., Sigafoos, J., Boccasini, A., La Martire, M. L., Perilli, V., & Spagnuolo, C. (2016a). Technology to support positive occupational engagement and communication in persons with multiple disabilities. *International Journal on Disabilities and Human Development*, 15, 111–116.

Lancioni, G. E., Singh, N., O'Reilly, M., Green, V. A., van der Meer, L., Alberti, G., Perilli, V., Boccasini, A., La Martire M. L., & Lang, R. (2016b). A speech generating device for persons with intellectual and sensory-motor disabilities. *Journal of Developmental and Physical Disabilities*, 28, 85–98.

Lancioni, G. E., Singh, N., O'Reilly, M., Sigafoos, J., Boccasini, A., La Martire, M. L., & Smaldone, A. (2016c). People with multiple disabilities use assistive technology to perform complex activities at the appropriate time. *International Journal on Disabilities and Human Development*, 15, 261–266.

Lancioni, G. E., Singh, N., O'Reilly, M., Sigafoos, J., Alberti, G., Perilli, V., Zimbaro, C., & Chiariello, V. (2017a). Supporting leisure and communication in people with visual and intellectual disabilities via a smartphone-based program. *British Journal of Visual Impairment*, 35(3), 257–263.

Lancioni, G. E., Singh, N. N., O'Reilly, M. F., Sigafoos, J., Boccasini, A., Perilli, V., & Spagnuolo, C. (2017b). Persons with multiple disabilities manage positive leisure and communication engagement through a technology-aided program. *International Journal of Developmental Disabilities*, 63, 148–157.

Lancioni, G. E., O'Reilly, M. F., Sigafoos, J., Campodonico, F., Perilli, V., Alberti, G., Ricci, C., & Miglino, O. (2018). A modified smartphone-based program to support leisure and communication activities in people with multiple disabilities. *Advances in Neurodevelopmental Disorders*, 2. doi: 10.1007/s41252-017-0047-z.

Lorah, E. R., Parnell, A., Schaefer Whitby, P., & Hantula, D. (2015). A systematic review of tablet computers and portable media players as speech generating devices for individuals with autism spectrum disorder. *Journal of Autism and Developmental Disorders*, 45, 3792–3804.

McMillan, J. M., & Renzaglia, A. (2014). Supporting speech generating device use in the classroom. Part two: Student communication outcomes. *Journal of Special Education Technology*, 29, 49–61.

Mechling, L. C. (2006). Comparison of the effects of three approaches on the frequency of stimulus activations, via a single switch, by students with profound intellectual disabilities. *Journal of Special Education*, 40, 94–102.

Meder, A. M., & Wegner, J. R. (2015). iPads, mobile technologies, and communication applications: A survey of family wants, needs, and preferences. *Augmentative and Alternative Communication*, 31, 27–36.

Mihailidis, A., Melonis, M., Keyfitz, R., Lanning, M., Van Vuuren, S., & Bodine, C. (2016). A nonlinear contextually aware prompting system (N-CAPS) to assist workers with intellectual and developmental disabilities to perform factory assembly tasks: System overview and pilot testing. *Disability and Rehabilitation: Assistive Technology*, 11, 604–612.

Mullennix, J., & Stern, S. (Eds.). (2010). *Computer Synthesized Speech Technologies: Tools for Aiding Impairment*. Hershey, NY: Medical Information Science Reference.

Pérez-Cruzado, D., & Cuestas-Vargas, A. I. (2017). Smartphone reminder for physical activity in people with intellectual disabilities. *International Journal of Technology Assessment in Health Care*, 33, 442–443.

Pierce, W. D., & Cheney, C. D. (2008). *Behavior Analysis and Learning* (4th edn.). New York: Psychology Press.

Plackett, R., Thomas, S., & Thomas, S. (2017). Professionals' views on the use of smartphone technology to support children and adolescents with memory impairment due to acquired brain injury. *Disability and Rehabilitation: Assistive Technology*, 12, 236–243.

Ricci, C., Miglino, O., Alberti, G., Perilli, V., & Lancioni, G. E. (2017). Speech generating technology to support request responses of persons with intellectual and multiple disabilities. *International Journal of Developmental Disabilities*, 63, 238–245.

Roche, L., Sigafoos, J., Lancioni, G. E., O'Reilly, M. F., & Green, V. A. (2015). Microswitch technology for enabling self-determined responding in children with profound and multiple disabilities: A systematic review. *Augmentative and Alternative Communication*, 31, 246–258.

Schepis, M. M., & Reid, D. H. (1995). Effects of a voice output communication on interaction between support personnel and an individual with multiple disabilities. *Journal of Applied Behavior Analysis*, 28, 73–77.

Scherer, M. J., Craddock, G., & Mackeogh, T. (2011). The relationship of personal factors and subjective well-being to the use of assistive technology devices. *Disability and Rehabilitation*, 33, 811–817.

Shih, C. H., Shih, C. T., Lin, K. T., & Chiang, M. S. (2009). Assisting people with multiple disabilities and minimal motor behavior to control environmental stimulation through a mouse wheel. *Research in Developmental Disabilities*, 30, 1413–1419.

Shih, C. H., Shih, C. J., & Shih, C. T. (2011). Assisting people with multiple disabilities by actively keeping the head in an upright position with a Nintendo Wii remote controller through the control of an environmental stimulation. *Research in Developmental Disabilities*, 32, 2005–2010.

Sigafoos, J., Green, V. A., Payne, D., Son, S. H., O'Relly, M., & Lancioni, G. E. (2009). A comparison of picture exchange and speech-generating devices: Acquisition, preference, and effects on social interaction. *Augmentative and Alternative Communication*, 25, 99–109.

Stasolla, F., Perilli, V., Di Leone, A., Damiani, R., Albano, V., Stella, A., & Damato, C. (2015). Technological aids to support choice strategies by three girls with Rett syndrome. *Research in Developmental Disabilities*, 36, 36–44.

Sutherland, D., van der Meer, L., Sigafoos, J., Mirfin-Veitch, B., Milner, P., O'Reilly, M. F., Lancioni, G. E., & Marschik, P. B. (2014). Survey of AAC needs for adults with intellectual disability in New Zealand. *Journal of Developmental and Physical Disabilities*, 26, 115–122.

Tam, G. M., Phillips, K. J., & Mudford, O. C. (2011). Teaching individuals with profound multiple disabilities to access preferred stimuli with multiple microswitches. *Research in Developmental Disabilities*, 32, 2352–2361.

Taylor, J. L., & Hodapp, R. M. (2012). Doing nothing: Adults with disabilities with no daily activities and their siblings. *American Journal on Intellectual and Developmental Disabilities*, 117, 67–79.

van der Meer, L., Kagohara, D., Achmadi, D., O'Reilly, M. F., Lancioni, G. E., & Sigafoos, J. (2012). Speech-generating devices versus manual signing for children with developmental disabilities. *Research in Developmental Disabilities*, 33, 1658–1669.

van der Meer, L., Matthews, T., Ogilvie, E., Berry, A., Waddington, H., Balandin, S., O'Reilly, M. F., Lancioni, G. E., & Sigafoos, J. (2017). Training direct-care staff to provide communication intervention to adults with intellectual disability: A systematic review. *American Journal of Speech-Language Pathology*, 26(4), 1279–1295.

6

Using Digital Photography to Support the Communication of People with Aphasia, Dementia or Cognitive-Communication Deficits

Karen Hux

Quality Living, Inc.

Carly Dinnes

Bowling Green State University

CONTENTS

Introduction 90
Aphasia 90
    Early Attempts to Use Photographs as Communication Supports 91
    Contextually Rich and Personally Relevant Photographs 91
    Incorporating Digital Images into Communicative Interactions 92
Dementia 93
    Reminiscence Therapy 94
    Storytelling 96
    Life Story Documentation 96
    Caveats for Consideration 97
Traumatic Brain Injury 98
    Supporting Memory 98
        Severe Memory Impairments 98
        Mild or Moderate Memory Impairments 100
    Supporting Writing 101
Future Directions 103
References 104

Introduction

The development of photography in the 1800s provided a powerful means of 'reality capturing' and 'memory preservation' (van Dijck, 2008, p. 62). Photography gave people a way of gathering images of geographic locations and historical happenings to share with others not present at the time. As camera technology and accessibility progressed, changes occurred in how and why people acquired, used and stored photographs. First, family photography emerged as a means of documenting important people and events to preserve personal heritage and autobiographical memories. Then, continued advances prompted a shift from displaying individual portraits in homes and storing collected photographs in albums to relying on digital scanning, display and storage techniques to facilitate access, transfer and retrieval of images regardless of location. With this technological advance, a shift occurred from using photographs to preserve memories to using them to support ongoing communicative interactions (Hanson, Beukelman, & Yorkston, 2013; Engebretson, Hartman, Beukelman, & Hux, 2014; van House, 2011).

The availability and ease with which people can capture and access photographs have heightened interest in their use as supports for people with communication challenges. Because photographs are visual symbols that do not require the sharing of a common language or culture to make them comprehensible, they represent a means of circumventing many communication barriers. The purpose of this chapter is to explain ways of using digital photography to help people with language and cognitive limitations resulting from acquired neurological disorders. The first section addresses communicative supports for people with aphasia – an acquired symbolic processing impairment that frequently results from strokes and other injuries to the language-dominant hemisphere of the brain. The second section extends the use of these supports to people struggling with both language and cognitive limitations because of progressive declines associated with dementia. The third section addresses the use of digital photography to support people with traumatic brain injury (TBI) who have impairment to the cognitive processes underlying communication.

Aphasia

People with aphasia are inefficient in accessing and using symbolic elements – such as spoken and written words – to understand and express communicative intents. The disorder extends to all symbol systems and communication modalities (i.e. speaking, listening, writing, reading and gesturing). As such, providing sets of icons, isolated pictures or drawings, gestures, written words or other abstract symbols as substitutes for individual words and expecting people with aphasia to string them together to form linguistic structures is not effective. Instead, people with aphasia need methods of compensating for their challenges that either (1) support residual language comprehension and production by providing redundancy in the form of multimodal contextual content or (2) minimize reliance on linguistic or symbolic processing. The purpose of this section is to explain how contextually rich photographs can support both of these compensatory methods and allow people with aphasia to understand and express novel content during conversational interactions.

Early Attempts to Use Photographs as Communication Supports

Traditional treatment efforts to restore language functioning to premorbid levels are often insufficient following the onset of aphasia. The result is that up to 60% of people who acquire aphasia experience it as a chronic condition interfering with full participation in daily communicative interactions (Laska, Hellblom, Murray, Kahan, & Von Arbin, 2001; Pedersen, Vinter, & Olsen, 2004). These communication challenges exist despite retained ability in other aspects of cognition. For example, people with aphasia typically have preserved visual-perceptual skills, facial recognition, intellect and autobiographical memory (Blake, 2005; Brookshire, 2003; McNeil, 1983). Taking advantage of retained skills while simultaneously minimizing reliance on impaired symbolic processing is central to the advantage digital photographs provide as supports to people with aphasia.

Early attempts to use images to support communication often involved grid-based displays showing pictures or drawings of isolated images (Beukelman, Hux, Dietz, McKelvey, & Weissling, 2015). Pointing to a depicted item can provide an alternative to verbalizing basic wants and needs. However, referencing isolated images does not suffice when the goal is to convey novel content typical of conversational exchanges, such as the sharing of personal stories and daily experiences. Because of the inadequacy of grid-based displays to meet needs associated with these types of interactions, professionals began exploring other ways of using images to support people with chronic aphasia.

Contextually Rich and Personally Relevant Photographs

Recognition of the limited benefit people with aphasia receive from accessing grids displaying isolated images prompted exploration of contextually rich and personally relevant photographs as communication supports. Contextually rich images are ones that 'depict situations, places, or experiences in ways that clearly represent relationships and interactions among important people or objects' (Hux, Buechter, Wallace, & Weissling,

2010, p. 644). They show the setting in which an event or activity occurs; relevant people, objects and actions associated with the event; and content that suggests relationships among the depicted people or objects. Wallace, Hux, Brown and Knollman-Porter (2014) established that the visual complexity of contextually rich images is not problematic for people with aphasia. Specifically, the researchers found the average performance of adults with aphasia when selecting contextually rich images to match spoken sentences conveying either main action, background or inferential information ranged from 71.50% to 86.75% even though some participants exhibited severe language deficits on standardized aphasia measures.

Personally relevant photographs are ones showing people and events relevant to an individual's autobiographical history. People with aphasia are more accurate when associating personally relevant photographs with words representing actions and events than they are with generic photographs or simple drawings (McKelvey, Hux, Dietz, & Beukelman, 2010). They also prefer personally relevant photographs to the other types of images (McKelvey et al., 2010).

Incorporating Digital Images into Communicative Interactions

Extant research gives credence to the idea that access to contextually rich, personalized photographs might provide better support to people with aphasia than access to displays of isolated images. This prompted exploration of methods of pairing personal photographs with written words and graphic scales to create both high- and low-technology communication supports. As an example, Hux et al. (2010) examined the effects of having access to contextually rich photographs and written text as a shared communication space with which a person with aphasia and another person could co-construct messages. Compared to conditions in which either one or both interactants could not reference the support materials, the researchers found that sharing the supplemental resources resulted in (1) a greater number of conversational turns; (2) the person with aphasia generating more content; (3) communication partners producing more conceptually complex utterances; and (4) the person with aphasia perceiving better information transfer, ease of interaction and partner understanding. Having access to contextually rich photographs and written text had a positive effect on the type and amount of information transferred between two people when one conversant had aphasia.

Another group of researchers – Ulmer, Hux, Brown, Nelms and Reeder (2016) – extended the idea of using contextually rich photographs to support conversations by having people with aphasia capture desired images themselves and then use them to support interactions with a novel communication partner. The participants with aphasia first captured as many or as few photographs as desired while observing other people perform a series of wellness activities (i.e. height and weight measurement, hearing screening, endurance testing, etc.); later, the participants could access the digital photographs on a laptop computer to reference or share with a communication partner while conversing about the observed activities. The number of captured photographs ranged from 0 to 95 across the five study participants despite all having received instruction in camera use and being told they could use the photographs to support later conversation. This variability suggests that some people with aphasia do not intuitively recognize the potential benefit of having photographs available as a language support and will need direct instruction about this strategy. Comparison of the conversational interactions by participants who did versus did not reference photographs revealed the following benefits of photographic supports: (1) generation of more content, (2) generation of content with greater specificity, (3) greater topic maintenance and (4) less frequent disability-related comments. Once again, referencing contextually rich photographs proved to be an effective method of compensating for acquired language impairment.

Dementia

People with dementia experience progressive decreases in cognitive functions that coincide with increasing communication challenges. The combination of cognitive and communication difficulties result in discourse limited in content and replete with repetitive statements; with disease progression, the amount and quality of verbalizations deteriorate. Because limitations in engaging in meaningful conversation contribute directly to declines in socialization, finding ways of supporting communication is critical to maximizing quality of life for people with dementia.

One of the most noticeable cognitive deteriorations associated with dementia is progressive worsening of the formation and retrieval of new memories. As a result, people with dementia typically exhibit poor recall of recent events. This impairment in forming new memories contrasts with slower degradation of memories from the distant past. Although a person with dementia may struggle to maintain and participate in conversations about recent happenings, he/she may converse at length about childhood recollections. This preserved recall of events from the remote past has spurred family members and professionals to engage people with dementia in activities involving reminiscence about the past, storytelling and documentation of life stories. All of these activities – as well as the concomitant development and implementation of memory supports – can be enhanced through the use of digital photography. The case example about Henry provides an example of how a person with dementia can use photography to support memory challenges and enhance social interactions.

CASE EXAMPLE: HENRY

Henry, an 83-year-old male with dementia, received speech-language therapy services during a short stay at a skilled nursing facility. Because he exhibited only mild deficits, Henry's treatment focused on supporting his return home. In addition to traditional therapy activities, Henry worked on identifying and implementing effective technology-based compensatory strategies to support memory.

Henry began using the camera on his cell phone to take photographs of staff members at the facility as one compensatory strategy. Viewing these images served as a reminder of which staff worked with him and the role each played in his daily care. Henry regularly reviewed the photographs during therapy sessions to verify his recall accuracy. He also used his cell phone camera to capture images of objects and events that interested him. These photographs promoted conversations with others. Referring to captured images, Henry could double-check information relating to specific conversational topics. He could also provide his communication partners with visual images to support their interactions.

Henry had a digital picture frame in his room at the facility that displayed images of friends, family and important life events. Henry spent time each day using the pictures to initiate conversations with others. This strategy provided Henry's communication partners with a visual referent and contextual information for the conversation. Henry also used the displayed photographs as part of a daily memory exercise during which he practised identifying key details.

Reminiscence Therapy

Reminiscence therapy is a type of interaction that promotes the discussion of past experiences, usually with the aid of tangible props such as photographs, newspaper clippings and musical recordings (Cotelli, Manenti, & Zanetti, 2012; Woods, O'Philbin, Farrell, Spector, & Orrell, 2018). Clinicians implementing reminiscence therapy identify important events and milestones in a person's life – such as academic achievements, military service, marriage ceremonies and holiday celebrations – and use them to scaffold conversational exchanges. Incorporating multisensory input in the form of tangible props supports recall. For example, props to support a conversation about the winter holidays might include traditional holiday decorations, music, winter outerwear and foods that provide sounds, smells, tastes, images and touch sensations that maximize the potential for recall of relevant past experiences. The addition of photographs as a tangible prop can play a particularly important role in promoting recall and stimulating language production, especially when the images are personally relevant ones depicting the individual him/herself or immediate family members (Andrews, 1997). Also important is the selection of photographs depicting people engaged in activities rather than portraits, depictions of scenes or pictures of isolated objects (Alm, Ellis, Astell, Dye, Gowans, & Campbell, 2004). However, because misinterpretations sometimes occur when people with dementia encounter visually complex photographs, balancing simplicity and transparency with contextual richness may be critical when selecting photographs for reminiscence purposes.

Engaging in reminiscence therapy in conjunction with referencing external memory aids supports interactions critical to fostering the maintenance of communicative and social interaction skills. Although empirical evidence about the beneficial effects of reminiscence therapy remains elusive (Cotelli et al., 2012; Woods et al., 2018), the activity has become a mainstay among professionals working with dementia populations. The technique may be particularly effective when supplemented with external supports such as memory wallets, memory books, reminder cards and memo boards. These supports – while flexible enough to serve different purposes depending on the content included – present obvious opportunities to incorporate photographs. For example, reminder cards and memo boards typically convey short written messages that may change on a regular basis, such as a note stating that a family member will visit later that day to participate in a scheduled reminiscence activity. Adding a photograph may foster understanding of the person referenced in the message or the purpose of the scheduled event. In contrast, memory wallets and memory books are effective for conveying fairly consistent information – such as biographical facts and important life experiences – about the person with dementia.

These aids serve as expressive communication supports and typically incorporate both text and images. The text provides a script to support initial conversational interactions; the inclusion of meaningful photographs promotes the likelihood a person with dementia will relate details about the topic and engage in multiple conversational turns rather than reading aloud only the provided written statement. Similarly, communication partners may find the text and photographs helpful when generating questions to foster continued conversation and reminiscence about the selected topic.

Astell and colleagues (Astell, Ellis, Alm, Dye, Campbell, & Gowens, 2004; Astell, Ellis, Alm, Dye, Gowens, & Campbell, 2005) combined reminiscence therapy with a communication aid on a multimedia computer system. The system – called CIRCA (computer-aided reminiscence and communication aid) – provides touchscreen accessing of photographs, music and video clips via an easily navigated interface. The researchers found that use of CIRCA supported greater conversational control by people with dementia than is typical of traditional reminiscence therapy. In particular, a shift occurred from a staff-directed question-and-answer format to one in which people with dementia assumed active roles in directing conversational interactions.

Storytelling

Storytelling is another activity that encourages conversation and promotes positive social interactions by people with dementia. Storytelling is a routine form of interaction among groups of people, and it persists as an important feature of communication throughout all life stages (Gubrium & Holstein, 1998; Langellier, 1989; van Dijk, 1997). By eliciting and analysing stories generated during one-on-one interactions, Fels and Astell (2011) found that people with dementia demonstrated command of basic storytelling components even when the disease had progressed to the severe stage. As such, engaging in storytelling may remain a viable means of communicative interaction despite the presence or severity of dementia.

Stories that are autobiographical in nature – often referred to as personal narratives – relate details about a person's lived experiences and can play a key role in establishing and maintaining relationships within families and social groups (Fivush, 1993). Storytelling is distinct from reminiscence therapy in that it occurs on a routine basis as a pastime rather than as a dementia-specific activity (Fels & Astell, 2011). Also, storytelling does not demand accuracy or truthfulness in the same manner that recounting events during reminiscence activities may (Fels & Astell, 2011). For example, when a person with dementia reminisces about life events, a family member may be tempted to interrupt and correct inaccuracies; the emphasis is on recalling and recounting the events as they happened rather than forming and maintaining relationships. This contrasts with the scenario created when a person assumes the role of storyteller; here, the emphasis is on interpersonal connections and making shared interactions enjoyable.

Fels and Astell (2011) suggest using generic rather than personal photographs when engaging people with dementia in storytelling. Both contextually rich photographs and pictures of isolated objects tied to a specific event (e.g. a birthday cake) can serve as prompting stimuli. The expectation is that stories will emerge relating only to a few of several presented photographs, and predicting which stimuli will spark stories is not possible. Furthermore, Fels and Astell caution that story themes may differ substantially from depicted content. They stress that this is not concerning given the intent to elicit storytelling behaviour rather than conversations about pre-specified topics; once again, keeping in mind that the benefit of storytelling is its role in building and maintaining relationships is key.

Life Story Documentation

Another activity that provides a means of facilitating social and conversational interactions with people with dementia is life story documentation. This activity involves having a person with dementia and/or family members of that person identify and record information about salient life events (McKeown, Clark, Ingleton, Ryan, & Pepper, 2010). Displaying the content can take many forms: a life storybook, a photo album with or without related written or auditory text, a memory box containing mementos or digital blogs or websites. As accessing and storing content on the Internet has become more common, the use of multimedia digital formats for developing and sharing biographical content central to life story documentation has increased. Life stories documented in this fashion are sometimes called multimedia biographies (Smith, Crete-Nishihata, Damianakis, Baecker, & Marziali, 2009). Using multimedia formats and assuming the disease process is not advanced, people with dementia can record themselves talking about life events to supplement digitized photographs, videos and background music.

A major focus of life story work is its use to promote person-centred care for people with dementia (Stenhouse, Tait, Hardy, & Sumner, 2013). The final product has the potential to promote respect towards and personhood for the person with dementia by providing a means of sharing – either verbally or non-verbally – life events. As with storytelling, this sharing of life stories is critical to forming and strengthening interpersonal relationships. Life story work also supports self-expression – a critical element given the loss of identity that occurs as cognitive decline progresses. A life story production provides a way for a person with dementia to connect to his/her past and, simultaneously, build and fortify new relationships with current peers and caregivers.

Caveats for Consideration

Certain caveats may limit the effectiveness of using digital photography with dementia populations. First, many elderly adults have personal photograph collections that are not in digital form. Although this likelihood will lessen in future years as people switch from physical to digital repositories, the collected photographs of many of today's elderly may exist exclusively as hard copies – some of which may have deteriorated in quality with age. Transferring cherished photographs to digital form is a project that family members may embrace as way of recalling and celebrating a person's life.

Another potential concern is a person's visual status. Evaluating visual acuity and processing are necessary when determining the feasibility of using digital photography to support communication for a person with dementia. Decreased visual acuity is relatively common among the elderly and can limit the extent to which a person benefits from visual supports. Similarly, visual processing deficits can co-occur with dementia and can contribute to misinterpretations of elements depicted in photographs.

Another concern about using digital photography to support the communication of people with dementia is familiarity with technology. Many digital cameras are relatively simple to operate, but the steps involved in saving, downloading, transferring and accessing stored photographs are likely to tax the cognitive skills of people with dementia, especially when the disease has progressed beyond the initial stages. Also, elderly people in general have less experience and confidence using technology than their younger counterparts. Having a family member or caregiver available to support the use of digital photography is essential when working with people with dementia.

Traumatic Brain Injury

People who sustain TBI often display cognitive-communication deficits as a chronic condition. Cognitive-communication deficits occur when diffuse damage to the brain interferes with cognitive processes underlying communicative functions (MacDonald & Shumway, 2002). Dysfunction in memory, attention, problem-solving, organization and/or executive functioning negatively affect communicative performance by resulting in expressive output lacking in detail, having abrupt topic shifts, having limited coherence and macrostructure, and including non-essential or tangentially related ideas in place of or in addition to relevant content (Coelho, 2007; Hux, Wallace, Evans, & Snell, 2008; MacDonald & Shumway, 2002; Togher et al., 2014).

Using photographs to support routine interactions following TBI is not typically warranted unless the person exhibits severe communication difficulties extending beyond cognitive-communication deficits – such as might be the case when concomitant aphasia affecting language processing or dysarthria affecting speech production occurs. However, two scenarios may arise for which implementing digital photography as a compensatory support can be an asset: (1) severe memory deficits that limit the recall of daily events (Jamieson, Cullen, McGee-Lennon, Brewster, & Evans, 2014; Svoboda, Richards, Leach, & Mertens, 2012) and (2) written language challenges that interfere with resuming academic, social and vocational endeavours (Dinnes & Hux, 2018; Dinnes, Hux, Holmen, Martens, & Smith, 2018; Ledbetter, Sohlberg, Fickas, Horney, & McIntosh, 2017). The purpose of this section is to explain how digital photography can support communication-based activities relating to these challenges.

Supporting Memory

Severe Memory Impairments

Memory deficits are among the most common and enduring complaints of people with TBI (Jamieson et al., 2014; Khan, Baguley, & Cameron, 2003; Ponsford et al., 2014; Svoboda et al., 2012; Velikonja, Tate, Ponsford, McIntyre,

Janzen, & Bayley, 2014). When memory problems are particularly severe, a person may fail to lay down any new memories about daily events. As a result, the only means of recalling salient happenings is through recording details about them as they occur. Methods of doing this include writing notes, making audio recordings of event summaries and capturing images digitally. The case example about Janet provides an account of how digital photography supported her engagement in daily living and social activities despite the severity of her memory deficits.

CASE EXAMPLE: JANET

Janet had severe memory impairment secondary to a burst aneurysm at age 15. Her injury resulted in near-complete amnesia for new experiences, although Janet could recognize and recall people she met both before and after injury. Being highly social, Janet enjoyed interacting with other people her age, but her only means of recalling what she had done with them was by relying on external memory supports. Writing remarks in a journal, day planner or on sticky notes became a necessary strategy for tracking activities. Janet also found that capturing photographs was effective for creating a tangible record of salient daily events. Furthermore, this procedure was much less time consuming and burdensome than constantly writing notes.

Capturing photographs was particularly important when Janet went shopping for clothing and entertainment items. Because Janet had limited funds, she needed to be diligent about recording expenditures and not buying the same or similar items multiple times. Janet tracked her expenses in a chequebook but also took pictures of purchases as she paid for them. By referencing photographs from recent shopping trips, she could be confident that she was not duplicating previous purchases.

Janet also found that taking digital photographs was a good way of sharing experiences with family members. Her parents and siblings were supportive of Janet's desire to engage in activities without them, but they wanted to know what she had done during time spent with friends. Capturing photographs of the people present and events occurring during outings provided a way for Janet to keep her family informed about her activities.

Using digital photography to support severe memory loss has several advantages over creating written or auditory notes. First, capturing photographs is faster than generating handwritten notes or recording auditory messages. Second, it requires less fine motor control than writing – another area of challenge for some survivors of severe TBI. Third, taking pictures with a digital camera is substantially less demanding on cognitive resources than listening to and processing ongoing events, translating that content into words and recording the resultant words, phrases and sentences either as spoken or written messages. Finally, most digital photography includes an option for including time and date stamps, so the resulting images automatically provide a record of when an event occurred and the temporal sequence of relevant happenings during a day.

Remembering to capture photographs may be a problem for people with particularly severe memory impairments. Just like with the cueing people with severe memory impairments often need to record written or auditory notes, assistance from another person may be necessary to provide reminders about taking photographs. Another problem is handling the camera with sufficient skill and efficiency to capture photographs at the moment critical events happen. Recent technology advances may hold the key to overcoming these particular challenges, however, because some glasses-mounted and hands-free cameras available for consumer purchase automatically capture photographs at specified time intervals. The type and extent of purposeful action required by the user to trigger photograph capture varies from one device to another. With purely automatic systems, a disadvantage is sacrificing control about the specific images captured; instead of framing a shot to ensure depiction of salient content, automatic photography captures whatever is happening directly in front of the person. Another problem is the potential for privacy invasion when images are taken at preset intervals; people in the surrounding area have not consented to having their picture taken and may not even realize it is happening. Yet another problem is that the sheer number of captured photographs may be overwhelming for the person with TBI; having to review, select and organize hundreds of captured images from a single day to determine which convey relevant content may require substantial time and exceed the cognitive abilities of some survivors.

Mild or Moderate Memory Impairments

Mild or moderate memory deficits secondary to TBI often present as unreliable recall of prospective events or critical information. Many people with TBI use a combination of strategies involving written notes, calendars and alarms to compensate for these challenges; capturing digital photographs can serve as a supplement or alternative to other strategies. Just as people without cognitive or communication challenges can use digital photography as an effective tool for supporting everyday memory, so can people with TBI. Capturing digital images is an easy and efficient way of recording pertinent visual information without taxing cognitive resources. Furthermore, having access to a photograph allows for repeated reference to material identical to that originally presented. This reduces the chances of recalling details inaccurately or incompletely.

Examples of ways in which people with memory challenges use digital photography as a compensatory support are numerous and reflect the many vocational, social and academic settings survivors routinely encounter. Digital cameras have become increasingly portable and accessible given technological advances promoting their inclusion in electronic devices such as cell phones, tablets and laptop computers. Because members of the general population routinely use these forms of technology, taking digital photographs does not draw attention or signal the presence of a disability. Students with TBI may find that taking photographs of instructors' handwritten diagrams or examples presented during lectures are advantageous for later review and study. People in work settings may capture images of written instructions or demonstrations of new procedures that they can later reference when trying to incorporate new tasks or skills into their work routines. Socially, people with TBI may find that posting images to social media sites serves as an alternative method of relaying information about recent events that eliminates the need for extended writing. As is true for people with severe memory impairments, capturing images of salient content in situations like these allows a person to focus fully on ongoing events rather than having to split attention among listening, processing, recalling and translating spoken words to written form to generate meaningful notes.

Supporting Writing

Written expression requires a complex interplay of cognitive-linguistic skills – such as word retrieval, language, memory and organization – to generate concise, cohesive and informative messages. The intricacy involved in recruiting and coordinating these skills makes writing particularly susceptible to TBI. Similar to the effect TBIs may have on spoken language, disruption to the cognitive skills underlying effective written communication can result in messages that are disorganized, repetitive and lacking in sufficient detail. Post-injury writing challenges may also include impairment in writing conventions (e.g. spelling, punctuation and grammar), which may increase message ambiguity. The combination of these difficulties can result in vague, imprecise writing or even complete failure to convey an intended message.

The impact of TBI on written communication remains largely unexplored despite the susceptibility of writing to the disruptive effects of acquired neurological damage. However, a recent qualitative study (e.g. Dinnes et al., 2018) highlighted the characteristics and consequences of TBI-related writing difficulties and some of the ways digital photography can serve as a writing support. The researchers interviewed 11 adults with TBI about their post-injury writing experiences, challenges and support strategies. Prior to injury, all were engaged in full-time work or academic activities and did not experience substantial writing problems. However, after injury, the majority reported writing difficulties and experienced multiple challenges with the writing process. Generating sufficient ideas, recalling details and translating ideas into coherent written messages were frequently highlighted as areas of particular challenge.

The people with TBI interviewed by Dinnes et al. (2018) discussed their routine implementation of strategies to promote success when performing writing activities. One strategy specifically involved the use of digital photography. Capturing digital photographs allowed for the creation of permanent records showing people, settings and event sequences. In this way, digital photographs served as reference materials to support the later generation of written accounts about recent events. As illustrated in the case examples of Beth and Eric, having photographs available for review while writing can promote idea generation, the addition of relevant details and the verification of information accuracy.

CASE EXAMPLE: BETH

Beth, a 36-year-old female, sustained a severe TBI in a car accident when she was 15 years old. She received extensive rehabilitation services to address her many post-injury challenges. Upon returning to school, Beth received academic accommodations to support persistent difficulties with cognitive and linguistic skills. She successfully completed high school and recently completed a Bachelor's degree. As part of her academic work, Beth regularly completed reading, writing and research assignments.

Beth actively sought and generated compensatory strategies to support persistent areas of challenge affecting her academic pursuits. Writing, in particular, was a difficult and frustrating task for Beth. She struggled to generate ideas and translate them into written form. Beth also struggled to recall information and noted that trying to remember an idea and the words to express that idea long enough to transcribe them was extremely challenging. Among the several strategies Beth implements to support her written communication, she has found that referencing photographs is one of the most effective.

For Beth, using a digital camera to take photographs provides support for generating ideas as well as an effective means of compensating for memory challenges. As she explained: 'If I take a picture, I can kind of come up with something. If I'm gonna write, I need a picture or… something I can reference cause it helps guide me….I still have a hard time…getting it [a thought] out, but at least with that picture, I can usually come back to that thought because it was something in the picture that showed me'.

CASE EXAMPLE: ERIC

Eric, a 58-year-old male, sustained a mild TBI in a car accident at age 17. Although the TBI exacerbated pre-injury difficulties with reading and writing and made subsequent academic work challenging, Eric successfully completed high school as well as two Associate's degrees and a Bachelor's degree. Eric currently works as a rehabilitation technology specialist evaluating individuals with disabilities, their homes and their work environments to determine technology-based supports that may be beneficial. Thorough documentation and report writing are key components of Eric's job responsibilities.

Eric has generated several strategies to support persisting areas of challenge resulting from his TBI. One of his more recent strategies is capturing digital photographs when completing assessments for work. Previously, Eric relied on taking written notes to record details about the home and work environments of his clients. However, he found converting his abbreviated notes into cohesive and formal written reports was difficult. This prompted him to switch to using a digital camera to take photographs during assessments.

Recalling details and generating reports is easier for Eric when he can reference a photograph rather than rely solely on field notes. Photographs often show details of an environment that Eric does not record in written notes. Thus, the photographs serve as a support for identifying and recalling critical information. Eric also incorporates the photographs into his written reports to provide more informative messages than is otherwise possible. His combined text and picture reports now serve as a template for documentation and work reports completed by other rehabilitation technology specialists in his company.

Future Directions

Digital photography provides several ways of supporting people with language and cognitive impairments resulting from aphasia, dementia or TBI. Although referencing photographs alone may not always be sufficient to compensate fully for substantial communication and memory impairments, the technique offers an alternative way of introducing content when cognitive or language barriers are present. Furthermore, text messaging and social media platforms such as Instagram and Snapchat have advanced the popularity of digital photography and established its role as a routine method of documenting and communicating about both ordinary and extraordinary events. This acceptance by the general public makes digital photography unobtrusive as a support strategy for people with disabilities. As technological advances continue to improve the quality of captured images, the amount of storage space available and the ease of taking, storing, organizing, transferring and accessing collections, new applications and methods of using digital photographs as compensatory supports are likely.

Applications of digital photography as a support mechanism are likely to expand to include digital videography in the future. Many commercially available digital cameras already have the capability of recording videos that can be transferred and shared as easily as photographs. Given this scenario, videography may soon emerge as a preferred method of supporting communication and memory. Indeed, digital videography already provides a means of documenting life stories for people with dementia. Extending this to other scenarios – such as providing instructions for completing specific tasks – may expand the potential for people with disabilities to function more independently and successfully in a variety of settings. However, before this can occur on a routine basis, a reduction in the amount of file space required for video storage will be necessary. Reliance on Graphics Interchange Formats (GIFs) may be a viable solution to this problem in some situations. GIFs are short videos that capture several seconds of visual information; the recordings loop to play repeatedly. Although GIFs do not include auditory content, short captions can be added and timed to appear at specific points during the playback. The advantages of GIFs are that they can capture more visual information than photographs and their short length reduces the amount of space they occupy in comparison with other video files.

Finally, future efforts need to determine best practices for teaching people with cognitive or communication impairments to benefit from digital photography supports. Although some people with disabilities appear to understand intuitively the potential benefits of accessing and referencing digital photographs, other people need direct instruction about these possibilities. Establishing best practices for providing this instruction to people with various types and severities of acquired cognitive and communication limitations needs to be the focus of future endeavours.

References

Alm, N., Ellis, M., Astell, A., Dye, R., Gowans, G., & Campbell, J. (2004). A cognitive prothesis and communication support for people with dementia. *Neuropsychological Rehabilitation*, *14*, 117–134. DOI: 10.1080/09602010343000147

Andrews, T. A. (1997). Effects of picture stimuli on language production of people with Alzheimer's Disease. (Unpublished master's thesis). University of Nebraska – Lincoln, Lincoln, NE.

Astell, A. J., Ellis, M., Alm, N., Dye, R., Campbell, J., & Gowens, G. (2004). Facilitating communication in dementia with multimedia technology. *Brain and Language*, *91*, 80–81. DOI: 10.1016.j.bandl.2004.06.043.

Astell, A. J., Ellis, M., Alm, N., Dye, R., Gowens, G., & Campbell, J. (2005). Using hypermedia to support communication in Alzheimer's disease: The CIRCA project. In D. D. Schmorrow (Ed.), *Foundations of augmented cognition*, Vol. 11 (pp. 758–767). Mahway, NJ: Lawrence Erlbaum Associates Publishers.

Beukelman, D. R., Hux, K., Dietz, A., McKelvey, M., & Weissling, K. (2015). Using visual scene displays as communication support options for people with chronic, severe aphasia: A summary of AAC research and future research directions. *Augmentative and Alternative Communication, 31*, 234–245. DOI: 10.3109/07434618.2015.1052152.

Blake, M. (2005). Right hemisphere syndrome. In L. LaPointe (Ed.), *Aphasia and related neurogenic language disorders* (pp. 213–224). New York, NY: Thieme Medical.

Brookshire, R. H. (2003). *Introduction to neurogenic communication disorders* (5th ed.). St. Louis, MO: Mosby.

Coelho, C. A. (2007). Management of discourse deficits following traumatic brain injury: Progress, caveats, and needs. *Seminars in Speech and Language, 28*, 122–135. DOI: 10.1055/s-2007-970570.

Cotelli, M., Manenti, R., & Zanetti, O. (2012). Reminiscence therapy in dementia: A review. *Maturitas, 72*(3), 203–205. DOI: 10.1016/j.maturitas.2012.04.008.

Dinnes, C. & Hux, K. (2018). A multicomponent writing intervention for a college student with mild brain injury. *Communication Disorders Quarterly, 39*(4), 490–500. DOI: 10.1177/1525740117716416.

Dinnes, C., Hux, K., Holmen, M., Martens, A., & Smith, M. (2018). Writing changes and perceptions after traumatic brain injury: "Oh, by the way, I can't write." *American Journal of Speech-Language Pathology, 27*, 1523–1538. DOI: 10.1044/2018_AJSLP-18-0025.

Engebretson, K., Hartman, R., Beukelman, D., & Hux, K. (2014). The role of photographs in face-to-face interactions involving younger and older neurotypical adults. *Perspectives on Augmentative and Alternative Communication, 233*(1), 82–89.

Fels, D. I., & Astell, A. J. (2011). Storytelling as a model of conversation for people with dementia and caregivers. *American Journal of Alzheimer's Disease and Other Dementias, 26*, 535–541. DOI: 10.1177/1533317511429324.

Fivush, R. (1993). Emotional content of parent–child conversations about the past. In C. A. Nelson (Ed.), *The minnesota symposia on child psychology*, Vol. 26, *Memory and Affect in Development* (pp. 39–77). Hillsdale, NJ: Erlbaum.

Gubrium, J. F. & Holstein, J. A. (1998). Narrative practice and the coherence of personal stories. *The Sociological Quarterly, 39*, 163–187.

Hanson, E., Beukelman, D., & Yorkston, K. (2013). Communication support through multimodal supplementation: A scoping review. *Augmentative and Alternative Communication, 29*, 310–321. DOI: 10.1080/02687030902869299.

Hux, K., Buechter, M., Wallace, S., & Weissling, K. (2010). Using visual scene displays to create a shared communication space for a person with aphasia. *Aphasiology, 24*, 643–660. DOI: 10.1080/02687030902869299.

Hux, K., Wallace, S. E., Evans, K., & Snell, J. (2008). Performing cookie theft picture content analyses to delineate cognitive-communication impairments. *Journal of Medical Speech-Language Pathology, 16*(2), 83–103.

Jamieson, M., Cullen, B., McGee-Lennon, M., Brewster, S., & Evans, J. J. (2014). The efficacy of cognitive prosthetic technology for people with memory impairments: A systematic review and meta-analysis. *Neuropsychological Rehabilitation, 24*(3–4), 419–444. DOI: 10.1080/09602011.2013.825632.

Khan, F., Baguley, I. J., & Cameron, I. D. (2003). 4: Rehabilitation after traumatic brain injury. *Medical Journal of Australia, 178*(6), 290–297.

Langellier, K. M. (1989). Personal narratives: Perspectives on theory and research. *Text Performance Quarterly, 9,* 243–276.

Laska, A.C., Hellblom, A., Murray, V., Kahan, T., von Arbin, M. (2001). Aphasia in acute stroke and relation to outcome. *Journal of Internal Medicine, 249,* 413–422. DOI: 10.1046/j.1365–2796.2001.00812.x.

Ledbetter, A. K., Sohlberg, M. M., Fickas, S. F., Horney, M. A., & McIntosh, K. (2017). Evaluation of a computer-based prompting intervention to improve essay writing in undergraduates with cognitive impairment after acquired brain injury. *Neuropsychological Rehabilitation,* 1–30. DOI: 10.1080/09602011.2017.1383272.

MacDonald, S. & Shumway, E. (2002). Preferred practice guidelines for cognitive-communication disorders. Publication of the College of Speech-Language Pathologists and Audiologists of Ontario (CASLPO).

McKelvey, M., Hux, K., Dietz, A., & Beukelman, D. (2010). Impact of personal relevance and contextualization on comprehension by people with chronic aphasia. *American Journal of Speech Language Pathology, 19,* 22–33. DOI: 10.1044/1058–0360(2009/08–0021).

McKeown, J., Clark, A., Ingleton, C., Ryan, T., & Pepper, J. (2010). The use of life story work with people with dementia to enhance person-centered care. *International Journal of Older People Nursing, 5,* 148–158.

McNeil, M. (1983). Aphasia: Neurological considerations. *Topics in Language Disorders, 3,* 1–19.

Pedersen, P., Vinter, K., & Olsen, T. S. (2004). Aphasia after stroke: Type, severity and prognosis. *Cerebrovascular Diseases, 17,* 35–43. DOI: 10.1159/000073896.

Ponsford, J. L., Downing, M. G., Olver, J., Ponsford, M., Acher, R., Carty, M., & Spitz, G. (2014). Longitudinal follow-up of patients with traumatic brain injury: outcome at two, five, and ten years post-injury. *Journal of Neurotrauma, 31*(1), 64–77. DOI: 10.1089/neu.2013.2997.

Smith, K. L., Crete-Nishihata, M., Damianakis, T., Baecker, R. M., & Marziali, E. (2009). Multimedia biographies: A reminiscence and social stimulus tool for persons with cognitive impairment. *Journal of Technology in Human Services, 27,* 287–306. DOI: 10.1080/15228830903329831.

Stenhouse, R., Tait, J., Hardy, P., & Sumner, T. (2013). Dangling conversations: Reflections on the process of creating digital stories during a workshop with people with early-stage dementia. *Journal of Psychiatric and Mental Health Nursing, 20,* 134–141. DOI: 10.1111/j.1365–2850.2012.01900.x.

Svoboda, E., Richards, B., Leach, L., & Mertens, V. (2012). PDA and smartphone use by individuals with moderate-to-severe memory impairment: Application of a theory-driven training programme. *Neuropsychological Rehabilitation, 22*(3), 408–427. DOI: 10.1080/09602011.2011.652498.

Togher, L., Wiseman-Hakes, C., Douglas, J., Stergiou-Kita, M., Ponsford, J., Teasell, R.,... & Turkstra, L. S. (2014). INCOG recommendations for management of cognition following traumatic brain injury, part IV: Cognitive communication. *The Journal of Head Trauma Rehabilitation, 29*(4), 353–368. DOI: 10.1097/HTR.0000000000000071.

Ulmer, E., Hux, K., Brown, J., Nelms, T., & Reeder, C. (2016). Using self-captured photographs to support the expressive communication of people with aphasia, *Aphasiology, 31,* 1183–1204. DOI: 10.1080/02687038.2016.1274872.

van Dijck, J. (2008). Digital photography: Communication, identify, and memory. *Visual Communication, 7,* 57–76. DOI: 10.1177/1470357207084865.

van Dijk, T. A. (1997). Discourse as interaction in society. In T. A. van Dijk (Ed.), *Discourse as social interaction* (pp. 1–37). London: Sage.

van House, N. A. (2011). Personal photography, digital technologies, and the uses of the visual. *Visual Studies, 26,* 125–134. DOI: 10.1080/1472586X.2011.571888.

Velikonja, D., Tate, R., Ponsford, J., McIntyre, A., Janzen, S., & Bayley, M. (2014). INCOG recommendations for management of cognition following traumatic brain injury, part V: Memory. *The Journal of Head Trauma Rehabilitation, 29*(4), 369–386. DOI: 10.1097/HTR.0000000000000069.

Wallace, S. E., Hux, K., Brown, J., & Knollman-Porter, K. (2014). High-context images: Comprehension of main, background, and inferential information by people with aphasia. *Aphasiology, 28,* 713–730. DOI: 10.1080/02687038.2014.891095.

Woods, B., O'Philbin, L., Farrell, E. M., Spector, A. E., & Orrell, M. (2018). Reminiscence therapy for dementia. *Cochrane Database of Systematic Reviews, 2018*(3), 1–130. DOI: 10.1002/14651858.CD001120.pub3.

7

Common and Assistive Technology to Support People with Specific Learning Disabilities to Access Healthcare

Dianne Chambers

University of Notre Dame Australia

Sharon Campbell

La Trobe University

CONTENTS

Introduction 109
Impacts of Learning Disabilities 111
Accessing Healthcare.. 112
    Hospital Admittance... 113
    Visiting a GP... 113
    Written Information 114
    Dosage Calculations.. 114
    Informed Consent 114
Everyday and Assistive Technology 115
Future Directions and Considerations for Healthcare Providers................. 119
References 120

Introduction

It has been identified that low levels of literacy in regards to health information leads to '…increased hospitalizations, greater emergency care use, lower use of mammography, lower receipt of influenza vaccine, poorer ability to demonstrate taking medications appropriately, poorer ability to interpret labels and health messages, and, among seniors, poorer overall health status and higher mortality' (AHRQ, 2011, p. 1). People with specific learning disabilities (sLDs), particularly those with low-literacy levels, are at increased risk of poor health outcomes if they are unable to access information and resources to support them in making sound health choices and decisions

(Agency for Healthcare Research and Quality (AHRQ), 2011; Kaphingst, Zanfini, & Emmons, 2009; Miller, McCardle & Hernandez, 2010). It is therefore necessary to consider the needs of people with a learning disability within the healthcare sector as these needs are varied and can be addressed in a variety of ways, often through the use of existing and assistive technology.

Learning disabilities are described by the Learning Disability Association of America (LDAA) (2018), as '...neurologically-based processing problems. These processing problems can interfere with learning basic skills such as reading, writing and/or math. They can also interfere with higher level skills such as organization, time planning, abstract reasoning, long or short term memory and attention' (para. 1). In some countries, the term 'learning disabilities' has historically been used to describe an intellectual disability. Until very recently (approximately 2014), the term 'learning disabilities' in the United Kingdom, for example, referred to students with a low IQ (below 70) and poor adaptive behaviours, which were evident in childhood (The British Psychological Society, 2015). Practitioners and clinicians in the United Kingdom are now using the term intellectual disability to describe people with these characteristics, consistent with terminology used in the United States and Australia. Research in the area of learning disabilities, therefore, needs to be viewed and interpreted with care to ensure that comparisons or characteristics are not extended to groups with differing features. People experiencing a sLD generally have the intelligence and motivation to succeed, but have a neurological difference that prevents them from reading, spelling, writing or comprehending maths (Peterson & Pennington, 2012; Reid Lyon, Shaywitz & Shaywitz, 2003).

Learning disabilities, sometimes known as sLDs, can impact areas beyond academic skills, in areas such as relationships and friendships with others, memory difficulties and the ability to plan effectively (Lavoie, Levine, Reiner & Reiner, 2005). There are a number of types of learning disability and they each manifest differently between individuals. The most common categories of diagnosed learning disability include dyslexia, dysgraphia and dyscalculia (Dyslexia SPELD Foundation, 2014). Dyslexia refers to a difficulty with language-related tasks, in particular reading, but also spelling, writing and pronunciation to some extent (Armstrong & Squires, 2015). It is estimated that approximately 5%–7% of people have dyslexia (Peterson & Pennington, 2012).

Dysgraphia impacts on a person's ability to acquire written language and how well the person is able to express their understanding through written mediums. Poor spelling can also be a characteristic of a person who has dysgraphia (Judd, 2012). Around 5%–20% of people are said to have some form of writing difficulty; however, it is not known how many of these would demonstrate the diagnostic criteria for dysgraphia (Phillips & Clark, 2013).

Dyscalculia consists of a wide variety of difficulties in the area of mathematics. The Dyslexia SPELD Foundation (2014) describe a person with dyscalculia as having difficulty with learning number concepts, manipulating numbers, learning facts and identifying mathematical patterns.

Butterworth, Varma and Laurillard (2011) describe dyscalculia as being the 'poor cousin' of dyslexia. Although it has a similar prevalence rate of 5%–7%, there has been less research and interest than in dyslexia.

sLDs are known as 'disabilities' as they often impact on learning, or inhibit other aspects of the person's everyday functioning, although some use the term specific learning differences to avoid the stigma of a 'disability'. While these issues are generally identified in childhood, some are not diagnosed until late adolescence, or even into adulthood, as the person may not have been effectively assessed, has masked their difficulties throughout their schooling or has withdrawn from schooling as a result of their struggle with learning. Learning disabilities are ongoing and persistent throughout a person's life, contrasting with learning problems or difficulties, which generally manifest as a result of a circumstance such as low-cognitive ability, injury, socioeconomic status and which may be addressed through appropriate intervention (Westwood, 2015).

As there are no external indicators that there is an underlying disability, learning disabilities are sometimes known as 'hidden disabilities' (LDAA, 2018). The hidden nature of the learning disability can cause difficulties for people trying to access healthcare, as there is often an assumed level of literacy/numeracy that they may not possess. There is great potential for the use of technology to support the needs of people with a learning disability in accessing health information, communicating effectively with health practitioners and in complying with health guidelines. With a thorough understanding of the needs of people with sLDs and the impacts of the disability, healthcare educators and practitioners can develop appropriate guidelines and strategies, along with the use of everyday and assistive technologies, to assist all people to access appropriate healthcare.

Impacts of Learning Disabilities

There are many ways to view the impacts of learning disabilities on the individual. Walker and Shaw (2018) discuss the model used to view disability as impacting on how people with learning disabilities are perceived. They suggest that using a medical model to describe sLD places an emphasis on something innate within the individual that is not functioning or is a deficit, whereas a social model lens places emphasis on how society creates expectations and potential barriers for people with sLD. The social model of disability permits an examination of society's attitudes, social conventions and organisational structures and how these impact on the ability of a person with sLD to navigate healthcare. Access to healthcare is inherently a social issue.

One of the main impacts of a learning disability as described in the literature is in the area of reading, not only evident in those with dyslexia, but also associated with other learning disabilities (Peterson & Pennington, 2012). Poor reading skills can lead to a person having low-literacy levels, particularly if they have not been provided with adequate support during their schooling. Berkman et al. (2004), in a report sponsored by the Agency for Healthcare Research and Quality (AHRQ) in the United States, suggest that people who have low levels of literacy are at greater risk of poor health outcomes, due to increased difficulty in navigating the healthcare system and accessing relevant information. A person with a learning disability is more likely to have difficulties with accessing content, not only due to possible low levels of literacy, but also due to the way that the content is organised or displayed. The complexity of the language used, including complicated medical terminology can also be a barrier to understanding content. Miller, McCardle and Hernandez (2010) state that not only do low levels of literacy impact on the health of adults, but may also affect their children, leading to multigenerational difficulties.

Dysgraphia may affect an individual's ability to appropriately convey information in written formats and spell appropriately (Judd, 2012; McCloskey & Rapp, 2017). Individuals are most impacted in a health setting when they are required to complete forms, or convey symptoms in a written format. Providing consent may also cause some concern. As with other sLDs individuals with dysgraphia may also have dyslexia or dyscalculia, compounding any difficulties they experience.

While there has been less research in the area of maths learning disability, or dyscalculia, the impacts on the individual are known to be just as significant as those known to effect people with dyslexia (Butterworth et al., 2011) and significantly impact upon the life outcomes for those who have dyscalculia. Some of the areas of difficulty identified in the literature include difficulty with simple number concepts, difficulty with arithmetic (counting or subitising), poor short- and long-term memory for mathematical facts, problems with learning number facts and procedures, poor time management and difficulty budgeting (Emerson, 2014; Iuculano, Tang, Hall, & Butterworth, 2008; Judd, 2012). Mathematical disabilities may impact on determining correct dosages for medication, result in time and spatial difficulties when attending appointments, and cause issues when filling out health forms and providing information for healthcare professionals.

Accessing Healthcare

Evidence exists in relation to the fact that people with disabilities, including those with sLDs can face significant disparities when trying to access healthcare when compared with peers who do not have a disability (Jones,

Morris & Deruyter, 2018). This lack of access can result in a reduced likelihood of receiving preventative healthcare services, a higher risk for poor health outcomes and engagement in unhealthy behaviours. There are a number of situations where people with learning disabilities need to access healthcare, including hospital admittance, visiting a local general practitioner (GP), accessing written health information in a variety of formats, providing informed consent for themselves or dependents, and calculating correct dosages for medications. There are specific demands on a person with a learning disability in each of these circumstances.

Hospital Admittance

Visiting or being admitted to a hospital in particular can be a daunting experience, especially in an emergency situation. There are many different people who will be involved in treatment, including a triage nurse; emergency department clerk; orderly, clinician and registrar, all in one visit. Additionally, the person may undergo multiple treatments, scans and other investigations. The difficulty for all people, and specifically those with a learning disability, lies in attempting to remember or follow what is occurring with his/her treatment and ongoing care. Those with chronic illness may provide large amounts of written information to hospital staff; however, information can be missed by busy clinicians, it may not be added to the hospital health record (due to hospital protocol) and there is the danger that it can be lost. The person may also be required to complete large amounts of paperwork, challenging them to be able to write and remember details effectively. Other impacts can include long waiting times and rushed assessments by medical staff that can create higher levels of anxiety. Health information managers (HIMs) in hospital settings are well placed to assist people with learning disabilities to navigate the necessary systems.

Visiting a GP

In order to visit a doctor, whether for a routine check-up or when ill requires that the person locates or knows where the surgery is located, makes an appointment, remembers to attend the appointment, has all of the medical information in a written format and can complete forms appropriately as needed. The person then needs to be able to provide medical insurance or coverage information to the receptionist and pay for the appointment. One or all of these tasks may be daunting for a person with a sLD, and yet they will need to be able to navigate these in order to ensure basic health is maintained. Providing supports to ensure people with learning disabilities are accessing routine healthcare can assuage trauma later on, or prevent higher costs in relation to medical care (Butterworth et al., 2011).

Written Information

Written information for people with learning disabilities may cause distress if the information cannot be understood, read easily or is confused in some way. Examples include a patient being late for an appointment or getting the day or time of their appointment wrong. Medical information may be presented in a variety of formats, for example, information sheets provided with medication detailing dosage and contraindications, websites on areas of concern, handouts from practitioners, booklets, pamphlets and doctors' notes. For those with reading issues, written information may represent an insurmountable barrier to accessing current, relevant and much needed information.

Dosage Calculations

People with dyslexia and/or dyscalculia may see numbers as transposed or reversed. This can create a dangerous situation when medication is prescribed. Pamphlets and information sheets for prescribed medications are often difficult to read and interpret, with extremely small and condensed text and highly technical information. In addition, patients have to keep track of their medication, knowing how often, what time of day and how much of the medication to take. Some people may have difficulty in ensuring medication adherence, which in turn, has the potential to negatively impact on their overall health outcomes.

Informed Consent

When consenting to a routine surgical procedure, or providing consent for a dependent, the person granting the consent has to be fully informed in relation to the procedure itself, intended outcomes, any risks involved and any potentially aversive outcomes that may be experienced as a result of the procedure. Gaining informed consent is a legal and moral necessity (Menendez, 2013; Miles, 2005). People with learning disabilities may need to be provided with information in a number of formats/modalities in order to ensure that they are fully informed and able to provide appropriate consent. Except in the case of a power of attorney, consent must be given by the patient and other adults cannot legally sign on their behalf. Therefore, it is critical that they fully understand and are able to give informed consent. Patients with dyslexia, for example, should not be provided with written information alone, but may also require a verbal and possibly pictorial representation of the procedure to ensure clarity for consent.

While the elements described in the previous paragraphs are common across patients, the way in which they are approached may need to be adjusted to ensure those with learning disabilities can effectively deal with them. There is a range of everyday and assistive technologies that are available to support people with learning disabilities. A small range of the technologies will be discussed, but the reader is also encouraged to seek out further technologies to support those who may struggle with health-related tasks.

Everyday and Assistive Technology

Everyday and assistive technology, in the context of healthcare, consists of devices or tools and software that allow a person to access written and verbal information and instructions, provide fully informed consent for medical procedures, and understand and organise medication for themselves and their dependents. The technology may be readily available and be in common use (everyday technology), or may be specifically designed to augment existing skills or bypass areas of difficulty for those who struggle with certain tasks (assistive technology). The technology should also ensure that the people with a learning disability are able to fully engage with health professionals and the information they are providing, and allow them to access all required information in a format suitable for their needs. For some people, this may include the use of pictorial cues or verbal information, while others may require organisational supports.

With the increasing proliferation of technologies in society, there are often solutions that may be low cost or free, that will address the needs of people with sLDs who are attempting to access healthcare or health-related information (Fett, 2000; UNICEF, 2015). Many of these technologies are already accessible to healthcare professionals including the use of devices such as computers, mobile devices or mobile telephones. If not already utilised, the technology required to support people with learning disabilities is available from a variety of sources.

Mobile healthcare (mHealth), for example, may assist in the development of better health literacy and management of chronic health conditions (Byambasuren, Sanders, Beller, & Glasziou, 2018; Morgan & Agee, 2012). Mobile healthcare, also known as mHealth, is used in the dissemination, delivery and facilitation of health information through multimedia and mobile telecommunication technology including smart phones, wireless infrastructure and tablet devices. There should be some caution in recommending apps, however, as there is often limited evidence of their effectiveness (Byambasuren, Sanders, Beller, & Glasziou, 2018), although this evidence will build over time, given appropriate research.

For people with sLDs commonly available apps such as Leo, which records and transcribes conversations, and Sonocent, which records and allows the user to add visual information, may be helpful when meeting with practitioners to ensure that they have effective notes of the conversation. For reading content on a webpage, ClaroSpeak, ClaroPDF or Voice Dream Reader will allow the person to use a text-to-voice function, with the ability to modify the speed and tone (voice), and highlight text as it is read. ClaroSpeak will also save the text as an audio file for later listening. Apps with an optical character recognition (OCR) feature (such as ClaroPDF, KNFB Reader or Prizmo) allow users to take a picture of the text and then read the text back to them. When determining an appropriate app to support the person with a learning disability, it is critical to focus on the function that is required, such as the need to read text easily, or a timer to remember appointments, rather than focusing on the disability.

In addition to apps that can be downloaded on smart phones and tablet devices, there are a range of extensions and add-ins for browsers that can be accessed when people with learning disabilities are browsing online for information using any operating system. For example, Chrome extensions that support people with reading difficulties include Read & Write for Google, Readability and Purify, which extract text from the website to avoid distracting elements such as advertisements, and read the text to the viewer. Beeline Reader allows extracts text from a webpage, and additionally displays the text in a line-by-line format that may make the text more accessible to the reader. If a person requires assistance with writing, apps such as Co: Writer, Ginger and Scrible may assist them with word prediction and writing supports, such as sticky notes and dictionary access. When completing online forms these extensions may be invaluable in supporting the person with a learning disability. These are just a sample of the many apps available and many more are being developed daily, which will enhance the ability of those with sLDs to engage in their healthcare.

The introduction of a personally controlled electronic health record, known as My Health Record in Australia, and a Qualified Electronic Health Record in the United States (Australian Digital Health Agency, n.d.; Office of the National Coordinator for Health Information Technology, n.d.), holds some promise for those with sLDs, as information trends can be devised from event summaries which may include diagnoses, investigations, adverse reactions, medications and immunisation records. This information is in a clear-type format, which will greatly assist clinicians to review the patient's past history (Australian Digital Health Agency, 2018). However, the electronic health record may not provide an immediate solution for those with sLD as the information may only be available in a specified format, which may not be accessible through some screen readers. The information, however, may be downloaded and read at a later date via electronic access. Medical information can also be downloaded onto several mHealth apps, which may assist in providing important information in an expedient manner. There have been some concerns with the security and privacy relating to electronic health records (Office of the Auditor General Western Australia, 2018), which will need to be addressed in any ongoing manner by health authorities.

Sources of good quality software that can be adapted by health professionals for a specific use are often found in free and open source software (FOSS). 'Free and open source software (FOSS) refers to software that has been designed by a person or group, openly modified and then distributed freely for use' (Chambers, Varoglu & Kasinskaite-Buddeberg, 2015, p. 13). Some of the FOSS that may be used includes text-to-speech programs, speech-to-text programs, conversion of text to an audio file, graphical organisation software, word prediction software, screen overlays or rulers and an online dictionary and thesaurus. Not only can this software be freely used, but also it is often available to be modified for specific health-related purposes. Table 7.1 highlights some FOSS that addresses these areas.

For many people with reading difficulties, including those with dyslexia, the use of text-to-speech software is necessary to ensure that information about healthcare is able to be read and understood. Comprehensibility of the information may also require that it is in plain English (Bates, 2011; Stodart, 2014), and at an appropriate level of complexity for the intended audience (Zamanian & Heydari, 2012). In the case of health information, there will often be words or phrases that are specific to the health condition or procedure that need to be used in the text. If this is the situation, then the

TABLE 7.1

FOSS to Assist People with Learning Disabilities Access Health Information

Title	Task	Link
Audacity	Creates an audio track from a written text	http://audacity.sourceforge.net/
Balabolka	Converts text to speech and creates a file which can be listened to at the person's leisure	http://balabolka.en.softonic.com/
FreeMind	A graphical mind-mapping tool for organising ideas and content	http://freemind.sourceforge.net/
LetMeType	Autocomplete words regardless of the program. Guesses a word after the first two or three letters	http://letmetype.en.softonic.com/
Powertalk	Speaks any text appearing in a Microsoft PowerPoint presentation	http://fullmeasure.co.uk/powertalk/
TBar	A coloured bar or block which acts like a coloured overlay	www.fx-software.co.uk/assistive.htm
VuBar	Provides an on-screen slotted ruler to highlight and limit the field of view to an area as small as a single line	http://download.cnet.com/VuBar/3000-2094_4-10730580.html
WordWeb	A one-click English thesaurus and dictionary for Windows	http://wordweb.info/free/
WordTalk	An add-in for Microsoft Word that reads and converts the text into an audio file	www.wordtalk.org.uk/home/

Source: Adapted from Chambers et al. (2015).

addition of links to an online dictionary would allow the person with the learning disability to access any information/words they did not know. This consideration also applies more broadly to people without learning disabilities who may be unfamiliar with the terminology used in the medical arena.

Accessibility of web-based content is an area that should be considered, and there are a number of tools that developers/website owners can use to ensure that they are meeting the needs of all users of a website. The World Wide Web Consortium (W3C) Web Accessibility Initiative (WAI) released updated guidelines, which include reference to the success criteria for people with learning disabilities (W3C WAI, 2018). The updated *Web Content Accessibility Guidelines* (WCAG) 2.1 suggest that developers include autocomplete features in commonly used fields, appropriate text spacing (or the ability to work with style sheets) in relation to line height, paragraph, letter and word spacing and provide timeout warnings for users. All of these considerations are relevant to people accessing healthcare on a computer or tablet device, including tasks such as making appointments and filling in electronic forms.

Websites can be assessed for accessibility using an online tool such as a Web accessibility evaluation tool (WAVE) (WebAIM, 2018). Any website address can be entered into this tool and a report is generated which identifies errors such as missing alternative text, empty links or broken links. The tool also highlights features and structural elements of the website, contrast errors or features and appropriate levels of headings. Ensuring that links are correct, headings are appropriate and the structure of the website is sound will support a person with a learning disability who may have issues with reading, or who is using a screen reader to access content. As websites and online content are increasingly being used to both convey and collect information, it is vital that they are fully accessible for people with learning disabilities.

There are many mHealth apps available for multiple devices that can remind people when they need to take medication (Shaw, Hines, & Kielly-Carroll, 2018). Apps that are currently available include Medisafe and Medication Reminder, along with standard calendar or reminder apps, such as To Do List and Google Assistant. Technology that has recently come onto the market includes automated pill dispensers, such as the TabTimer pill dispenser or e-Pill automatic pill dispenser, which allows the user to set up controlled dosage release, set automatic alarm reminders and provides an electronic notification link to carers or others if required. This type of system also ensures that the correct dose is provided and reduces the risk of overdosing. The aim of the automatic pill dispensers is to ensure adherence to medication as prescribed by a physician, and can assist if tracking time and memory are not strong skills of the patient.

Healthcare providers may also wish to consider adding pictorial or video cues to verbal or written information on websites or in other health information content (Berkman et al., 2004). In addition, a visual array to represent dosages may be beneficial. Although the use of pictorial and visual cues has mostly been used to support people with an intellectual disability, they also have the potential to support and contextualise content for someone who has issues with written content.

Future Directions and Considerations for Healthcare Providers

There are many instances where a patient with a learning disability would approach a healthcare professional for assistance. It might be as part of a standard GP visit, as a patient undergoing a medical procedure, or when attending an emergency department. Each of these situations has specific demands, which may be placed on a person with a learning disability. The need to provide a range of options for the person is key to ensuring that all needs are catered for. For example, when attending a surgery to see a GP, the patient has to first make an appointment. For people with verbal issues this can sometimes be a confronting scenario. With the increase (in Australia in particular) of the ability to book an appointment online, the need to formulate responses rapidly to a busy receptionist may be somewhat alleviated. Online booking also allows data to be saved reducing the need to re-enter the same information.

While there are available technologies that can be utilised to support people with sLDs to access health information and healthcare, associated healthcare professionals may require additional training in available technologies and in meeting the needs of people with sLDs. Alternatively, some further resources such as websites or written works could be developed to provide additional information for this somewhat 'hidden' group. Further education and research in regards to the efficacy of the technologies is also required to determine which of the technologies meet particular needs best, and to ensure that practitioners and healthcare workers are aware of, and competent in using, technology to support their patients.

The large range of common and assistive technology available to support people with sLDs to access health information and healthcare needs to be applied in a consistent and appropriate manner to a range of healthcare situations, such as hospital admissions, visiting a GP and providing informed consent. The technology is often readily available and is constantly being refined and enhanced to meet the needs of all users in the health arena. Access to quality healthcare and health-related information should be available to all people who require it, and applied appropriately; technology may be a key player in this field.

References

Agency for Healthcare Research and Quality. (2011). Health literacy interventions and outcomes: An updated systematic review. Retrieved October 1, 2018 from www.ahrq.gov/downloads/pub/evidence/pdf/literacy/literacyup.pdf.

Armstrong, D., & Squires, G. (2015). *Key perspectives on dyslexia: An essential text for educators.* London, UK: Routledge.

Australian Digital Health Agency. (n.d.). My health record. Retrieved October 6, 2018 from www.myhealthrecord.gov.au/.

Australian Digital Health Agency. (2018). Sample event summary. Retrieved October 5, 2018 from www.digitalhealth.gov.au/files/assets/cdaExamples/CDAEventSummary.html.

Bates, J. (2011). Plain english. *Nursing Standard, 25*(28), 25.

Berkman, N., Dewalt, D., Pignone, M., Sheridan, S., Lohr, K., Lux, L., et al. (2004). Literacy and health outcomes: Evidence Report/Technology Assessment No. 87 (AHRQ Pub. No. 04-E007-2). Rockville, MD: Agency for Healthcare Research and Quality. Retrieved October 9, 2018 from http://citeseerx.ist.psu.edu/viewdoc/download?doi=10.1.1.210.2733&rep=rep1&type=pdf.

Butterworth, B., Varma, S., & Laurillard, D. (2011). Dyscalculia: From brain to education. *Science, 332*(6033), 1049–1053.

Byambasuren, O., Sanders, S., Beller, E., & Glasziou, P. (2018). Prescribable mHealth apps identified from an overview of systematic reviews. *npj Digital Medicine, 1,* Article 12. DOI: 10.1038/s41746-018-0021-9

Chambers, D., Varoglu, Z., & Kasinskaite-Buddeberg, I. (2015). Learning for all: Guidelines on the inclusion of learners with disabilities in open and distance learning. Retrieved September 9, 2018 from http://unesdoc.unesco.org/images/0024/002443/244355e.pdf.

Dyslexia SPELD Foundation. (2014). *Understanding learning difficulties: A practical guide.* Perth, Western Australia: DSF Literacy Services.

Emerson, J. (2014). The enigma of dyscalculia. In S. Chinn (Ed.), *The Routledge International handbook of dyscalculia and mathematical learning difficulties* (pp. 217–227). London, UK: Routledge.

Fett, M. (2000). Technology, health and health care. Retrieved October 10, 2018 from www.health.gov.au/internet/main/publishing.nsf/Content/DA8177ED1A80D332CA257BF0001B08EE/$File/ocpahfsv5.pdf.

Iuculano, T., Tang, J., Hall, C. W. B., & Butterworth, B. (2008). Core information processing deficits in developmental dyscalculia and low numeracy. *Developmental Science, 11*(5), 669–680. DOI: 10.1111/j.1467-7687.2008.00716.x

Jones, M., Morris, J., & Deruyter, F. (2018). Mobile healthcare and people with disabilities: Current state and future needs. *International Journal of Environmental Research and Public Health, 15*(3), 515–527. DOI: 10.3390/ijerph15030515

Judd, S. J. (Ed.). (2012). *Learning disabilities sourcebook* (4th ed.). Detroit, MI: Omnigraphics.

Kaphingst, K.A., Zanfini, C. J., & Emmons, K. M. (2009). Accessibility of web sites containing colorectal cancer information to adults with limited literacy (United States). *Cancer Causes and Control, 17*(2), 147–151.

Lavoie, R. D., Levine, M. D., Reiner, R., Reiner, M. (2005). *It's so much work to be your friend: Helping the child with learning disabilities find social success.* New York, NY: Simon & Schuster.

Learning Disabilities Association of America [LDAA]. (2018). Types of learning disabilities. Retrieved September 14, 2018 from https://ldaamerica.org/types-of-learning-disabilities/.

McCloskey, M., & Rapp, B. (2017). Developmental dysgraphia: An overview and framework for research. *Cognitive Neuropsychology, 34*(3–4), 65–82. DOI: 10.1080/02643294.2017.1369016

Menendez, J. B. (2013). Informed consent: Essential legal and ethical principles for nurses. *JONA's Healthcare Law, Ethics, and Regulation, 15*(4), 140–144. DOI: 10.1097/NHL.0000000000000015

Miles, S. H. (2005). *The hippocratic oath and the ethics of medicine.* New York, NY: Oxford University Press.

Miller, B., McCardle, P., & Hernandez, R. (2010). Advances and remaining challenges in adult literacy research. *Journal of Learning Disabilities, 43*(2) 101–107. DOI: 10.1177/0022219409359341

Morgan, S. A., & Agee, N. H. (2012). Mobile healthcare. *Frontiers of Health Services Management, 29*(2), 3–10.

Office of the Auditor General Western Australia. (2018). Information systems audit report 2018. Retrieved October 12, 2018 from https://audit.wa.gov.au/wp-content/uploads/2018/08/report2018_14-IS-GCC-App-Pass.pdf.

Office of the National Coordinator for Health Information Technology. (n.d.). The health information technology for economic and clinical health (HITECH) act of 2009. Retrieved October 10, 2018 from www.healthit.gov/topic/laws-regulation-and-policy/health-it-legislation.

Peterson, R. L., & Pennington, B. F. (2012). Developmental dyslexia. *Lancet, 379*(9830), 1997–2007. DOI: 10.1016/S0140-6736(12)60198-6

Phillips, L. A., & Clark, E. (2013). Dysgraphia. In C. R. Reynolds, K. J. Vannest, & E. Fletcher-Janzen (Eds.), *Encyclopedia of special education: a reference for the education of children, adolescents, and adults with disabilities and other exceptional individuals* (4th ed.). Hoboken, NJ: Wiley. Retrieved from http://ipacez.nd.edu.au/login?url=https://search.credoreference.com/content/entry/wileyse/dysgraphia/0?institutionId=1939

Reid Lyon, G., Shaywitz, S. E., & Shaywitz, B. A. (2003). A definition of dyslexia. *Annals of Dyslexia, 53*(1), 1–14.

Shaw, T., Hines, M., Kielly-Carroll, C. (2018). *Impact of digital health on the safety and quality of health care.* Sydney: Australian Commission on Safety and Quality in Health Care.

Stodart, K. (2014). Speaking plainly about cancer. *Nursing New Zealand, 20*(11), 30.

The British Psychological Society. (2015). Guidance on the assessment and diagnosis of intellectual disabilities in adulthood. Retrieved September 14, 2018 from www1.bps.org.uk/system/files/Public%20files/DCP/guidance_on_the_assessment_and_diagnosis_of_intellectual_disabilities_in_adulthood.pdf.

UNICEF. (2015). Assistive technology for children with disabilities: Creating opportunities for education, inclusion and participation. Retrieved October 5, 2018 from www.unicef.org/disabilities/files/Assistive-Tech-Web.pdf.

Walker, E. R., & Shaw, S. C. K. (2018). Guest editorial: Specific learning difficulties in healthcare education: The meaning in the nomenclature. *Nurse Education in Practice, 32*, 97–98. DOI: 10.1016/J.NEPR.2018.01.011

WebAIM. (2018). Web accessibility in mind. Retrieved September 19 2018 from https://webaim.org/

Westwood, P. (2015). *Commonsense methods for children with special educational needs* (7th ed.). London, UK: Routledge.

World Wide Web Consortium (W3C) Web Accessibility Initiative (WAI). (2018). Web Content Accessibility Guidelines (WCAG) 2.1. Retrieved October 9 2018 from www.w3.org/WAI/standards-guidelines/wcag/.

Zamanian, M. & Heydari, P. (2012). Readability of texts: State of the art. *Theory and Practice in Language Studies, 2*(1), 43–53. DOI: 10.4304/tpls.2.1.43–53

8

Pervasive and Emerging Technologies and Consumer Motivation

David Banes

David Banes Access and Inclusion Services Ltd

CONTENTS

Introduction – Disability Trends 123
Trends in User Behaviour 124
Understanding Disruption 125
Emerging Technologies and the Lives of People with a Disability.............. 127
Independent Living 127
Mobility 128
Communication... 129
Health and Well-being.. 130
Proactive and Responsive Delivery.. 132
Impact of Disruptive Innovation on AT Services 133
Changing Role of AT Services – Escalation, Curation and
Self-Determination.. 133
Implications for Services Development.. 135
Public Policy 135
Awareness 136
Assessment and Evaluation of Needs.. 137
Provision of Assistive Technology.. 138
Training... 139
Support 140
Research and Development 140
Conclusion 141
References 141

Introduction – Disability Trends

The World Health Organization (2018) estimates that by 2050 there will be two billion people globally who require assistive technologies. The growth of numbers emphasises a corresponding increased demand for accessible and assistive technology due to an ageing population, improved healthcare and the increased expectations of inclusive communities. They also estimate that only one in ten people with a disability have access to the tools they need,and that in low to middle income countries the figure is still lower, for instance, only 3% of those who would benefit from hearing aids having access to a solution.

Within wealthy countries, the provision of assistive technology services and products is under pressure to meet demands at reduced cost; often access to services is limited to urban settings with far more limited access in rural and sparsely populated areas. In response to the influence of changing demographics, economics and geography and the evolution of technology, models of escalated services have been identified including the GREAT summit in Geneva in 2017 (Banes, 2017) and the proposed assistive technology (AT) passport in Ireland (DFI and Enable Ireland, 2016). Both models are founded around a pyramid of provision where those with the greatest needs receive intensive interventions and those characterised as having high incidence needs requiring common solutions were located at the base and foundation of any escalation. To address the needs of those within the bottom tier of the pyramid, new approaches to service delivery have been identified including the introduction and implementation of user-led processes of both self-identification of needs and the provision of solutions (Banes, 2018, AAATE workshop).

Trends in User Behaviour

The demand for innovation reflects the changing behaviour and aspirations of people with disability in the face of rapid change. The continual struggle experienced to gain access reinforces a natural tendency to protect dearly won progress, and to embrace change with care. Such reticence is reflected when we consider the implementation of emerging and disruptive technologies. For those who are reliant upon solutions such as commercial screen-readers, there is anxiety about updating an operating system, or upgrading hardware, in case products prove to be incompatible and rendered unusable. Similarly, as smartphones became ubiquitous, the disabled community took time to embrace the technology with concerns discussed and shared in online forums such as AppleVis (2012). Users described how they remained loyal to the Nokia brand long after others shifted to Apple and Android products, but having made that leap, they could not envisage returning to their previous technology. At times, the disability community has taken time to grasp the potential of innovation, as was the case of the Amazon Kindle e-book reader upon its release.

The Kindle rapidly became a must-have device for the mass market offering access to a huge, diverse and affordable library and bookstore. Now sometimes cited as a cause of a demise of traditional bookstores and raising questions about the future of traditional books, the Kindle offered opportunities for those with a physical need who struggled to manipulate traditional books, or those with low vision or dyslexia, found that the variable text and font choices reduced the need to buy special editions. The integrated online dictionary and thesaurus provided instant support for readers who struggled with the vocabulary.

However, the debate around the use of the Kindle in education, and by people with a disability, was dominated by the challenge of the availability and implementation of text to speech and is well documented by the U.S. National Federation for the Blind (2015). With hindsight, the barriers experienced by one community, dominated and overshadowed discussion of the opportunities for others; a theme, which is echoed as we explore the potential impact of current emerging technologies. These technologies are often referred to as 'Disruptive'. One of the best-known and recent examples, with an impact upon both people with a disability and those without is Uber.

Uber offers an alternative to traditional taxi services. Through an app, riders with smartphones are connected to drivers to book journeys. The company has been widely criticised by both the blind community and by wheelchair users including a lawsuit filed in the U.S. state of California on 9 September 2014 by the state chapter of the National Federation of the Blind. The lack of availability of wheelchair accessible vehicles has been much commented upon, including complaints to the Human Rights Commission in New York (Bhuiyan 2016), leading to the introduction of additional services to meet the needs of wheelchair users, as reported in 2016 in *The Guardian* under the brand of 'UberWav,' which was widely welcomed by disability groups. However, little has been said about the benefits to other communities of people with a disability, however unanticipated or unplanned. Uber introduced an easy to use graphical interface to book a ride, with real-time information on estimated time of arrival, and the capacity to enter destination details easily. For those with a speech disability or hearing loss, such an interface was valuable allowing communication with drivers by text through the app. The success of this for many of the deaf communities led to the recruitment of drivers with hearing loss as partners, creating new employment opportunities as reported by Uber themselves (Metcalfe, 2015).

Clearly, disruption can have unanticipated outcomes, offering new opportunities for inclusion in employment or education that were not part of any original business concept or plan.

Understanding Disruption

Technology usage drives innovation and as technology evolves, there has been an increase in disruption to traditional businesses and services, wiping the slate clean and offering new solutions to old problems. For instance, the advent of digital photography and mobile phone photography is both influenced by and responds to both consumer behaviour and changing business models for photographic products and services. Some observers suggest that 'disruption' is merely a 'buzzword' that is synonymous with 'innovation'. This represents a misunderstanding. Disruption refers not just to technological innovation, but is also concerned with impact upon behaviour, attitudes and business as Schmidt (2013) suggests 'The screen that you want to apply about technology is not what technologies are interesting, because there are so many that are interesting. You want to look at which ones have a chance of having a volume impact on many, many people, or large segments of the society'.

Al Jaber (2016) summarises this relationship between technical innovation and business change, leading to disruption in addressing disruption within healthcare:

> Technology innovations are those that are exponentially increasing in power and scale while reducing in cost; building blocks for today and tomorrow; and those that are reshaping industries and markets over the next ten years. Examples of these technology innovations include networking and communications, sensing, artificial intelligence (AI) and machine learning, advanced robotics, 3D printing, and bioinformatics and synthetic biology.... When we combine technology innovation with social and business model innovation, we get industry disruption, and entirely new business opportunities are created.

Disruption suggests more than 'value for money'. It may be the way businesses and services survive and thrive, bringing both winners and losers as suggested in observations on the impact of the Mp3 format upon creative professionals by Democracy in America (2014). Disruption may have been driven initially by consumer choice and preferences, but over time may force consumers into specific paths and potentially reduce available options:

> New technologies have network effects that tend to force people to gradually buy in, whether they like it or not. The growth of online retailers selling books and groceries drives bookstores and grocers out of business, forcing more of us to shop online. Late adopters come to fear the tyranny of early adopters. One becomes reluctant to invest in a platform, buying a home music system, learning a software package, out of a sense that the next big thing will come along soon and destroy the value of the investment.

Such innovation is equally valid in the domains of rehabilitation and access for people with a disability. Understanding the opportunities and risks created by emerging technologies and service user expectations will be vital to respond effectively to the influence of demographics and economics through the design of future services and including the distribution of aids and devices.

Emerging Technologies and the Lives of People with a Disability

It is difficult to remember a time where the diversity of change and pace of change has been so great and emerging technologies are already impacting upon the lives of people with a disability.

Independent Living

Many people with a disability are already making use of the availability of smart homes, featuring home automation and control through a range of natural interfaces. People with a physical disability and those with vision loss are using voice or gestures via a smartphone, tablet or smart speaker to control their immediate environment and maximise their personal independence not only at homes but also in hotels, restaurants, schools and the workplace. Devices such as Amazon's Echo are being rapidly adopted by people with disabilities featuring an inclusive design using voice recognition, to search for information online or provide a means to control smart home features such as lighting, entrance doors and heating. Many of the technologies needed to establish such control are widely available to purchase online or in the high street, installation is simple and maintenance low cost. As a result, many such personal accommodations are being made by people with a disability themselves, their friends or family without necessarily seeking advice from the traditional environmental control industry.

Similarly, the direct provision of social care within the home is changing. By combining the technology of home automation with machine learning and AI, technologies prepare a home by anticipating needs. The systems may adjust heating or lighting in readiness for rising, can recognise that a carer will visit between 7 and 8 am and activate their personal door code for those hours. Such home automation reduces the need for human support for mundane tasks, allowing personal support to be used in far more social and communicative interactions.

For both carers and professionals, the technology facilitates their attention upon the person, rather than a task to be completed. Ensuring that systems are working well and that any safeguards are in place when technology stops working are likely to be a much greater part of their role currently.

As a result, for some therapists and other professionals there are challenges to define and refine their new role. In this context, their knowledge and experience retain value, but individual consultation is not a necessity for each potential user.

Mobility

Those trends that are impacting upon our capacity to support independent living have an equal capacity to impact upon mobility solutions. Major companies are working towards the development of autonomous vehicles, which have the potential to hugely increase the independent mobility of people with a range of needs. Early testing by Google and Tesla demonstrated how a blind person could use a self-driving car without the need for a sighted driver present, fully autonomous vehicles offer the greatest single potential for enhanced mobility for disabled people. Reports and reviews by people with a range of needs including hearing, vision and physical needs have been well received, with the technology reducing dependence on public transport or upon other people to assist.

These technologies can also transfer to a new generation of smart and semi-autonomous wheelchairs (Scudellari, 2017). The sensor technologies and AI developed for mass market vehicles are being introduced into the design of smart wheelchairs allowing greater use of chairs by those with physical needs where control of a chair is impacted by fatigue or tremor, or simply where existing control mechanisms require a degree of motor control that is beyond the capability of an individual.

As autonomous vehicles become widely accepted, so our concepts of the skills and abilities required for personal mobility will require revision. Establishing and maintaining such independence will be less about physical skill, the techniques of mobility, but much more about using a familiar interface to make decisions and establishing the parameters of the journey. The skills we learned to use navigation and orientation technologies that support people with disabilities to use GPS outdoors and beacons indoors and installed already in public places such as theme parks, football stadiums, museums and shopping malls are the skills needed to 'drive' such a mobility device. Such systems, such as those in use at Walt Disney World are integrated to locate the user, provide highly specific location information such as directions and orientation, obstacle avoidance, queue times, transport updates and offers orders from nearby kiosks and vendors.

To deliver such a machine-enhanced mobility solution, the services supporting implementation will need to draw upon new skill sets and approaches, most notably from computer sciences. Rehabilitation professionals will find that they can look much more closely at ensuring the comfort and safety of the person using a chair, as positioning for control may be less essential when the technology has the capacity to offer the fine levels of control required.

The levels of automation technologies that will support both independent living and mobility have many other implications including new applications for both robotics and drones. Robotic devices are already used to support people with a disability in a variety of forms including:

- humanoid robots for communication with children with autism.
- mechanical 'arms' and robots for self-care needs of those with physical needs such as eating or shaving.
- robotic-enhanced prosthetics that assist those with physical needs such as walking by replacing traditional models.
- remote presence of robots offering a physical presence in settings that the person with a disability is unable to travel to.

But as drones and robotics become increasingly widespread, so new opportunities for disabled people emerge. Drones have already been trialled in rural areas delivering goods from Amazon, offering greater flexibility of delivery time and reduce anxiety about opening doors to strangers to offer a greater sense of security. Drones offer opportunities for the rapid delivery of medications or spare parts for aids and appliances to rural communities and to those for whom traditional distribution channels are expensive or difficult. Similar innovative opportunities are also emerging in the use of robotics to create a physical presence in remote locations. These have value where a user is unable to interact with peers in school, at work or socially due to a health crisis and may have equal value for those who find social inclusion challenging because of conditions such as chronic fatigue or pain.

Such innovation through emerging technology will drive a reappraisal of our definitions of 'inclusion' which will address some current barriers and drive new challenges. For some, inclusion in the workplace, education or social settings may be less dependent upon our physical location and much more related to connectivity and the ways in which groups interact.

Communication

The integration of the virtual domain into the ways in which groups communicate is already widespread. Notions of face-to-face communication become blurred when online technology becomes both portable and pervasive, increasingly our physical interactions with whom we share interests are established, organised and at to some extent delivered by technology. Text analysis allows the technology to predict the responses that someone might wish to make, based on previous interactions and our personal preferences. Users of communication (AAC) software can access context-specific grids loaded up based upon their location and the language most used the last time they were at the same location. It is likely that the range of communications used at the supermarket will be 80% similar each time visited, and this can speed up communication.

AI, which analyses our behaviour to support independence at home and when travelling, has the capacity to perform the same function within interactions, helping to increase the speed of communication dialogue, selecting communication media most appropriate for the interaction, such as speech, text, graphics or emoji and directing the communication through the channel that best meets the person initiating the communication and those receiving it. A group in discussion may each get the message 'I'm happy with that' in a different format where the concept is consistent, but the message in a form that they can most consume, based on their needs, setting and preferences.

For those active in supporting the language needs of those with a disability, the new fluidity of communication requires less focus upon form 'how to say this' and much more upon content 'what we want to say'.

Health and Well-being

The use of technology to support health and well-being of a community including those with a disability has grown considerably. Wearable technologies have demonstrated significant growth in recent years with fitness trackers and smartwatches achieving considerable sales across many parts of the world. The value of wearable technologies has been championed by early adopters who speak positively about the experience of using a wearable, supporting communication, access to information, navigation and to give and receive notifications and alerts.

Current consumer technologies, recognising the ageing market, provide tools for maximising independent living. 'Sound Sentry' allows those with hearing loss to monitor the environment for specific sounds such as fire alarms, crying children and doorbells and to translate those into text and tactile alerts delivered to a wearable, whilst new features in the Apple Watch 4 include fall detection, triggering alerts to emergency services, friends and family.

The integration of sensors into the environment, or as a wearable, has provided the basis of new business offerings, which connect sensors to a smartphone where a trusted carer can monitor activity and act if required. The integration of the technologies during rehabilitation, at a consumer-level cost increases the ability of professionals to offer the ageing population and those recovering from trauma tools that reduce risk and mitigate impact, reducing dependence upon specialist care services and increasing a transition or return to independent and assisted living.

Such transition may also require the people affected to follow direction and advice to seek to improve specific functions. New forms of connected technology may allow such programs and recommendations to be available to the person with a disability on demand or coupled with alerts to take medication or complete a set of actions.

Making such direction and information readily available can be enhanced through emerging technologies such as heads-up displays for use with augmented and virtual reality systems. These are increasingly available as consumer items with popular headsets being available for gaming consoles and stand-alone models such as Hololens. Such devices can support people with a disability. Virtual reality is used with stroke victims, learning to become independent in a safe setting, whilst learning to drive a powered wheelchair in a virtual environment.

In 2016 Pokémon Go was released: the first truly mass market-augmented reality game based on smartphones. The technology was credited for encouraging large numbers of young people to walk and participate in searches for rare Pokémon. The release of the game illustrated the potential of the technology for everyday use offering a glimpse of highly usable 3D navigation and the integration of augmented reality data onto a screen displaying the view from the camera.

Some suggested applications for the technologies included the development of low-cost multisensory virtual environments for those with complex needs, simulations of wheelchair driving to practice skills and integration with the Seeing AI application as a means of providing those with a visual impairment the capability of interpreting environment in real time.

For the professionals, the pervasive, on-demand nature of the innovations offers the capacity to allow technology to 'do some of the lifting', reminders, training materials, guides and advice can all be delivered not only as required, but also at a time and location where the individual is most receptive to the prompt, increasing their motivation to respond, but gathering data if the programmes developed by the therapist are not being easily followed.

Access to information and advice may be further enhanced through the emerging use of 3D printing offering an alternative model of distribution for hardware devices and identified as a significant opportunity in developing countries and emerging markets. Maker communities such as ATmakers.org offer a capability to store and share designs online, through a bespoke repository or social networks of designs and instructions. Simple technologies that are easily fabricated such as switch-adapted toys and devices are distributed this way, those using such printed assistive technologies will be easily able to download and print spare parts for devices that have become unusable or to adjustments to a design with a remote professional to increase ease of use. Such printed components can be fabricated and shipped immediately. In some cases, such parts may even be printed and fitted at home in the near future.

The use of social media such as Facebook groups and Pinterest also provide useful ways of distributing safe and effective designs. Organisations such as 'Enabling the Future'[1] have successfully distributed designs and instructions for the 3D printing of prosthetics mostly targeted at emerging AT markets, but the principle can be applied more widely.

The impact of these emerging technologies and their successful implementation will be driven not only by the commitment of professionals to such change, but also by the behaviour of people with a disability themselves, and with such a diversity of sources, it will be increasingly important that the principles of curation be applied to such resources.

Proactive and Responsive Delivery

Underlying much of the emerging technology described is the use of AI. AI allows people with a disability to gather and share data through consumer devices and represent it in different formats. It is used to transform data between one medium to another such as auto captioning on YouTube or face recognition on Facebook. Seeing AI, produced by Microsoft, is an app using a phone camera input to describe the world; pointed at a person, it can say who he/she is and guess how he/she is feeling; pointed towards a product, it can describe it using AI running locally on the device. The technology has many applications but has been welcomed by the visually impaired community amongst others.

Such technologies reduce dependency on people. Future iterations of the technology are likely to be integrated into augmented reality wearable technologies to facilitate real-time interpretation of the environment and hence greater independence.

Our physical and virtual actions produce large amounts of data, recording the ways in which we interact that can be used to anticipate our behaviour and needs, analysed through machine learning as the basis of AI-enhanced services and used to support disabled people by anticipating their preferences either from location, time or planned activity. Using such data sets with the potential of comparing and contrasting options with others with similar needs and preferences will drive forward the ways in which services will be delivered to effectively implement the emerging technologies.

---

[1] http://enablingthefuture.org/upper-limb-prosthetics/.

Impact of Disruptive Innovation on AT Services

In recent years, the assistive technology industry has responded to innovations such as cloud-based computing, portable devices and the explosion of 'apps' and gradually technology is both enhancing and replacing some direct services. The convergence of accessible and assistive technologies has led to access features becoming an indivisible part of operating systems and the application of universal design principles upon mainstream products has helped them become assistive devices with many people benefiting from enhanced functionality and ease of use without awareness of the added value to those with disabilities.

The WHO GATE Priority Assistive Products list (WHO, 2016) identified 50 products that are essential to the well-being of people with a disability. Of these, the functionality of 24 can already be delivered as apps on smartphones and tablets and a further 10 could be also be delivered through emerging technologies or could be fabricated locally using open design and 3D printing. Whilst such change may encounter some initial resistance amongst both professionals and some with a disability, trends in user behaviour suggest that such change is inevitable. Professionals are challenged to remain abreast of current and emerging solutions as trusted products become unavailable, and hence new approaches to professional development will be required to maximise the impact of innovation. Responding to the sale of demand requires new approaches to delivery, the assistive technologies themselves will not bring about such change unless the ways in which implementation takes place adapt and change at the same pace as products. This will impact across all aspects of delivery and provision of assistive technology products and services made available to those with a disability.

Changing Role of AT Services – Escalation, Curation and Self-Determination

Traditionally the market for accessible technologies has been characterised by a range of specialist goods and services, designed predominantly for the use of people with a disability. Some technologies have shifted between mainstream and specialist markets, driven by opportunity to increase market share rather than a desire for fundamental change to business models. Current technology provides for direct and on-demand access to products and services including transport, accommodation or restaurants; these may be the products that are technically accessible, which are integrated with an inclusive business model.

The design of delivery models is responding to multiple influences. Demographic change is reflected in the growing number of people living with a disability and requiring accommodation and support. Simultaneously, economic necessity has impacted on our ability to meet that demand through traditional models of intervention and the technologies available to us, and our access to those technologies has evolved rapidly. Such a shift cuts deeply. Software is no longer downloaded or purchased from the developer's website, instead available through the operating system 'store' with business models that shape customer expectations including free and low-cost solutions, 'freemium' products and subscription-based models. Distribution is via a closed ecosystem related to the operating system or manufacturer, for instance those wishing to purchase communication software for the iPad are limited to a single source, the Apple online app store, significantly different to purchasing software for a computer, with different expectations of the price point for products and to the concept of ownership. Consumers no longer purchase applications with a perpetual license for use with free updates and discounted pricing for upgrades with a significant upfront cost and lower costs over time to maintain the product. Today the reverse is true.

Such change has implications for models of delivery, with escalation processes becoming established to link levels of intervention to need. Assessments, traditionally delivered through individual, personal interactions on-site or at clinics, comprising of professional observation, review and recommendation are likely to be reserved for those with the most complex needs. For others, a shift from direct intervention to mediation and curation supporting self-determination is taking place. In this scenario, the user self-identifies their own needs and challenges, and professionals are less concerned with making a direct recommendation, but instead seek to guide, mentor and share resources to help reach an informed decision. As AI evolves such guidance becomes automated and integrated with the curation of information.

Similar escalation routes using technology are being applied to services including awareness, training, distribution and technical support. In each, users make decisions based upon navigating curated knowledge. Curation is a field of endeavour involved with assembling, managing and presenting some type of collection. Curators of galleries and museums, research, select and acquire pieces for' collections and oversee interpretation, displays and exhibits. Curated AT information assists users to make decisions having considered the factors that influence success, helping shape the questions that need to be asked to provide options and potential answers.

Curation is about more than storing information randomly, it requires a set of competencies ensuring that stored information is accessible and useful including:

- Aggregation – the gathering and sharing of relevant content.
- Filtering – sharing only the most relevant and valuable resources.

- Elevation – recognising underlying trends in the mass of data.
- Mashups – combining two or more pieces of content to form new messages.
- Timelines – organising pieces of content in chronological order to demonstrate evolution of ideas.
- Communication – clearly and effectively with a variety of audiences, including users, creators, managers, researchers and collaborators.

Competencies in managing such a volume of data are quite different to those upon which job descriptions of AT professionals have been based in the past and increasingly further technologies will emerge that fulfil some of these functions on behalf of services releasing AT professionals to focus on the greatest needs and to offer creativity and insight to resolving complex challenges.

Implications for Services Development

Innovation and the implementation of emerging and disruptive technologies, both products and services will not take root unless nurtured. Creating an environment that is receptive to such innovation is based around actions that are integrated and mutually supportive. Coordinated actions for service delivery include activity that relates to policy, awareness, assessment of needs, provision, training, technical support and accessible content. These also inform and shape any future research and development agenda.

Emerging technologies have an important role in bringing about such change in service delivery processes.

Public Policy

Effective policy underpins the development of assistive technology services in many parts of the world. Policy that promotes inclusion of disabled people and explicitly outlines the right to access, whilst clarifying the roles and responsibilities of providers and public bodies, creates conditions that increase demand for, and availability of, accessible products. Technology can be applied to facilitate the engagement of people with a disability with the policymaking process. Online tools such as polls, town halls, forums and social listening offer new ways for the voices of those with a disability to be heard, whilst emerging technologies such as Blockchain secure the data produced by those voices as well as any transactions and records of identified needs or solutions.

As services develop in line with any model of escalation, rehabilitation and disability services will need to seek new ways to monitor impact and effectiveness, both to shape their own practice and moreover to inform any future policy initiative. The tools outlined allows input not only form past and current users of services, but also from those not directly engaged.

Awareness

Developing a programme to increase awareness of assistive technology and its impact on the quality of life of people with disabilities is important in promoting access to people with disabilities. Awareness is driven by many stakeholders and can encompass a range of activities with messages tailored to different audiences. A range of strategies have been employed in assistive technology and accessibility awareness campaigns, ranging from activities that are fun (such as accessible video gaming) to those which have evoked strong emotional responses from the audience to call for change.

Any approach to raising awareness of assistive technologies needs to be based upon the ways in which the target audiences are consuming information. In research undertaken by the author, it was found that disabled people using assistive technologies consumed information differently to those who were not. Far less information was available, with fewer sources and a greater dependency on traditional media or friends, families and professionals to share information with them.

This bubble effect was much discussed during elections in the United States and United Kingdom, and might suggest that reuse and sharing of information by disabled people online may only reach existing users of assistive technologies. In seeking to reach a wider audience, a different strategy may be required.

One of the best examples of the use of new technologies to engage in awareness raising has been demonstrated by #axschat delivered through social media channels. #axschat records an interview with a person of interest every week, that interview can be viewed live on Facebook or is archived for later viewing. Within the week following the interview a series of questions for discussion are posted based upon the interview and are the subject of online debate and discussion on twitter. Alongside such events, we are seeing the emergence of 'virtual' conferences that replace or enhance physical events, making events accessible where cost or transport are a barrier to physical attendance.

For those seeking to raise awareness there are multiple tools now available to communicate. However, customising any message to the needs of a specific audience, delivered through preferred channels is a complex task; services may have to include much greater resource into this area, especially if they wish to reach underserved communities and groups.

Assessment and Evaluation of Needs

Successful use of assistive technology is based upon effective identification of a solution that meets the needs of an individual. Traditionally, this is undertaken on an individual basis in clinic or within the community, seeking to identify whether an individual can use a solution and whether it is likely to have the desired outcomes.

Services are often positioned within public services. Their specific placement is influenced by several factors, including the assistive products to be provided, the responsibility for provision, and the business model applied. In some cases, assistive technology services are established independently of the health sector, with provision offered according to setting, such as employment or education.

Research suggests that people with disabilities benefit from support to choose the solution that best fits their needs. Some with disabilities have the capacity and desire to carry out self-assessment, and access online peer support via online information. Whilst assessment criteria emphasise the need for assistive technology recommended to be fit for purpose, there is an awareness that the cost of assessment should be proportionate to product costs, assessment costs should not excessively exceed those of the equipment. To achieve this, intervention within the escalated model, can include self-help, whereby large numbers of people support themselves using limited resource, freeing up resources for those with the most complex requirements, needing intensive services.

Self-help services are dependent upon the availability of independent advice and information, which can be used to make informed decisions. Digital hubs of information have been created, often by NGOs with public funding including:

- Assistive Technology Infor Map for Africa[2]
- Assistive Technology Australia[3]
- GARI (Mobile Manufacturers Forum).[4]

---

[2] https://assistivetechmap.org/.
[3] http://at-aust.org/.
[4] www.gari.info.

Each comprises a range of 'knowledge artefacts' such as information sheets, videos, audio files and images. The need to plan for sustainability has been highlighted especially where any business model is founded upon grants and state funding. Such portals are further enhanced by online newsletters distributed via email and social media.

Machine learning can be applied to the process of selection and identification of assistive technologies such as 'ATvisor', a digital platform to aid rehabilitation professionals and people with disabilities to source and match assistive technology products to needs. Each user creates a profile detailing needs, tasks and setting which leads to recommendations based upon the data in that profile. Early results appear to be promising in giving disabled people much greater control over assistive technology decision-making.[5]

Such tools allow professionals to carry details of a wide variety of products to support the assessment process, far more than has previously been possible, linking directly to a variety of sources of provision, best prices can be found, and first interventions rapidly made. Moreover, as the technology supports decision-making, it is far easier for carers and family members to undertake a shared assessment with the person with a disability, reducing the lead times and wait for access to a therapist.

Provision of Assistive Technology

In many parts of the world, provision of assistive technology is fragmented and reliant on local services, which may vary according to the needs of the individual or the age or setting in which they wish to use the technology. Many people with disabilities understand their needs and also how those needs might be met. In Ireland (Enable Ireland/DFI, 2016), proposals have been made for an 'Assistive Technology Passport' which provides a record of the equipment, training and funding history of an individual user of assistive technology. The passport is owned by the AT user, giving autonomy over assistive technology needs. It can transition with the person, across school, college and work, allowing freedom of movement on a par with anyone else, without fear of losing funding, support or training on the assistive technology they use.

Solutions continue to evolve; smart technologies are increasingly integrated into traditional products as a fusion of low and high technology. Mobility canes for those with vision loss incorporate enhancements that detect obstacles beyond the reach of the cane and emit a tone to offer additional alerts, whilst mainstream technologies, based upon inclusive design, offer an alternative to traditional specialised products.

---

[5] www.atvisor.com/.

Decisions will need to be made about the model of provision of low-cost products such as apps for phones and tablets recognising the ease of accessing such products directly. Such solutions may be most appropriately provided through direct payments, with changing funding models and user behaviour. Increasingly, small purchases for personal use are made directly by the user without reference to funding sources and the threshold of personal cost acceptable to individuals will increase, as beneficial technologies are increasingly available through mainstream sources.

The integration of access technologies with mainstream solutions challenges existing models of funding and the process delivering assistive products. Traditional sourcing models are challenged by the business model through which apps are provided for mobile and portable technologies. AT services need to provide information streamline funding requests, recognising the variety of forms of licence under which solutions may be distributed, greater understanding of licences will help peers to offer meaningful advice.

Training

Increasingly, professionals are accessing information and learning through online connectivity as a means of acquiring knowledge and participating in debate and discussion. Global connections assist in understanding of diverse perspectives and different experiences of delivery. Assistive technology professionals report that access to social networks broadens their understanding of approaches and professionals are contributing to debate and discussion through collaborative online platforms, often referred to as communities of practice such as those offered by Cecops,[6] DoIT[7] and Supports to Families.[8] Both popular and professional social media platforms offer examples of supplier, professional and user resources that are shared and discussed encouraging professional debate and discussion.

The emergence of freely available massive open online courses (MOOCs) that are grant funded for their development and dissemination such as the Digital Accessibility: Enabling Participation in the Information Society[9] and those offered by OCALI,[10] offering structured lessons in assistive technologies with free access to content, but with fees charged for the provision of continuing education credits or certification. Such innovation offers a greater diversity of provider options for learners.

---

[6] www.cecops.org.uk/at-hub/.
[7] www.washington.edu/doit/resources/communities-practice.
[8] http://supportstofamilies.org/tag/assistive-technology/.
[9] www.futurelearn.com/courses/digital-accessibility.
[10] www.atinternetmodules.org/user_mod.php.

Successful use of technology often requires training for users and any carers and online and mobile learning in assistive products is widely reported and accessed on demand supporting solutions and settings where a refresh of knowledge is needed. Preferences for on-demand resources reflect the widespread change in behaviour in consuming entertainment including television, music and films.

Online resources, including the training units proposed by the WHO Gate initiative, support those engaged in implementing assistive products including how to clean, assemble, charge, install or update products depending on the technology and setting, whilst learning materials can be accessed by disabled people and professionals through platforms such as YouTube where both developers and services have created playlists of tutorials supporting solutions that are freely available.

Support

Effective implementation of assistive technologies requires that technical support is available throughout the lifetime of the use of the product. Support may be essential both before first use and to maintain use. Online resources include those related to implementation including fitting, installation and customisation, and ranging from adjustments in positioning devices to customising software, and the ongoing updating and upkeep of products, including what to do when solutions stop working.

There are further opportunities to address the need for technical support during rapid change to the industry. Where users opt for direct purchase of solutions a market will emerge for 'extended warranties' offering maintenance and after sales service independently of the vendor.

Technicians and therapists may embrace the growth of online service marketplaces such as Fiverr to offer competitive support services for assistive technology. Vendors would require assistive technology knowledge combined with competence and ease in communicating with those with a disability to ensure services are user centred and responsive to needs.

Research and Development

Over many years, instruments have been developed to assess the quality of services and the outcomes of assistive products. Many need to be translated to other languages and to be tested in a variety of a range of settings. The data produced by online services, reaching millions of people forms a vast pool of users; analysis of their behaviour and needs has value to those planning future products and services. The data gathered by way-finding systems used by people with a disability suggests variations in the travel habits of those with a disability and their peers when compared to the general population. Correlated with accessibility data of the built environment, a case for investment in access can be identified.

Machine learning and analysis of user behaviour related to initiatives across the areas of the UNCRPD has been advocated, where technology matches initiatives to UNCRPD commitments and ultimately to quality of life measures. Reporting on quality of life introduces a measure of real change in the daily experience of people with a disability. Such analysis can track impact from the point of implementation of policy across both short medium and long term.

Conclusion

Services face a challenge to ensure that access technologies are available to an increasingly diverse and growing body of users. Numbers are growing across the world and traditional approaches to delivery cannot fulfil demand resulting from demographic pressures and costs. Simultaneously, user behaviour and expectations are changing, and AT services can anticipate that a role will evolve of trusted intermediary, increasingly removed from direct contact and intervention for much of the population.

Emerging technologies provide a means by which people with a disability can access the support they require for their immediate and anticipated needs. Such products, when fully implemented will further disrupt services, by offering greater reach and value. Effective services will both respond to and anticipate such disruption and hence will find new ways to fulfil demand.

References

Al Jaber, H. (2016) Healthcare disruption is already happening—policymakers in our region can't ignore it. Retrieved from www.linkedin.com/pulse/healthcare-disruption-already-happening-our-region-cant-al-jaber, October 26 2018.

AppleVis (2012) How many blind people use iPhones. Retrieved from www.applevis.com/forum/app-development/how-many-blind-people-use-iphone, October 26 2018.

Banes, D. (2016) How disruptive technology is reshaping access. Retrieved from http://tech.newstatesman.com/enterprise-it/disruptive-technology-shaping-assistive, October 26 2018.

Banes, D. (2017) Qatar and Beyond: WHO Great Summit Geneva.

Banes, D. (2018) The growth of self determination in Assistive Technology at AAATE Workshop at ICCHP 2018 Linz.

Bhuiyan, J. (2016) Disability rights advocate files discrimination complaint against Uber. Retrieved from www.buzzfeednews.com/article/johanabhuiyan/ disability-rights-advocate-files-discrimination-complaint-ag, October 26 2018.

Christensen, C. M. (1997) *The Innovator's Dilemma: When New Technologies Cause Great Firms to Fail.* Boston, MA: Harvard Business School Press, ISBN 978-0-87584-585-2.

Cook, A. M. and Polgar, J. M. (2007) *Cook and Hussey Assistive Technologies: Principles and Practice.* St. Louis, Mo: Mosby.

Democracy in America (2014) Negative externalities the economist. Retrieved from www. economist.com/blogs/democracyinamerica/2014/07/disruptive-innovation, October 26 2018.

Enable Ireland and Disability Federation of Ireland (2016) Assistive Technology for people with disabilities and older people – A discussion paper DFI.

Metcalfe, B. (2015) App updates for deaf and hard-of-hearing partners. Retrieved from www.uber.com/newsroom/app-updates-for-deaf-and-hard-of-hearing-parvtners, October 26 2018.

National Federation for the Blind (2015) Make kindle Ebooks accessible. Retrieved from https://nfb.org/kindle-books, October 26 2018.

Price Waterhouse and Cooper (2017) Six technologies that are transforming infrastructure. Retrieved from www.pwc.com/gx/en/industries/capital-projects-infrastructure/publications/six-technologies-that-are-transforming-infrastructure.html, May 21 2018.

Scherer, M. (ed.) (2002) *Assistive Technology: Matching Device and Consumer for Successful Rehabilitation.* Washington, D.C.: American Psychological Association.

Schmidt, E. (2013) The impact of disruptive technology: An interview with Eric Schmidt McKinsey Global Institute. Retrieved from www.mckinsey.com/ industries/high-tech/our-insights/the-impact-of-disruptive-technology-a-conversation-with-eric-schmidt, October 26 2018.

Scudellari, M. (2017) Lidar-equipped autonomous wheelchairs roll out in Singapore and Japan IEEE Spectrum.

Wheeler, S. (2011) Social impact of disruptive technology. Retrieved from www. steve-wheeler.co.uk/2011/01/social-impact-of-disruptive-technology.html.

WHO (2016) Priority assistive products list World Health Organisation.

World Health Organisation (2018) Assistive technology. Retrieved from www.who. int/news-room/fact-sheets/detail/assistive-technology, August 22 2018.

Zabala, J. (2005) Using the SETT framework to level the learning field for students with disabilities. Retrieved from www.joyzabala.com, October 26 2018.

Zichermann, G. and Cunningham, C. (2011) Preface. In *Gamification by Design: Implementing Game Mechanics in Web and Mobile Apps,* 1st edn. Sebastopol, CA: O'Reilly Media, pp. ix, 208, ISBN 1-4493-1539-9. Retrieved from November 25 2012.

9

Feedback-Based Technologies for Adult Physical Rehabilitation

Leanne Hassett and Natalie Allen
The University of Sydney

Maayken van den Berg
Flinders University

CONTENTS

Introduction 144
Reasons for Using Feedback-Based Technology in Rehabilitation 144
Feedback-Based Technologies and Motor Learning 146
    Content 147
    Modality 148
    Schedule 149
    Attentional Focus 150
Examples of Feedback-Based Technologies 151
    VR Gaming Technologies 151
        Recreational Gaming Technologies 151
        Rehabilitation–Specific Gaming Technologies 152
    Wearable Devices 153
    Tablet and Smartphone Applications 153
    Combined Technologies 155
Effectiveness of Using Feedback-Based Technologies in Rehabilitation 156
    VR Gaming Technologies 156
    Wearables 157
    Tablet and Smartphone Apps 158
    Mixed Technologies 158
Therapist Acceptability for Using Technology 159
Patient Acceptability for Using Technology 160
Implementing Technology into Clinical Practice 161
Considerations for Future Technology Development 164
Acknowledgements 165
References 165

Introduction

Many types of technologies are widely available for use in rehabilitation. Technologies that provide extrinsic feedback to the user about their performance, or the dose of practice completed, have been shown to facilitate engagement in exercise (Lewis and Rosie, 2012) and enhance motor learning (van Vliet and Wulf, 2006; Boyd et al., 2010). These technologies, which we will refer to as 'feedback-based technologies', include virtual reality (VR) gaming technologies (recreational and rehabilitation-specific), wearable devices (e.g. activity monitors), tablet and smartphone applications and combined technologies (e.g. VR treadmill systems).

Reasons for Using Feedback-Based Technology in Rehabilitation

Feedback-based technology can increase effectiveness, sustainability and efficiency of rehabilitation interventions through increasing, optimising and monitoring performed exercise. The dose of exercise can be increased using technologies that are engaging and motivating, and that can be used in a variety of settings, such as the clinic and the home. The quality of exercise performed can be optimised through the delivery of feedback to facilitate motor learning and the provision of an enriched environment, which delivers both physical and cognitive challenges. Technologies can also be used to monitor exercise programmes by collecting information about activity performance and adherence to prescribed programmes.

Exercise-based rehabilitation programmes are known to be effective for improving activity performance in people with impairments related to a variety of neurological, orthopaedic and age-related conditions (French et al., 2016; Tomlinson et al., 2012; Diong et al., 2016; Handoll and Sherrington, 2007; Rietberg et al., 2005). Evidence suggests that optimal rehabilitation programmes are likely to involve higher doses of exercise, including task-specific repetitive exercise (Lohse et al., 2014; Veerbeek et al., 2014; Schneider et al., 2016; Sherrington et al., 2017; Carr and Shepherd, 2010; French et al., 2016; Keus et al., 2014). Despite this, people in inpatient rehabilitation units often spend little time exercising (West and Bernhardt, 2012; Smith et al., 2008; Hassett et al., 2018) and many people with mobility limitations living in the community are less active than the already sedentary general population (Hassett et al., 2015; Ellis and Motl, 2013; van Nimwegen et al., 2011; Motl et al., 2005; English et al., 2014). Repetitive exercise can be tedious and boring, and therefore difficult to sustain over time. Gaming technologies can provide a fun, engaging and motivating way for people to complete high doses of exercise, including large numbers of repetitions (Lewis and Rosie, 2012; Allen et al., 2017; Natbony et al., 2013; Schoene et al., 2013), with participants reporting games to be a more engaging way to complete exercise than standard rehabilitation (McNulty et al., 2015; Wingham et al., 2015; Housman et al., 2009). This is because gaming technologies use interactive environments, which change during gameplay and can be adjusted to maintain appropriate levels of challenge (Lewis and Rosie, 2012). Competitive and social aspects of games can also encourage people undertaking rehabilitation to try to improve their score or to beat other players (Lewis and Rosie, 2012; Wingham et al., 2015).

Various feedback-based technologies can be used across different environments, including the clinic and the home. People undergoing rehabilitation often require long-term exercise programmes tailored to their health condition, and most healthcare systems are not able to provide these costly ongoing services. Home-based programmes with intermittent monitoring from therapists are a more cost-efficient method of providing long-term therapy. Research has shown that home-based use of gaming technologies is safe and feasible in patients undertaking upper-limb exercise following stroke (Thomson et al., 2014) and with Parkinson's disease (Allen et al., 2017). Similarly, they have also been used successfully for home-based balance and stepping exercise in appropriately selected older adults at risk of falls (Schoene et al., 2013), and in people with mobility limitations from neurological and non-neurological health conditions (Hassett et al., 2016; Song et al., 2018; Hoang et al., 2016). Tailored therapist prescription of these home-based technologies is important to ensure that patients can engage with the technology correctly and safely (Hamilton et al., 2018b). It remains to be seen if unsupervised practice is as effective as practice supervised by a therapist. Nonetheless, the provision of these technologies in the home environment is likely to provide exercise options that are affordable, sustainable, accessible and acceptable to patients (Barry et al., 2014), therefore, facilitating long-term exercise adherence and motivation (Keshner, 2004).

The feedback provided by feedback-based technologies is another important factor in optimising rehabilitation programmes. Feedback that focuses on successful performance can serve to increase motivation (Wulf et al., 2010; van Vliet and Wulf, 2006) and may encourage persistence (Solmon and Boone, 1993). Additionally, feedback can serve to focus attention on specific aspects of task performance (Lewis and Rosie, 2012) and provides information that can be used to improve performance (Schmidt and Wrisberg, 2008; Magill and Anderson, 2014). In this way, feedback-based technologies can assist patients in completing their practice as effectively as possible, without the need for continual therapist involvement. More detailed discussion regarding the role of feedback-based technologies in motor learning is provided next in this chapter.

The enriched environments provided by feedback-based technologies can also optimise rehabilitation. Enriched environments are those that provide enhanced physical, sensory, cognitive and social stimulation (Janssen et al., 2010). A systematic review of studies using animal models of ischaemic stroke found that animals exposed to enriched environments, had improved neurobehavioural functioning and learning compared with those in standard laboratory environments (Janssen et al., 2010). A trial in humans undergoing inpatient rehabilitation following stroke reported increased participation in activities likely to promote recovery when participants were in an enriched environment, which included ready access to a variety of activities including a Nintendo Wii system (Janssen et al., 2014). The use of feedback-based technologies is a way of providing such an enriched environment. Additionally, bringing aspects of the outdoor environment into therapy allows people who are unable to participate in activities in the community, such as crossing the road to perform preparatory practice for real-life scenarios safely in a controlled environment (Tieri et al., 2018).

Finally, feedback-based technologies have the added benefit of automatically documenting the practice performed (Skjaeret et al., 2016; Sveistrup, 2004; Tieri et al., 2018). Therapists use information about exercise adherence and performance to optimise exercise prescriptions and tailor self-management programmes. Traditionally, therapists have relied on patients documenting their unsupervised practice to provide this information. However, the validity, reliability and accuracy of self-report measures for unsupervised practice are unclear (Bollen et al., 2014; Prince et al., 2008; Frost et al., 2016). Feedback-based technologies provide therapists with accurate information about the amount of exercise that has been completed each day (e.g. number of steps taken, number of games played), and in some cases can also report information which may reflect the standard of the performance (e.g. scores in a game). The instantaneous feedback to the patient aids in self-monitoring (Voth et al., 2016) and allows for electronic two-way communication between the patient and therapist. In this way, exercise adherence can be facilitated as programmes can be remotely monitored and progressed, patients can report difficulties and therapists can provide ongoing support and encouragement (Hamilton et al., 2018a).

Feedback-Based Technologies and Motor Learning

The feedback delivered by technologies used in rehabilitation can play an important role in motor learning. Motor learning refers to the acquisition, reacquisition or improvement of motor skills and is associated with physiological changes that occur following practice or experience (Schmidt and Wrisberg, 2008; Magill and Anderson, 2014). Clearly, motor learning is a key component of rehabilitation programmes, and studies have shown that people with neurological conditions are able to learn motor skills (Tomassini et al.,

2011; van Vliet and Wulf, 2006; Nackaerts et al., 2013). There is a continuum of motor learning from implicit (i.e. learning without conscious awareness) to explicit (i.e. learning with a high degree of awareness of the process and outcomes) (Magill and Anderson, 2014). Feedback facilitates motor learning by providing the learner with information that can be used to improve performance (Schmidt and Wrisberg, 2008; Magill and Anderson, 2014). Intrinsic feedback (i.e. feedback automatically occurring as part of the movement) can be supplemented by extrinsic feedback (i.e. feedback provided by an outside source, such as a game) (Schmidt and Wrisberg, 2008; Magill and Anderson, 2014). There is evidence that people with neurological conditions have impaired implicit learning and difficulty using intrinsic feedback, meaning that learning will be better if it is more explicit (Verschueren et al., 1997; Nieuwboer et al., 2009; van Vliet and Wulf, 2006). This can be achieved through extrinsic feedback. However, the delivery of this feedback needs to be carefully considered in order to optimally facilitate learning rather than just short-term improvements in performance (Wulf et al., 2010), so that improved performance is retained and transferable to other situations.

Extrinsic feedback takes the form of knowledge of results (KR) and/or knowledge of performance (KP) (Schmidt and Wrisberg, 2008; Magill and Anderson, 2014). KR provides information about the outcome of an action (e.g. the score achieved in a video game) whereas KP gives information about the characteristics of the movement that led to the outcome (e.g. a graph in a video game indicating the player's centre of pressure movement in relation to the required movement). Much is known about the best way to deliver extrinsic feedback for learning in the general population, and it seems likely that many of the same principles will apply to people in rehabilitation, particularly in those who are neurologically intact. However, people with neurological conditions may require some modifications to the way feedback is delivered. The following paragraphs use a framework based on that of van Vliet and Wulf (2006), to discuss the influence of the content, modality, schedule and attentional focus of extrinsic feedback provided by feedback-based technologies.

Content

Both KR and KP are important and effective forms of extrinsic feedback (Schmidt and Wrisberg, 2008; Magill and Anderson, 2014). Feedback-based technologies usually provide both KR and KP, and so are likely to provide feedback that can be used to improve motor skills. In particular, the KR can easily be used to set goals and provide a motivating record of improvement (Lewis and Rosie, 2012). However, the KP provided by these technologies can be inaccurate (Deutsch et al., 2011). For example, when the technology provides a visual representation of movement based on information from a force platform (e.g. Nintendo Wii), the movement represented may not match the actual movement. This is of concern as patients can be making unwanted compensatory movements but receive KP feedback that their movement is successful, thereby reinforcing the unwanted movement pattern. Additionally, patients may be motivated by achieving a higher point score, at the expense of a better movement strategy (Lewis et al., 2011). Given that randomised controlled trials suggest that in people following stroke, KP may be more potent, leading to better motor learning outcomes and retention than KR feedback (Cirstea et al., 2006; Cirstea and Levin, 2007), therapists need to monitor the movement strategies being used by patients during video games and ensure that patients understand the desired movement. The use of motion capture technologies can improve the accuracy of KP feedback as the technology displays kinematic information captured from the player. Rehabilitation-specific gaming systems that can be customised also have the potential to direct the player's attention to the most important features of the movement by presenting only the critical kinematic information, thereby improving not only the accuracy of the KP, but also its clinical utility (Yates et al., 2016).

Extrinsic feedback can serve to encourage and motivate the learner (Wulf et al., 2010; van Vliet and Wulf, 2006; Solmon and Boone, 1993) as well as provide information to assist them to improve their performance (Schmidt and Wrisberg, 2008). Rehabilitation-specific gaming technologies generally provide appropriate, encouraging feedback. However, the multimodal feedback of recreational systems has not been designed with the rehabilitation market in mind. While it may be useful to enhance performance in some people undergoing rehabilitation, it can also be experienced as negative and discouraging, reminding people of their impairments (Forsberg et al., 2015; Plow and Finlayson, 2014). For example, the Nintendo Wii Fit games provide an overall description of performance accompanied by a star rating at the end of each game. Performance may be described in negative terms, e.g. 'unbalanced' and the standard set to achieve a high star rating is relatively difficult, with the intervals between each rating such that patients are likely to have difficulty progressing (Deutsch et al., 2011). Patients may therefore receive feedback that they have performed poorly, even when their performance relative to their own goals was good. As well as information indicating the success or failure of a movement (i.e. descriptive feedback), technologies should optimally provide patients with information about what to change to improve their next attempt (i.e. prescriptive feedback) (Schmidt and Wrisberg, 2008). While video games often provide instructions on how to play the game, these often are not linked or tailored to the player's actual performance. Therapists should, therefore, be mindful that they may need to provide additional feedback to correct negative feedback, or to provide prescriptive feedback if patients are unsure of which features of their movement they need to modify (Deutsch et al., 2011).

Modality

Extrinsic feedback can be visual, auditory or haptic (i.e. via touch). Most technologies use a combination of these, with some recreational gaming technologies providing constant and overlapping feedback from different modalities (Deutsch et al., 2011). People in the general population and those with neurological impairments show improved learning of motor skills when any modality of extrinsic feedback is provided compared to no feedback (Schmidt and Wrisberg, 2008; Magill and Anderson, 2014; Mak and Hui-Chan, 2008; Sackley and Lincoln, 1997; Hebert et al., 1998). However, studies with people following stroke suggest that auditory feedback may be particularly important for them (Cirstea and Levin, 2007; Maulucci and Eckhouse, 2001; Secoli et al., 2011). Most gaming technologies used in rehabilitation provide KR using both visual and auditory feedback. Visual feedback often takes the form of pictures and text indicating the level of success, whereas auditory feedback takes the form of sounds indicating if the outcome was successful or unsuccessful. However, KP is typically provided as visual feedback only, using graphs to illustrate characteristics of the movement, an avatar on the screen representing the user's movements or an object responding to the user's movements.

Schedule

The schedule at which external feedback is delivered is known to influence motor learning. In the general population, learning is better when feedback is delivered after some trials (e.g. 50%–66%) compared to all trials (Winstein and Schmidt, 1990; Weeks and Kordus, 1998). Additionally, feedback that is delivered concurrently with the movement, or immediately at the end of the movement can be detrimental to learning compared to feedback that is delivered after a few seconds delay (Schmidt and Wulf, 1997; Swinnen et al., 1990). This is thought to be because the learner may come to rely on the external feedback rather than learning to utilise intrinsic feedback, leading to a decrement in performance once the external feedback is removed (Weeks and Kordus, 1998; van Vliet and Wulf, 2006; Nackaerts et al., 2013). There is some evidence that people with neurological impairments might also learn simple motor skills better with a reduced frequency of feedback (Winstein and Schmidt, 1990; Onla-or and Winstein, 2008; Chiviacowsky et al., 2010). However, there may be an interaction between the ideal scheduling of feedback and the relative task complexity (Wulf and Shea, 2002), with more frequent feedback preferable for learning more complex tasks (Wulf and Shea, 2002; van Vliet and Wulf, 2006). Given that any given task is likely to be relatively more complex for a person with neurological impairments (van Vliet and Wulf, 2006), as well as the added difficulties people with neurological impairment can have with accessing intrinsic feedback (Verschueren et al., 1997; Nieuwboer et al., 2009; van Vliet and Wulf, 2006), concurrent feedback may be more important for this population (Magill and Anderson, 2014). It seems likely that gradually reducing (i.e. fading) feedback could facilitate motor learning (Magill and Anderson, 2014; Nackaerts et al., 2013), as more frequent feedback is provided in the early stages of learning, followed by a reduction in feedback as the learner improves. Consequently, the learner is encouraged to utilise intrinsic feedback and learn from their errors. This is supported by trials with participants following stroke, where trial and error was superior to errorless learning (Mount et al., 2007), and concurrent but faded feedback resulted in better learning than terminal, summary feedback (Cirstea et al., 2006; Cirstea and Levin, 2007).

Recreational gaming technologies tend to provide large amounts of feedback both concurrently and terminally, which can enhance engagement in and enjoyment of the game. However, the feedback often contains KP and KR, and can be visual, auditory and haptic, resulting in a large amount of rapidly changing and complex information which can then be difficult for the player to use effectively (Lewis and Rosie, 2012; Deutsch et al., 2011). Although much of this feedback is likely to be redundant, it cannot be faded to a schedule that would be more optimal for motor learning. Rehabilitation-specific gaming technologies usually provide less complex feedback, though it typically is still delivered both concurrently and terminally and cannot be faded. Therapists can assist patients to use the feedback more effectively by directing their attention to specific features, or by removing the auditory feedback (e.g. by turning the volume down).

Attentional Focus

During motor learning, the learner can be directed to focus on specific aspects of the bodily movement (i.e. an internal focus of attention) or to focus on the outcome of the movement (i.e. an external focus of attention) (Schmidt and Wrisberg, 2008). Studies have shown that an external focus of attention is superior for learning motor skills for people in the general population (Wulf and Prinz, 2001), and are likely to be superior for people with neurological conditions (van Vliet and Wulf, 2006; Wulf et al., 2009; Shafizadeh et al., 2013). This may particularly be the case for people with Parkinson's disease, where movement automaticity is impaired and cueing strategies (i.e. strategies that provide an external trigger or target for movement) assist with motor learning (Nieuwboer et al., 2009; Nackaerts et al., 2013). Feedback-based gaming technologies typically provide an external focus of attention, as the player seeks to interact with the virtual environment. Occasionally, however, games may present the player with a choice of an external or internal focus of attention. For example, games that involve shifting weight on a force platform can provide KP where the player attempts to match their centre of pressure to a graph (internal focus of attention) while also interacting with the objects in the game (external focus of attention). While patients may benefit from practice with both forms of attention, to attempt to use both during one game is likely to lead to deterioration in performance. Therapists should, therefore, direct the patient's attention according to the feedback that is likely to be the most helpful at that time, with most practice completed using an external focus of attention.

Examples of Feedback-Based Technologies

VR Gaming Technologies

There has been a rapid growth in the use of interactive video games for rehabilitation purposes. Generally, VR gaming technologies are based on the concept of avatar motor learning, providing KP by mirroring the player's movement on the screen. The use of the avatar allows the patient to benefit from action-observation, as well as from extrinsic feedback. The avatar emulates the exercise, according to the body movements of the player, and provides feedback on the correctness of the movement (KP). VR gaming technologies include both recreational systems (commercially available, used by the general public) and systems developed specifically for rehabilitation (commercially available and bespoke creations).

Recreational Gaming Technologies

Two examples of commonly used recreational gaming technologies are the Nintendo Wii (*Nintendo*, Kyoto, Japan) and Xbox Kinect (*Microsoft* Redmond Campus, Redmond, Washington, United States). Both these technologies use body motion to control game play. The Wii uses haptic sensor-based hand-held controllers, which measure changes in direction and acceleration, plus a balance board and a kinetic force plate containing four pressure sensors allowing for centre of pressure measures, which translate the movement of the player onto the screen. The Wii Fit and Wii Sports games are the most commonly used games in the clinic. One example is the Wii Fit Penguin Slide game. The player is required to shift their weight side-to-side on the balance board to tilt an iceberg upon which a penguin is standing to guide the penguin to catch fish. Feedback is provided by visual (score, iceberg tilting) and auditory (when fish caught) modes concurrently and terminally. In rehabilitation, the purpose of using this game is to practice lateral horizontal pelvic shift; however, rapid lateral flexion of the trunk is likely to achieve a higher score and more positive feedback than a slower more correct movement of the pelvis.

The Xbox Kinect uses cameras and depth sensors to enable gesture recognition, using full-body 3D motion data, and does not require handheld controllers or a balance board. The user interacts with the games through a virtual avatar created by the system. In addition, the system guides the user with audio and visual feedback (Türkbey et al., 2017). All games use whole body movements and may require stepping, bending and jumping. Xbox Kinect Adventures and Sports are commonly used in the clinic. One example from the Adventures games is 20,000 leaks. The player performs reaching and stepping movements to plug the holes created by various sea creatures in an ocean glass tank. Feedback is provided during (KP) and after the game (KR). Both auditory and visual feedback is provided when the player plugs a leak (visually displaying the body part that plugged the leak). The score is shown during and at the end of the game.

The clinical use of technologies like the Nintendo Wii and the Xbox Kinect is limited by the fact that settings cannot be customised to meet the needs of people undertaking rehabilitation. Often the games are too fast and they do not take quality of movement into account (Pirovano et al., 2016), and feedback may not be clinically appropriate. The design of rehabilitation-specific gaming technologies intends to overcome these shortcomings.

Rehabilitation–Specific Gaming Technologies

Rehabilitation-specific gaming technologies are growing in number, partly due to high-quality technology components, such as sensors becoming more affordable. Several of the more affordable systems use the Microsoft Kinect sensor paired with software that can be customised to better suit a range of patients and settings. The systems often include options for assessment, basic exercises and interactive games that can be customised in different ways (e.g. dose, level of difficulty, direction of movement) to match the patient's needs. Examples of current commercially available systems using the Kinect sensor include VirtualRehab (*Evolv* rehabilitation technologies, London, United Kingdom), Jintronix (*Jintronix*, Seattle, United States) and Fysiogaming (*Doctor Kinetic*, Netherlands) (see Figure 9.1).

Other rehabilitation-specific systems use sensors attached to the person to detect movement. Sensors may be attached directly on the skin or applied, for example, within a glove on the hand. IREX (*GestureTek, Inc*, Toronto, Canada) is an example of this type of system that uses sensors as well as

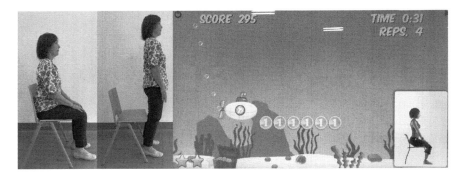

FIGURE 9.1
Fysiogaming, *Doctor Kinetic* sit to stand game. Games can be customised from easy (level 1) to difficult (level 30) as can number of repetitions, sets and rest period between sets. An ocean ground is displayed on the screen. The player must stand up and sit down to move the submarine up (standing up) and down (sitting down) to collect the coins. A virtual trainer is provided on the screen for the patient to follow as they stand up and sit down, which enables learning by imitation. Concurrent audio feedback is provided when coins are collected, and visual feedback provides the score. Terminal feedback includes score, medals and photos of performance.

video capture technology to display a mirror image of the player on the screen. Visual and auditory input generated by the system provide feedback on KP, such as speed, body position and direction of movement, and KR, e.g. game score and error rate (Glegg et al., 2014).

In addition to video gaming systems, immersive technologies, using 3D displays such as head-mounted displays or cave systems have recently been introduced. Head-mounted displays have now become commercially available, e.g. Oculus Rift, HTC Vive and Samsung Gear VR. These systems place the patient inside the virtual environment creating a sense of immersion and can be used in conjunction with treadmill walking (in a harness) or activities performed while seated.

Wearable Devices

Wearables are designed to monitor and provide feedback on health-related activities, such as physical activity, sleep and heart rate. The simplest and cheapest wearable sensor is the pedometer, which uses a switch mechanism to detect steps taken. Activity monitors, which detect acceleration of objects in motion, provide additional feedback on velocity, intensity and frequency of movement. Examples of commonly used, commercially available, activity monitors in rehabilitation include different models of Fitbit (*Fitbit Inc.*, San Francisco, California, United States) (see Figure 9.2a), ActiGraph (*ActiGraph Corp*, Pensacola, Florida, United Sates) and Stepwatch (*modus health llc*, Edmonds, Washington, United States). Feedback from these devices, usually through a downloaded companion app, include data such as step count, distance travelled, time spent active and inactive, goal achievement and some include GPS location, heart rate, sleep time and provide haptic feedback to encourage movement or indicate goal achievement (see Figure 9.2b). Choice of which monitor to use with patients may vary according to purpose, preference, cost and accuracy (Treacy et al., 2017).

Heart rate monitors with chest straps or an optical wrist sensor are another common wearable used in rehabilitation; however, many wrist-worn activity monitors nowadays also have built-in optical heart rate monitors. Wireless headphones have now also been introduced to measure pulse (e.g. *Jabra GN*, Copenhagen, Denmark). All these devices provide instant feedback through a connected device, allowing the user to stay within or reach a certain target heart rate zone, which is important in rehabilitation as part of cardiorespiratory fitness training programmes.

Tablet and Smartphone Applications

Most smartphones can also be used as activity monitors, as they have built-in motion sensors such as accelerometers and gyroscopes. With a physical activity app on the smartphone (e.g. Runkeeper, *FitnessKeeper Inc.*, Boston, Massachusetts, United States), real-time feedback on the amount

(a)

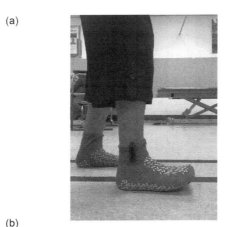

(b)

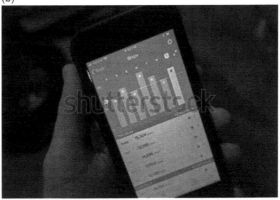

FIGURE 9.2
Fitbit activity monitor. Step count goal can be customised to match current physical activity level. Concurrent feedback is provided on number of steps provided as well as other variables such as number of stairs climbed. (a) The Fitbit can be attached to the person's sock or shoe for greater accuracy in slower walkers (Treacy et al., 2017). (b) Fitbit companion app can be downloaded to a smartphone, tablet or computer. Feedback on step count (and other variables) and goal achievement can be viewed graphically for different time periods.

and intensity of physical activity and GPS tracking for outdoor location can be provided. Smartphone applications (and activity monitors) have been designed to set goals and include tools such as reminders and real-time alerts (through a message, vibration or a noise) when a user has been inactive for a certain period of time or has met a goal. Goal setting, feedback and rewards have been described as important elements for behaviour change (Glynn et al., 2013; Lynch et al., 2018; Sullivan and Lachman, 2016; Yang and Hsu, 2010) which may be important when encouraging physical activity as part of rehabilitation programmes.

Apart from apps designed to monitor and promote physical activity, other apps have been developed for smartphones and tablets to deliver rehabilitation exercises (e.g. PhysioTherapy eXercises www.physiotherapyexercises.com) and to provide feedback for mobility training (e.g. haptic feedback for balance training (Lee et al., 2012)). Tablets have also been used for interactive gaming systems, for example, for arm-hand training in stroke survivors, providing patients with visual and auditory feedback on performance (Jacobs et al., 2013).

Combined Technologies

Recent research has focused on maximising rehabilitation outcomes by combining technologies such as VR with treadmill walking (e.g. C-Mill, *Motek*, Netherlands) and/or robotics (e.g. Lokomat, *Hocoma AG*, Volketswil, Switzerland; see Figure 9.3), providing environments which include problem-solving as well as physical challenges. This combination enables multisensory (visual and auditory) feedback to train motor-cognitive aspects

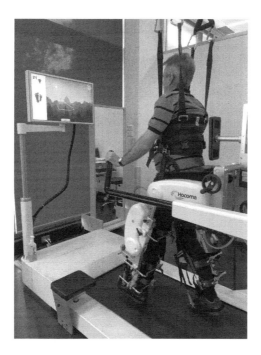

FIGURE 9.3
Combined technology of VR with robotic treadmill walking, Lokomat, *Hocoma, AG*, thirsty hiker stepping game. The player follows the trajectory to reach the water bottle and must control the shoe on the screen that appears along the path. Lokomat settings can be customised (speed, guidance force and body weight support), as well as play time, focus selection (left leg, right leg or both), step length, step height and exercise level (easy, medium or hard). Concurrent visual (focus selection, score, number of steps taken, distance walked and time left) and auditory feedback (when reaching the water bottle) is provided. The score is displayed during (displaying a trophy) and at the end (with a star rating) of the game.

such as dual tasking, executive function and obstacle negotiation in combination with treadmill training, even for people unable to walk independently. These combined systems tend to come with a large price tag and although there are some studies demonstrating effectiveness (Nam et al., 2017; Bruni et al., 2018), little has been examined on the cost-effectiveness compared to cheaper technologies.

Effectiveness of Using Feedback-Based Technologies in Rehabilitation

VR Gaming Technologies

VR gaming technologies (recreational, rehabilitation-specific and combined technologies) are the most commonly evaluated feedback-based technologies with safety, feasibility and effectiveness of VR interventions evaluated in various patient populations.

In people with stroke, VR interventions have been found to be similarly effective as usual care rehabilitation in improving upper-limb function (Laver et al., 2017). However, there is low-quality evidence that VR interventions in addition to usual care, result in improved arm function (Laver et al., 2017). VR interventions focused on balance and gait in people with stroke have shown significant improvements when compared to conventional therapy (Corbetta et al., 2015; de Rooij et al., 2016). Another systematic review (Palma et al., 2017) explored how VR interventions affect outcomes in people with stroke, according to the International Classification of Function, Disability and Health. Positive results on body functions and structures were found (e.g. upper-limb structure and function); however, evidence to support the effects across the domains of activity and participation remained inconclusive.

In people with Parkinson's disease, a systematic review incorporating eight studies (263 people with Parkinson's disease) (Dockx et al., 2016) demonstrated that clinical effectiveness of VR in rehabilitation is still unclear. Low-quality evidence showed that VR interventions may lead to moderate improvements in step and stride length compared to traditional physiotherapy, but was no more effective in improving gait, balance and quality of life (Dockx et al., 2016). Similar findings have been reported in people with multiple sclerosis. A recent systematic review (Casuso-Holgado et al., 2018) showed that VR interventions and traditional physiotherapy interventions have similar effects on outcomes of gait and balance. In a randomised controlled trial designed to assess feasibility ($n=25$), VR in combination with treadmill training demonstrated greater improvements in gait kinematics and kinetics compared to treadmill training alone; however, there were no differences between groups in gait and balance measures (Peruzzi et al., 2017).

In older adults, VR interventions have been used mainly to target balance and fear of falling, and have been found superior to conventional therapy. VR interventions have also demonstrated positive effects on mobility when compared to no intervention (Neri et al., 2017). In combination with treadmill training, VR has been used to train cognition and mobility outcomes in older adults with high risk of falls, including those with a history of idiopathic falls, those with cognitive impairment and those with Parkinson's disease. A 6-month combined intervention significantly decreased fall rates when compared to treadmill training alone and this effect was maintained during a 6-month follow-up period (Mirelman et al., 2016).

Generally, the literature has demonstrated large variability in intervention delivery. A variety of VR systems and training protocols have been used. Most studies have used solely one device, or games targeting one physical function only. Positive effects have been found limited to the specific functions trained during VR gaming, without generalising to other functions. The diversity of approaches has also been highlighted by large differences in intensity, frequency and duration of interventions. Typically, studies in this area have been rated as low quality with poor reporting (Laver et al., 2017). Small-sample size has led to studies frequently being underpowered to assess effectiveness. Adequately powered, high-quality randomised controlled trials that include a follow-up period and adequate description of the intervention protocols are required.

Wearables

In inactive older people, those receiving step count feedback from a pedometer have been found to increase their physical activity (Bravata et al., 2007; Kolt et al., 2012; Snyder et al., 2011). But in people after stroke, this has not yet been demonstrated. A recent systematic review (Lynch et al., 2018) summarised the evidence of using activity monitors (including pedometers) in people with stroke in hospital or living in the community. The four low-quality included trials did not show a clear effect of the use of an activity monitor in combination with another intervention, such as with inpatient rehabilitation or a walking programme, on physical activity levels in people with stroke. One of the included studies also showed that incorporating activity monitor feedback in the goal-setting process of people with stroke did not increase the overall amount of walking in the inpatient setting; however, participants did demonstrate an increased cadence, translating into increased walking speed (Mansfield et al., 2015).

Wearable biofeedback technologies have also been investigated in rehabilitation populations. Smartwatches have been used to provide feedback on falls in the elderly, to help people with Alzheimer's disease to recognise people, and to monitor activity in people with stroke and Parkinson's disease (Lu et al., 2016). A systematic review demonstrated audio and visual feedback on weight distribution, muscle activity or gait parameters from a range of technologies (many wearable technologies such as sensors) improved lower-limb activity significantly better than therapist instruction alone in people after stroke (Stanton et al., 2017). In adults after traumatic brain injury, audio and visual feedback from heart rate monitors did not increase the intensity of exercise in a circuit class group; however, the use of monitors was seen as important to monitor the intensity and duration of exercise to ensure sufficient dose of cardiorespiratory fitness training (Hassett et al., 2012).

Tablet and Smartphone Apps

Tablet and smartphone applications have been found feasible in assisting elements of home rehabilitation programmes. The evaluation of a hospital rehabilitation service using a combination of tablets, videoconferencing software, exercise and rehabilitation applications showed that telerehabilitation could be delivered using off-the-shelf applications. The devices delivered feedback through incorporating fitbits (Fitbit Inc., San Francisco, California, United States) and using real-time feedback, such as through using the Bandicam screen recorder (Bandicam Company, Seoul, Korea). Participants felt comfortable with the technology and clinicians were positive about its usefulness (Crotty et al., 2014). In people with Parkinson's disease, a personalised smartphone application using wearable sensors, providing audio biofeedback and external cueing, was found effective in improving gait and balance (Ginis et al., 2016).

Mixed Technologies

Two recent studies have investigated the use of a suite of feedback-based technologies to improve mobility and physical activity in a mixed rehabilitation population (Hassett et al., 2016; van den Berg et al., 2016). The first (van den Berg et al., 2016) showed improvements in balance but not overall mobility when a range of VR gaming technologies and activity monitor were prescribed in a circuit exercise programme, in addition to usual care inpatient rehabilitation for 2 weeks. The second study (Hassett et al., 2016) involved physiotherapists selecting the most appropriate feedback-based technologies (VR gaming technologies, activity monitors and tablet and smartphone applications) to address mobility limitations and increase physical activity. Technologies were progressed and changed as required and were provided in addition to usual care for a 6-month period and were compared to usual care alone. Significant improvements were observed in mobility at 3 weeks and 6 months after randomisation in the technology plus usual care group, compared to the usual care only group. Physical activity outcomes were mixed with no difference in measured upright time; however, significant differences in self-reported planned physical activity were observed.

Therapist Acceptability for Using Technology

The decision to accept use of a new technology in practice is influenced by many factors. An early study conducted in a business setting found two key influencers: perceived usefulness and perceived ease of use (Davis, 1989). Perceived usefulness is the belief that the new technology will enhance performance, make the job more efficient, or improve functionality. Perceived ease of use is the belief that using the new technology will be free from effort. Out of the two, perceived usefulness was a stronger driver, with users able to accept some complexity within the system if the technology enhanced performance.

Similar drivers for technology acceptability have been reported by therapists when considering use of technology in rehabilitation. A recent systematic review synthesising ten qualitative studies of therapists' experiences of using feedback-based technologies in rehabilitation found that the benefits of using the technology (i.e. perceived usefulness) and the design of the technology (i.e. perceived ease of use) were key themes (Hamilton et al., 2018a). Therapists reported benefits of technology use including patient functional improvements similar to traditional therapy, however, with the added benefits of increased motivation and enjoyment, the potential for competition and social interaction, and practicing real-life tasks in a safe environment. In addition, therapists reported benefits for themselves including increased productivity, time saving and digital recording of dose of practice. Ease of use features included wanting reliable systems that were quick to set up and easy to transport between settings, and easy for the users to follow instructions and navigate through menus. Therapists also identified the importance of support to both purchase and use technologies, including training and resources as well as support to manage technical problems. Another key finding was that therapists were accepting of using the technology; however, they perceived it as an adjunct to usual rehabilitation care and they needed to be intimately involved in technology prescription, training and monitoring of patient practice to ensure therapeutic benefit.

Survey data from 1,325 physiotherapists, occupational therapists and speech pathologists who may or may not have used technology in practice identified patient factors and larger organisational factors as other drivers for therapists deciding to purchase and use technology in practice (Chen and Bode, 2011). The three most important considerations when purchasing new technologies were the initial cost, the ability to bill for services, and to have sufficient appropriate patients to use the technology with. When deciding to use a technology, therapists were influenced by patient acceptance, the suitability of the therapy setting and logistics such as scheduling, set-up time and the amount of assistance required to use the technology. Therapists were also influenced by key stakeholders, e.g. rehabilitation physicians in the inpatient setting and family members in the home setting.

Patient Acceptability for Using Technology

An important factor influencing therapists' decisions to use technology in practice is patient acceptability. Studies investigating patient acceptability of using technology as part of their rehabilitation have had mixed, but overall positive results. In a study of older (mean age 85 years) hospitalised patients who used the Nintendo Wii for 6 sessions, participants indicated a stronger preference for traditional therapy (Laver et al., 2011b). In contrast, other studies in community-based participants have reported positive findings. One feasibility study (participant mean age 76 years; fallen at least once in the previous 12 months) used the Nintendo Wii twice weekly for 12 weeks and reported good compliance, enjoyment and acceptability of the intervention (Williams et al., 2010). In people after stroke, a systematic review evaluated their experiences of using recreational gaming systems such as Nintendo Wii as part of upper-limb rehabilitation (Thomson et al., 2014). Overall, participants were positive about games being fun, engaging and challenging; however, they did report frustration when games were too quick for their ability and suggested that recreational gaming systems may be better suited later in rehabilitation once more movement had been achieved.

Patient experiences and acceptability of using VR technologies in neurorehabilitation have been investigated in a review incorporating 3 qualitative studies and 18 quantitative studies (Lewis and Rosie, 2012). The majority of participants reported positive experiences of using VR, particularly enjoying the cognitive and physical challenge, and reported it to be more engaging and fun than traditional therapy. Participants liked the feedback they received from systems, particularly positive feedback and high scores, plus an ability to see improvements. Participants also clearly identified that the games needed to meet their rehabilitation needs as well as being enjoyable. Technical difficulties and difficulty manipulating devices led to frustrations and less positive experiences. A consistent finding was the need for a large selection and variety of games to enhance enjoyment.

A recent qualitative study (Hamilton et al., 2018b) investigated the experiences of 20 mixed diagnoses aged-care and neurological rehabilitation patients using a range of affordable feedback-based technologies as part of the AMOUNT rehabilitation trial discussed in the previous section (Hassett et al., 2016). Participant interviews identified two key conditions to optimise patient experience of using technology: support and perceived benefit. Participants needed to have sufficient support to use the technology, either from the therapist or family members. This support could entail physical support to use the technology, motivational support to encourage use and educational support to learn to use the technologies and interpret feedback. Participants also needed to perceive benefit from using the technology to initiate and sustain engagement with it. Benefits included providing variety, novelty, enjoyment and distraction for exercise, cognitive challenge, provision of additional exercise, convenience of use, feedback on performance and opportunity for social interaction.

Implementing Technology into Clinical Practice

When health organisations are planning change, such as implementing technology-based rehabilitation, they need to consider their patient population and how rehabilitation is delivered. By appropriately matching the technology with the organisation, the technology should suit the rehabilitation philosophy, match the rehabilitation delivery mode (e.g. clinic versus home) and be useful for the types of patients managed by the organisation. Organisations should also consider the support available to successfully use technology by assessing whether the service has or is able to acquire sufficient IT capabilities to support technology use. Finally, organisations should look how best to integrate the technology into existing practices. For example, if the gym is usually set up in the morning by the therapy assistant, turning on and preparing the technology at this time may be a successful strategy to facilitate its use in practice.

It is important to involve patients (Laver et al., 2011c) and staff in the planning and development when implementing technology-based rehabilitation, taking into consideration the experiences of technology use of both therapist and patient. Having a variety of technologies available allows a therapist to choose a technology that matches each patient's impairments and activity limitations, goals, technology experience and personal preferences. Table 9.1 provides a list of technology attributes identified from the literature and our team's research findings that are perceived as important considerations from the therapist, patient and contextual perspective. This table could be used as a checklist for therapists and organisations when purchasing or trialling a new technology in practice.

It is important that therapists feel confident in the use of the technologies available to them. Implementation research (and similar findings from Davis (1989)) demonstrates that therapist behaviour is unlikely to change if the new behaviour is more difficult than current practice, unless therapists perceive substantial benefits (French et al., 2012). Furthermore, patients are more engaged and therapeutic benefit is likely to be optimised when therapists are proficient at using technology, and can combine these skills with clinical reasoning to ensure the right activities are practiced with the right level of challenge (Hamilton et al., 2018a,b). To enable proficiency, therapists require sufficient time to familiarise themselves with the technology, and to receive training. This training can include case studies with examples of technology prescription for therapeutic benefit including how to modify game play (see Figure 9.4). Therapists then need ongoing resources such as simple, easy to

TABLE 9.1

Technology Attributes to Consider when Selecting New Technology for a Clinical Setting and for Future Technology Development

Attribute[a]	Description
Therapeutic Prescription	
Evidence	What is the evidence to support use of this technology in clinical practice
Customisation	How much the technology can be customised to match the needs of the patient e.g. time of practice, time between games/sets, level of difficulty, avatar/user profile and amount, direction and repetition of movement
Population	Whether the technology is appropriate for rehabilitation patients with different health conditions and of different ages and stages of rehabilitation
Type of practice	Whether the technology can be used for different aspects of training e.g. upper limb, lower limb, impairment, activity and participation-level training
Dose of practice	How much extra active practice time the technology enables the patient to have
Risk and safety	How safe is the technology for use in the planned setting, e.g. risk of falls
Data	How is data about the dose and type of therapy stored, exported and presented
Time to learn how to use the technology	How much time it takes for a typical rehabilitation therapist to become proficient at using the technology. How much training, resources and support is provided
Therapeutic Prescription/Patient Engagement	
Additional benefits	Whether there are additional benefits to using technology above usual care rehabilitation, e.g. physical, cognitive, social and self-efficacy
Feedback	Modality (i.e. visual, auditory and/or haptic), schedule, content (KR, KP, Motivational), focus of attention and whether it can be customised
Reliability of system	Reliability of the system to detect movement accurately in the patient group it is being used
Patient Engagement	
Variety	How many games/exercises there are to choose from in the technology
Enjoyment	How fun and engaging the technology is to use
Time to understand the game/exercise requirements	How well the technology provides instruction/demonstration to enable a patient to understand the requirements of the game/exercise, e.g. the movement required, objective of the game
Patient set up	How easy or difficult it is for the patient to learn to set up the technology independently
Independent use	Whether the technology is easy to use so that for most patients they would be able to use it independently

(Continued)

TABLE 9.1 (*Continued*)

Technology Attributes to Consider when Selecting New Technology for a Clinical Setting and for Future Technology Development

Attribute[a]	Description
Contextual Factors	
Time to set up technology	How long it takes to set up the technology each time it is going to be used (repeat patient, new patient)
Time to learn how to use the technology	How well the technology provides instruction/demonstration to non-therapists, e.g. therapy assistant, volunteers, caregivers to assist the person in rehabilitation to use the technology
Cost	Whether the cost of purchasing the technology is prohibitive or affordable for patients or organisations
Setting/portable	Whether the technology can be used in different settings, e.g. clinic, home, etc., and how easy it is to move, pack away and set up each time
IT support	Whether or not the technology has an IT support system in place for troubleshooting

[a] There is no current evidence to support the order of importance of attributes.

access instructions and protocols for using the technology. Some resources exist for recreational gaming systems with games analysis and recommendations for the best games for therapeutic benefit (Harvey and Ada, 2012; Levac et al., 2015, 2018).

To implement technology in practice, organisations and therapists need to consider their patient population as feedback-based technology will not be suitable for all people undertaking rehabilitation. People with visual or

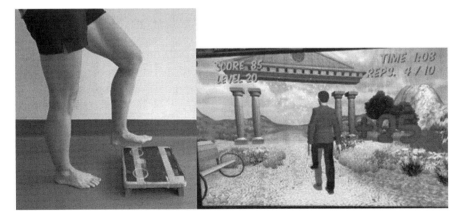

FIGURE 9.4
Fysiogaming, *Doctor Kinetic* knee flexion game. The player performs alternate knee lifts to build a coliseum. Game play can be modified to better match common rehabilitation exercises prescribed such as touching a block in front with alternate feet to practice shifting weight side-to-side.

severe cognitive impairments, for example, are less suited for this type of intervention and recreational technologies will not be suitable for people with severe physical impairments. In addition, older people have reported less enthusiasm for using computer-based technologies than younger people in rehabilitation (Laver et al., 2011c). This finding is likely due to unfamiliarity and lack of self-efficacy of older people using these technologies (Scanlon et al., 2015). Over time, this is likely to change as future generations become increasingly familiar with technology (Laver et al., 2011c).

Considerations for Future Technology Development

Although there are now rehabilitation-specific technologies commercially available, there is still a need for further technology development to meet all stakeholders needs (i.e. organisations, therapists and patients). For future development, it is essential that technology experts, such as software engineers, work collaboratively with the other stakeholders to ensure that new technologies meet the needs of all involved. Rehabilitation therapists need to be engaged early in the process to ensure that designed games and exercises are of therapeutic benefit and can be customised appropriately for a range of people with different health conditions at different stages and settings of rehabilitation (Laver et al., 2011a). Rehabilitation therapists can provide clear guidance regarding movements to be required or avoided in the games/exercises, how to grade tasks to make them easier or more challenging, and to ensure that a comprehensive set of games/exercises is provided.

The different stakeholders have varying perspectives, which need to be considered when developing new technologies. Organisations are interested in the cost of the technology and its applicability to their service. For example, technologies that incorporate clinic and home versions of a system, or therapist and patient modes, may be viewed favourably. Therapists need to perceive the usefulness of the device to provide therapeutic benefit for a range of patients. It needs to be reliable and not too difficult to use and there needs to be sufficient training and IT support for use. Most importantly, therapists need to be satisfied that it will be acceptable to their patients with appropriate support. Patients require the technology to be enjoyable and engaging, but still address their rehabilitation goals. Table 9.1 can be used as a checklist to consider therapist, patient and contextual attributes when designing a new technology.

Thinking into the future, a key requirement of technology in rehabilitation is to increase dose of practice. This means ensuring systems can be set up for use by patients independently or supported by therapy assistants or caregivers where appropriate. A notable gap in currently available technologies is the lack of home-based rehabilitation-specific technologies. Given the increasing demand for rehabilitation globally and that rehabilitation in some countries is only provided in the home setting, greater work should focus on developing reliable, home-environment friendly technologies that enable remote communication and exchange of data between the therapist and patient, allowing the therapist to monitor rehabilitation and intercede when required.

In summary, while feedback-based technologies such as VR gaming technologies can provide an enjoyable way for patients to complete high doses of exercise, therapists play a vital role in prescribing, teaching and progressing the technology. It is important that therapists choose the correct technology to meet each individual's rehabilitation needs and personal preferences. With a wide variety of ever-evolving technologies available, both rehabilitation-specific and recreational, therapists should be adaptable and open to trialling different technologies and should consider the different technology attributes when deciding the appropriateness of new technologies. While for some patients, recreational technologies may be suitable, for others, these may be too fast and complex, or may be too difficult to manipulate. Future technology development requires close collaboration with all stakeholders to ensure it can be customised to suit a large range of patients and that it is therapeutically beneficial and relatively easy and intuitive to use.

Acknowledgements

The authors would like to acknowledge that much of their understanding of this topic has been developed through collaborative work with their research students and research teams. In particular, staff, students and investigators on the AMOUNT rehabilitation trial and research students Caitlin Hamilton (University of Sydney), Sarah Brown (University of Sydney) and Sally White (Flinders University).

References

Allen, N. E., Song, J., Paul, S. S., Smith, S., O'Duffy, J., Schmidt, M., Love, R., Sherrington, C. & Canning, C. G. 2017. An interactive videogame for arm and hand exercise in people with Parkinson's disease: A randomized controlled trial. *Parkinsonism Relat Disord*, 41, 66–72.

Barry, G., Galna, B. & Rochester, L. 2014. The role of exergaming in Parkinson's disease rehabilitation: A systematic review of the evidence. *J NeuroEng Rehabil*, 11, 33.

Bollen, J. C., Dean, S. G., Siegert, R. J., Howe, T. E. & Goodwin, V. A. 2014. A systematic review of measures of self-reported adherence to unsupervised home-based rehabilitation exercise programmes, and their psychometric properties. *BMJ Open*, 4, e005044.

Boyd, L. A., Vidoni, E. D. & Wessel, B. D. 2010. Motor learning after stroke: Is skill acquisition a prerequisite for contralesional neuroplastic change? *Neurosci Lett*, 482, 21–5.

Bravata, D. M., Smith-Spangler, C., Sundaram, V., Gienger, A. L., Lin, N., Lewis, R., Stave, C. D., Olkin, I. & Sirard, J. R. 2007. Using pedometers to increase physical activity and improve health: A systematic review. *JAMA*, 298, 2296–304.

Bruni, M. F., Melegari, C., de Cola, M. C., Bramanti, A., Bramanti, P. & Calabro, R. S. 2018. What does best evidence tell us about robotic gait rehabilitation in stroke patients: A systematic review and meta-analysis. *J Clin Neurosci*, 48, 11–7.

Carr, J. H. & Shepherd, R. B. 2010. *Neurological Rehabilitation: Optimizing Motor Performance*, 2nd edn. Philadelphia, PA, Elsevier.

Casuso-Holgado, M. J., Martín-Valero, R., Carazo, A. F., Medrano-Sánchez, E. M., Cortés-Vega, M. D. & Montero-Bancalero, F. J. 2018. Effectiveness of virtual reality training for balance and gait rehabilitation in people with multiple sclerosis: A systematic review and meta-analysis. *Clin Rehabil*, 32(9), 1220–1234.

Chen, C. C. & Bode, R. K. 2011. Factors influencing therapists' decision-making in the acceptance of new technology devices in stroke rehabilitation. *Am J Phys Med Rehabil*, 90, 415–25.

Chiviacowsky, S., Campos, T. & Domingues, M. R. 2010. Reduced frequency of knowledge of results enhances learning in persons with Parkinson's disease. *Front Psychol*, 1, 226.

Cirstea, C. M., Ptito, A. & Levin, M. F. 2006. Feedback and cognition in arm motor skill reacquisition after stroke. *Stroke*, 37, 1237–42.

Cirstea, M. C. & Levin, M. F. 2007. Improvement of arm movement patterns and endpoint control depends on type of feedback during practice in stroke survivors. *Neurorehabil Neural Repair*, 21, 398–411.

Corbetta, D., Imeri, F. & Gatti, R. 2015. Rehabilitation that incorporates virtual reality is more effective than standard rehabilitation for improving walking speed, balance and mobility after stroke: A systematic review. *J Physiother*, 61, 117–24.

Crotty, M., Killington, M., van den Berg, M., Morris, C., Taylor, A. & Carati, C. 2014. Telerehabilitation for older people using off-the-shelf applications: Acceptability and feasibility. *J Telemed Telecare*, 20, 370–6.

Davis, F. D. 1989. Perceived usefulness, perceived ease of use, and user acceptance of information technology. *MIS Q*, 13, 319–40.

de Rooij, I. J., van de Port, I. G. & Meijer, J.-W. G. 2016. Effect of virtual reality training on balance and gait ability in patients with stroke: Systematic review and meta-analysis. *Phys Ther*, 96, 1905–18.

Deutsch, J. E., Brettler, A., Smith, C., Welsh, J., John, R., Guarrera-Bowlby, P. & Kafri, M. 2011. Nintendo Wii sports and Wii fit game analysis, validation, and application to stroke rehabilitation. *Top Stroke Rehabil*, 18, 701–19.

Diong, J., Allen, N. & Sherrington, C. 2016. Structured exercise improves mobility after hip fracture: A meta-analysis with meta-regression. *Br J Sports Med*, 50, 346–55.

Dockx, K., Bekkers, E. M., van den Bergh, V., Ginis, P., Rochester, L., Hausdorff, J. M., Mirelman, A. & Nieuwboer, A. 2016. Virtual reality for rehabilitation in Parkinson's disease. *Cochrane Database Syst Rev*, 12, CD010760.

Ellis, T. & Motl, R. W. 2013. Physical activity behavior change in persons with neurologic disorders: Overview and examples from Parkinson disease and multiple sclerosis. *J Neurol Phys Ther*, 37, 85–90.

English, C., Manns, P. J., Tucak, C. & Bernhardt, J. 2014. Physical activity and sedentary behaviors in people with stroke living in the community: A systematic review. *Phys Ther*, 94, 185–96.

Forsberg, A., Nilsagård, Y. & Boström, K. 2015. Perceptions of using videogames in rehabilitation: A dual perspective of people with multiple sclerosis and physiotherapists. *Disabil Rehabil*, 37, 338–44.

French, B., Thomas, L. H., Coupe, J., McMahon, N. E., Connell, L., Harrison, J., Sutton, C. J., Tishkovskaya, S. & Watkins, C. L. 2016. Repetitive task training for improving functional ability after stroke. *Cochrane Database Syst Rev*, 11, CD006073.

French, S. D., Green, S. E., O'Connor, D. A., McKenzie, J. E., Francis, J. J., Michie, S., Buchbinder, R., Schattner, P., Spike, N. & Grimshaw, J. M. 2012. Developing theory-informed behaviour change interventions to implement evidence into practice: A systematic approach using the Theoretical Domains Framework. *Implement Sci*, 7, 38.

Frost, R., McClurg, D., Brady, M. & Williams, B. 2016. Optimising the validity and completion of adherence diaries: A multiple case study and randomised crossover trial. *Trials*, 17, 489.

Ginis, P., Nieuwboer, A., Dorfman, M., Ferrari, A., Gazit, E., Canning, C. G., Rocchi, L., Chiari, L., Hausdorff, J. M. & Mirelman, A. 2016. Feasibility and effects of home-based smartphone-delivered automated feedback training for gait in people with Parkinson's disease: A pilot randomized controlled trial. *Parkinsonism Relat Disord*, 22, 28–34.

Glegg, S. M., Tatla, S. K. & Holsti, L. 2014. The GestureTek virtual reality system in rehabilitation: A scoping review. *Disabil Rehabil Assist Technol*, 9, 89–111.

Glynn, L. G., Hayes, P. S., Casey, M., Glynn, F., Alvarez-Iglesias, A., Newell, J., Olaighin, G., Heaney, D. & Murphy, A. W. 2013. SMART MOVE - a smartphone-based intervention to promote physical activity in primary care: Study protocol for a randomized controlled trial. *Trials*, 14, 157.

Hamilton, C., Lovarini, M., McCluskey, A., Folly de Campos, T. & Hassett, L. 2018a. Experiences of therapists using feedback-based technology to improve physical function in rehabilitation settings: A qualitative systematic review. *Disabil Rehabil*, DOI: 10.1080/09638288.2018.1446187.

Hamilton, C., McCluskey, A., Hassett, L., Killington, M. & Lovarini, M. 2018b. Patient and therapist experiences of using affordable feedback-based technology in rehabilitation: A qualitative study nested in a randomized controlled trial. *Clin Rehabil*, 32, 1258–70.

Handoll, H. H. & Sherrington, C. 2007. Mobilisation strategies after hip fracture surgery in adults.[update of Cochrane Database Syst Rev. 2004;(4):CD001704; PMID: 15495015]. *Cochrane Database of Syst Rev*, 18(4), CD001704.

Harvey, N. & Ada, L. 2012. Suitability of Nintendo Wii Balance Board for rehabilitation of standing after stroke. *Phys Ther Rev*, 17, 311–21.

Hassett, L. M., Moseley, A. M., Harmer, A. & van der Ploeg, H. P. 2015. The reliability, validity, and feasibility of physical activity measurement in adults with traumatic brain injury: An observational study. *J Head Trauma Rehabil*, 30, E55–61.

Hassett, L. M., Moseley, A. M., Whiteside, B., Barry, S. & Jones, T. 2012. Circuit class therapy can provide a fitness training stimulus for adults with severe traumatic brain injury: A randomised trial within an observational study. *J Physiother*, 58, 105–12.

Hassett, L. M., van den Berg, M., Lindley, R. I., Crotty, M., McCluskey, A., van der Ploeg, H. P., Smith, S. T., Schurr, K., Killington, M., Bongers, B., Howard, K., Heritier, S., Togher, L., Hackett, M., Treacy, D., Dorsch, S., Wong, S., Scrivener, K., Chagpar, S., Weber, H., Pearson, R. & Sherrington, C. 2016. Effect of affordable technology on physical activity levels and mobility outcomes in rehabilitation: A protocol for the Activity and MObility UsiNg Technology (AMOUNT) rehabilitation trial. *BMJ Open*, 6, e012074.

Hassett, L. M., Wong, S., Sheaves, E., Daher, M., Grady, A., Egan, C., Seeto, C., Hosking, T. & Moseley, A. 2018. Time use and physical activity in a specialised brain injury rehabilitation unit: An observational study. *Brain Inj*, 32, 850–7.

Hebert, E., Landin, D. & Menickelli, J. 1998. Videotape feedback: What learners see and how they use it. *J Sport Peda*, 4, 12–28.

Hoang, P., Schoene, D., Gandevia, S., Smith, S. & Lord, S. R. 2016. Effects of a home-based step training programme on balance, stepping, cognition and functional performance in people with multiple sclerosis--a randomized controlled trial. *Mult Scler*, 22, 94–103.

Housman, S. J., Scott, K. M. & Reinkensmeyer, D. J. 2009. A randomized controlled trial of gravity-supported, computer-enhanced arm exercise for individuals with severe hemiparesis. *Neurorehabil Neural Repair*, 23, 505–14.

Jacobs, A., Timmermans, A., Michielsen, M., Vander Plaetse, M. & Markopoulos, P. 2013. Contrast: Gamification of arm-hand training for stroke survivors. *CHI'13 Extended Abstracts on Human Factors in Computing Systems*, ACM, Paris, France, 415–20.

Janssen, H., Ada, L., Bernhardt, J., McElduff, P., Pollack, M., Nilsson, M. & Spratt, N. J. 2014. An enriched environment increases activity in stroke patients undergoing rehabilitation in a mixed rehabilitation unit: A pilot non-randomized controlled trial. *Disabil Rehabil*, 36, 255–62.

Janssen, H., Bernhardt, J., Collier, J. M., Sena, E. S., McElduff, P., Attia, J., Pollack, M., Howells, D. W., Nilsson, M., Calford, M. B. & Spratt, N. J. 2010. An enriched environment improves sensorimotor function post-ischemic stroke. *Neurorehabil Neural Repair*, 24, 802–13.

Keshner, E. A. 2004. Virtual reality and physical rehabilitation: A new toy or a new research and rehabilitation tool? *J NeuroEng Rehabil*, 1, 8.

Keus, S., Munneke, M., Graziano, M., Paltarnaa, J., Pelosin, E., Domingos, J., Bruhlmann, S., Ramaswamy, B., Prins, J., Struiksma, C., Rochester, L., Nieuwboer, A., Bloem, B. & On Behalf of the Guideline Development Group. 2014. European physiotherapy guideline for Parkinson's disease. KNGF/ParkinsonNet, the Netherlands.

Kolt, G. S., Schofield, G. M., Kerse, N., Garrett, N., Ashton, T. & Patel, A. 2012. Healthy steps trial: Pedometer-based advice and physical activity for low-active older adults. *Ann Family Med*, 10, 206–12.

Laver, K. E., Lange, B., George, S., Deutsch, J. E., Saposnik, G. & Crotty, M. 2017. Virtual reality for stroke rehabilitation. *Cochrane Database Syst Rev*, 11, CD008349.

Laver, K., George, S., Ratcliffe, J. & Crotty, M. 2011a. Virtual reality stroke rehabilitation--hype or hope? *Aust Occup Ther J*, 58, 215–9.

Laver, K., Ratcliffe, J., George, S., Burgess, L. & Crotty, M. 2011b. Is the Nintendo Wii Fit really acceptable to older people? A discrete choice experiment. *BMC Geriatr*, 11, 64.

Laver, K., Ratcliffe, J., George, S., Lester, L., Walker, R., Burgess, L. & Crotty, M. 2011c. Early rehabilitation management after stroke: What do stroke patients prefer? *J Rehabil Med*, 43, 354–8.

Lee, B. C., Kim, J., Chen, S. & Sienko, K. H. 2012. Cell phone based balance trainer. *J NeuroEng Rehabil*, 9, 10.

Levac, D., Espy, D., Fox, E., Pradhan, S. & Deutsch, J. E. 2015. "Kinect-ing" with clinicians: A knowledge translation resource to support decision making about video game use in rehabilitation. *Phys Ther*, 95, 426–40.

Levac, D. E., Pradhan, S., Espy, D., Fox, E. & Deutsch, J. E. 2018. Usability of the 'Kinect-ing' with clinicians website: A knowledge translation resource supporting decisions about active videogame use in rehabilitation. *Games Health J*, 7, 362–68.

Lewis, G. N. & Rosie, J. A. 2012. Virtual reality games for movement rehabilitation in neurological conditions: How do we meet the needs and expectations of the users? *Disabil Rehabil*, 34, 1880–6.

Lewis, G. N., Woods, C., Rosie, J. A. & McPherson, K. M. 2011. Virtual reality games for rehabilitation of people with stroke: Perspectives from the users. *Disabil Rehabil Assist Technol*, 6, 453–63.

Lohse, K. R., Lang, C. E. & Boyd, L. A. 2014. Is more better? Using metadata to explore dose-response relationships in stroke rehabilitation. *Stroke*, 45, 2053–8.

Lu, T. C., Fu, C. M., Ma, M. H., Fang, C. C. & Turner, A. M. 2016. Healthcare applications of smart watches. A systematic review. *Appl Clin Inform*, 7, 850–69.

Lynch, E. A., Jones, T. M., Simpson, D. B., Fini, N. A., Kuys, S. S., Borschmann, K., Kramer, S., Johnson, L., Callisaya, M. L., Mahendran, N., Janssen, H., English, C. & Collaboration, A. C. 2018. Activity monitors for increasing physical activity in adult stroke survivors. *Cochrane Database Syst Rev*, 7, CD012543.

Magill, R. A. & Anderson, D. 2014. *Motor Learning and Control: Concepts and Applications*, 10th edn. New York, NY: McGraw-Hill Education.

Mak, M. K. & Hui-Chan, C. W. 2008. Cued task-specific training is better than exercise in improving sit-to-stand in patients with Parkinson's disease: A randomized controlled trial. *Mov Disord*, 23, 501–9.

Mansfield, A., Wong, J. S., Bryce, J., Brunton, K., Inness, E. L., Knorr, S., Jones, S., Taati, B. & McIlroy, W. E. 2015. Use of accelerometer-based feedback of walking activity for appraising progress with walking-related goals in inpatient stroke rehabilitation: A randomized controlled trial. *Neurorehabil Neural Repair*, 29, 847–57.

Maulucci, R. A. & Eckhouse, R. H. 2001. Retraining reaching in chronic stroke with real-time auditory feedback. *Neurorehabil*, 16, 171–82.

McNulty, P. A., Thompson-Butel, A. G., Faux, S. G., Lin, G., Katrak, P. H., Harris, L. R. & Shiner, C. T. 2015. The efficacy of Wii-based movement therapy for upper limb rehabilitation in the chronic poststroke period: A randomized controlled trial. *Int J Stroke*, 10, 1253–60.

Mirelman, A., Rochester, L., Maidan, I., Del Din, S., Alcock, L., Nieuwhof, F., Rikkert, M. O., Bloem, B. R., Pelosin, E., Avanzino, L., Abbruzzese, G., Dockx, K., Bekkers, E., Giladi, N., Nieuwboer, A. & Hausdorff, J. M. 2016. Addition of a non-immersive virtual reality component to treadmill training to reduce fall risk in older adults (V-TIME): A randomised controlled trial. *Lancet*, 388, 1170–82.

Motl, R. W., McAuley, E. & Snook, E. M. 2005. Physical activity and multiple sclerosis: A meta-analysis. *Mult Scler*, 11, 459–63.

Mount, J., Pierce, S. R., Parker, J., Diegidio, R., Woessner, R. & Spiegel, L. 2007. Trial and error versus errorless learning of functional skills in patients with acute stroke. *Neurorehabil*, 22, 123–32.

Nackaerts, E., Vervoort, G., Heremans, E., Smits-Engelsman, B. C., Swinnen, S. P. & Nieuwboer, A. 2013. Relearning of writing skills in Parkinson's disease: A literature review on influential factors and optimal strategies. *Neurosci Biobehav Rev*, 37, 349–57.

Nam, K. Y., Kim, H. J., Kwon, B. S., Park, J. W., Lee, H. J. & Yoo, A. 2017. Robot-assisted gait training (Lokomat) improves walking function and activity in people with spinal cord injury: A systematic review. *J NeuroEng Rehabil*, 14, 24.

Natbony, L. R., Zimmer, A., Ivanco, L. S., Studenski, S. A. & Jain, S. 2013. Perceptions of a videogame-based dance exercise program among individuals with Parkinson's disease. *Games Health J*, 2, 235–9.

Neri, S. G., Cardoso, J. R., Cruz, L., Lima, R. M., de Oliveira, R. J., Iversen, M. D. & Carregaro, R. L. 2017. Do virtual reality games improve mobility skills and balance measurements in community-dwelling older adults? Systematic review and meta-analysis. *Clin Rehabil*, 31, 1292304.

Nieuwboer, A., Rochester, L., Muncks, L. & Swinnen, S. P. 2009. Motor learning in Parkinson's disease: Limitations and potential for rehabilitation. *Parkinsonism Relat Disord*, 15(Suppl 3), S53–8.

Onla-or, S. & Winstein, C. J. 2008. Determining the optimal challenge point for motor skill learning in adults with moderately severe Parkinson's disease. *Neurorehabil Neural Repair*, 22, 385–95.

Palma, G. C., Freitas, T. B., Bonuzzi, G. M., Soares, M. A., Leite, P. H., Mazzini, N. A., Almeida, M. R., Pompeu, J. E. & Torriani-Pasin, C. 2017. Effects of virtual reality for stroke individuals based on the International Classification of Functioning and Health: A systematic review. *Top Stroke Rehabil*, 24, 269–78.

Peruzzi, A., Zarbo, I. R., Cereatti, A., Della Croce, U. & Mirelman, A. 2017. An innovative training program based on virtual reality and treadmill: Effects on gait of persons with multiple sclerosis. *Disabil Rehabil*, 39, 1557–63.

Pirovano, M., Surer, E., Mainetti, R., Lanzi, P. L. & Borghese, N. A. 2016. Exergaming and rehabilitation: A methodology for the design of effective and safe therapeutic exergames. *Entertain Comput*, 14, 55–65.

Plow, M. & Finlayson, M. 2014. A qualitative study exploring the usability of Nintendo Wii Fit among persons with multiple sclerosis. *Occup Ther Int*, 21, 21–32.

Prince, S. A., Adamo, K. B., Hamel, M. E., Hardt, J., Connor Gorber, S. & Tremblay, M. 2008. A comparison of direct versus self-report measures for assessing physical activity in adults: A systematic review. *Int J Behav Nutr Phys Act*, 5, 56.

Rietberg, M. B., Brooks, D., Uitdehaag, B. M. & Kwakkel, G. 2005. Exercise therapy for multiple sclerosis. *Cochrane Database Syst Rev*, 25(1), CD003980.

Sackley, C. M. & Lincoln, N. B. 1997. Single blind randomized controlled trial of visual feedback after stroke: Effects on stance symmetry and function. *Disabil Rehabil*, 19, 536–46.

Scanlon, L., O'Shea, E., O'Caoimh, R. & Timmons, S. 2015. Technology use and frequency and self-rated skills: A survey of community-dwelling older adults. *J Am Geriatr Soc*, 63, 1483–4.

Schmidt, R. A. & Wrisberg, C. A. 2008. *Motor Learning and Performance: A Situation-Based Learning Approach*. Champaign, IL: Human Kinetics.

Schmidt, R. A. & Wulf, G. 1997. Continuous concurrent feedback degrades skill learning: Implications for training and simulation. *Hum Factors*, 39, 509–25.

Schneider, E. J., Lannin, N. A., Ada, L. & Schmidt, J. 2016. Increasing the amount of usual rehabilitation improves activity after stroke: A systematic review. *J Physiother*, 62, 182–7.

Schoene, D., Lord, S. R., Delbaere, K., Severino, C., Davies, T. A. & Smith, S. T. 2013. A randomized controlled pilot study of home-based step training in older people using videogame technology. *PLoS One*, 8, e57734.

Secoli, R., Milot, M. H., Rosati, G. & Reinkensmeyer, D. J. 2011. Effect of visual distraction and auditory feedback on patient effort during robot-assisted movement training after stroke. *J NeuroEng Rehabil*, 8, 21.

Shafizadeh, M., Platt, G. K. & Mohammadi, B. 2013. Effects of different focus of attention rehabilitative training on gait performance in Multiple Sclerosis patients. *J Bodyw Mov Ther*, 17, 28–34.

Sherrington, C., Michaleff, Z. A., Fairhall, N., Paul, S. S., Tiedemann, A., Whitney, J., Cumming, R. G., Herbert, R. D., Close, J. C. & Lord, S. R. 2017. Exercise to prevent falls in older adults: An updated systematic review and meta-analysis. *Br J Sports Med*, 51, 1750–8.

Skjaeret, N., Nawaz, A., Morat, T., Schoene, D., Helbostad, J. L. & Vereijken, B. 2016. Exercise and rehabilitation delivered through exergames in older adults: An integrative review of technologies, safety and efficacy. *Int J Med Inform*, 85, 1–16.

Smith, P., Galea, M., Woodward, M., Said, C. & Dorevitch, M. 2008. Physical activity by elderly patients undergoing inpatient rehabilitation is low: An observational study. *Austr J Physiother*, 54, 209–13.

Snyder, A., Colvin, B. & Gammack, J. K. 2011. Pedometer use increases daily steps and functional status in older adults. *J Am Med Dir Assoc*, 12, 590–4.

Solmon, M. A. & Boone, J. 1993. The impact of student goal orientation in physical education classes. *Res Q Exerc Sport*, 64, 418–24.

Song, J., Paul, S. S., Caetano, M. J. D., Smith, S., Dibble, L. E., Love, R., Schoene, D., Menant, J. C., Sherrington, C., Lord, S. R., Canning, C. G. & Allen, N. E. 2018. Home-based step training using videogame technology in people with Parkinson's disease: A single-blinded randomised controlled trial. *Clin Rehabil*, 32, 299–311.

Stanton, R., Ada, L., Dean, C. M. & Preston, E. 2017. Biofeedback improves performance in lower limb activities more than usual therapy in people following stroke: A systematic review. *J Physiother*, 63, 11–16.

Sullivan, A. N. & Lachman, M. E. 2016. Behavior change with fitness technology in sedentary adults: A review of the evidence for increasing physical activity. *Front Public Health*, 4, 289.

Sveistrup, H. 2004. Motor rehabilitation using virtual reality. *J NeuroEng Rehabil*, 1, 10.

Swinnen, S. P., Schmidt, R. A., Nicholson, D. E. & Shapiro, D. C. 1990. Information feedback for skill acquisition: Instantaneous knowledge of results degrades learning. *J Exp Psychol Learn Mem Cogn*, 16(4), 706–16.

Thomson, K., Pollock, A., Bugge, C. & Brady, M. 2014. Commercial gaming devices for stroke upper limb rehabilitation: A systematic review. *Int J Stroke*, 9, 479–88.

Tieri, G., Morone, G., Paolucci, S. & Iosa, M. 2018. Virtual reality in cognitive and motor rehabilitation: Facts, fiction and fallacies. *Expert Rev Med Devices*, 15, 107–17.

Tomassini, V., Johansen-Berg, H., Leonardi, L., Paixao, L., Jbabdi, S., Palace, J., Pozzilli, C. & Matthews, P. M. 2011. Preservation of motor skill learning in patients with multiple sclerosis. *Mult Scler*, 17, 103–15.

Tomlinson, C. L., Patel, S., Meek, C., Herd, C. P., Clarke, C. E., Stowe, R., Shah, L., Sackley, C., Deane, K. H., Wheatley, K. & Ives, N. 2012. Physiotherapy intervention in Parkinson's disease: Systematic review and meta-analysis. *BMJ*, 345, e5004.

Treacy, D., Hassett, L., Schurr, K., Chagpar, S., Paul, S. S. & Sherrington, C. 2017. Validity of different activity monitors to count steps in an inpatient rehabilitation setting. *Phys Ther*, 97, 581–8.

Türkbey, T. A., Kutlay, Ş. & Gök, H. 2017. Clinical feasibility of Xbox KinectTM training for stroke rehabilitation: A single-blind randomized controlled pilot study. *J Rehabil Med*, 49, 22–9.

van den Berg, M., Sherrington, C., Killington, M., Smith, S., Bongers, B., Hassett, L. & Crotty, M. 2016. Video and computer-based interactive exercises are safe and improve task-specific balance in geriatric and neurological rehabilitation: A randomised trial. *J Physiother*, 62, 20–8.

van Nimwegen, M., Speelman, A. D., Hofman-van Rossum, E. J., Overeem, S., Deeg, D. J., Borm, G. F., van der Horst, M. H., Bloem, B. R. & Munneke, M. 2011. Physical inactivity in Parkinson's disease. *J Neurol*, 258, 2214–21.

van Vliet, P. M. & Wulf, G. 2006. Extrinsic feedback for motor learning after stroke: What is the evidence? *Disabil Rehabil*, 28, 831–40.

Veerbeek, J. M., van Wegen, E., van Peppen, R., van der Wees, P. J., Hendriks, E., Rietberg, M. & Kwakkel, G. 2014. What is the evidence for physical therapy poststroke? A systematic review and meta-analysis. *PLoS One*, 9, e87987.

Verschueren, S. M., Swinnen, S. P., Dom, R. & de Weerdt, W. 1997. Interlimb coordination in patients with Parkinson's disease: Motor learning deficits and the importance of augmented information feedback. *Exp Brain Res*, 113, 497–508.

Voth, E. C., Oelke, N. D. & Jung, M. E. 2016. A theory-based exercise app to enhance exercise adherence: A pilot study. *JMIR mHealth uHealth*, 4, e62.

Weeks, D. L. & Kordus, R. N. 1998. Relative frequency of knowledge of performance and motor skill learning. *Res Q Exerc Sport*, 69, 224–30.

West, T. & Bernhardt, J. 2012. Physical activity in hospitalised stroke patients. *Stroke Res Treat*, 2012, 813765.

Williams, M. A., Soiza, R. L., Jenkinson, A. & Stewart, A. 2010. EXercising with Computers in Later Life (EXCELL) - pilot and feasibility study of the acceptability of the Nintendo® WiiFit in community-dwelling fallers. *BMC Res Notes*, 3, 238.

Wingham, J., Adie, K., Turner, D., Schofield, C. & Pritchard, C. 2015. Participant and caregiver experience of the Nintendo Wii Sports after stroke: Qualitative study of the trial of Wii in stroke (TWIST). *Clin Rehabil*, 29, 295–305.

Winstein, C. J. & Schmidt, R. A. 1990. Reduced frequency of knowledge of results enhances motor skill learning. *J Exp Psychol Learn Mem Cogn*, 16, 677–91.

Wulf, G., Landers, M., Lewthwaite, R. & Tollner, T. 2009. External focus instructions reduce postural instability in individuals with Parkinson disease. *Phys Ther*, 89, 162–8.

Wulf, G. & Prinz, W. 2001. Directing attention to movement effects enhances learning: A review. *Psychon Bull Rev*, 8, 648–60.

Wulf, G. & Shea, C. H. 2002. Principles derived from the study of simple skills do not generalize to complex skill learning. *Psychon Bull Rev*, 9, 185–211.

Wulf, G., Shea, C. & Lewthwaite, R. 2010. Motor skill learning and performance: A review of influential factors. *Med Educ*, 44, 75–84.

Yang, C. C. & Hsu, Y. L. 2010. A review of accelerometry-based wearable motion detectors for physical activity monitoring. *Sensors (Basel)*, 10, 7772–88.

Yates, M., Kelemen, A. & Sik Lanyi, C. 2016. Virtual reality gaming in the rehabilitation of the upper extremities post-stroke. *Brain Inj*, 30, 855–63.

10

Engaging Young Children in Speech and Language Therapy via Videoconferencing

Stuart Ekberg and Sandra Houen
Queensland University of Technology

Belinda Fisher
University of Queensland

Maryanne Theobald and Susan Danby
Queensland University of Technology

CONTENTS

Introduction 175
Data and Methods... 177
Analysis 180
    Using Objects Solely in a Therapist's Possession 180
    Using Identical Objects in Both a Therapist's and Client's Possession.... 185
Discussion 187
Acknowledgement... 189
Funding 189
References 189

Introduction

An estimated 9.92% of children meet contemporary diagnostic criteria for a language disorder (Norbury et al., 2016). Without intervention, children who have persistent language difficulties are more likely to encounter challenges in education and employment in later life (Conti-Ramsden et al., 2018). These problems can continue into adulthood and encompass reading, writing, focusing, thinking, calculating, communicating, mobility, self-care, education, employment and interpersonal relationships with acquaintances, family and authority figures (McCormack et al., 2009, 2011). Language difficulties affect children's peer relationships, as they may not be able to be understood or understand what others are saying to them, which may cause difficulties with social interactions. The effects of language difficulties can increase the likelihood of mental illness and reduce quality of life (van den Bedem et al., 2018; Eadie et al., 2018). Childhood language difficulties are also associated with increased healthcare costs in childhood (Cronin et al., 2017). Identifying and addressing speech and language difficulties in early childhood is one proactive way to address the diverse implications of these difficulties. Everyday technologies, such as videoconferencing, afford opportunities to promote access to specialist services for the treatment of these difficulties. Four types of technologies are used for current telehealth practice. These range from technologies that enable synchronous (i.e. 'real time') interaction, asynchronous (sometimes referred to as 'store and forward') interaction, remote patient monitoring and mobile health. The chapter focuses on synchronous audio-visual communication technologies, which are best suited for the clinical treatment of young children (Mashima and Doarn, 2008; Wilson et al., 2002; Dunkley et al., 2010).

In geographically dispersed countries, such as Australia, a particular challenge for children with speech and language difficulties is access to specialist services. Their geographical isolation in rural and remote areas means they can wait for many years to access treatment, if they are able to access treatment at all (O'Callaghan, 2005; Theodoros, 2008; Wilson et al., 2002). Telehealth offers a possible solution to ameliorating this and other barriers to access (Manzanares and Kan, 2014; Theodoros, 2008; Mashima and Doarn, 2008; Waite et al., 2010b and 2012). With early intervention widely recognised as having positive impacts on children's developmental trajectories and health outcomes (Campbell et al., 2014; Doyle et al., 2009), the opportunities created by telehealth services are relevant for very young children, particularly those who are geographically isolated.

Although evidence supports its use for diagnosis of speech and language difficulties (Waite et al., 2010a,b, 2012; Sutherland et al., 2016), only a handful of studies have considered the use of telehealth for the ongoing treatment of these difficulties (Hill and Miller, 2012; Ekberg et al., 2019; Wales et al., 2018). As the need for telehealth grows, training programmes are increasingly incorporating instruction about telehealth. A recent survey of the student therapists and educators revealed that the most important telehealth clinical skills that students required were the appropriate choice of clinical materials and how to engage clients across different telehealth media (Overby, 2018). This finding indicates the need to better understand how therapists adapt their therapeutic interactions to suit telehealth, how to plan for the session, including the types of therapy materials appropriate for telehealth settings, and how to integrate and use everyday technologies to effectively support and improve therapeutic outcomes for children and families. This chapter contributes to these goals by exploring the materials and strategies used by speech and language therapists (hereafter referred to as 'therapists') and service users (both child clients and their families) to facilitate engagement in therapeutic interventions via telehealth.

As shown previously (Ekberg et al., 2019), modes of therapy delivery make possible different affordances and challenges. In physically co-present (i.e.

'face-to-face') therapy, therapists use objects, including toys, as a way to encourage child clients to produce a specific target behaviour (usually an utterance). When the target behaviour is produced, the therapist makes available to the client access to the object. This strategy of making an object physically available is not always possible in telehealth sessions that rely upon videoconferencing. For this reason, the therapist has to identify and use alternate strategies to promote engagement with physical objects. By showing how the ways that objects are used occur 'through specific sites and associated practices' (Suchman, 2005: 381–382), this chapter builds on previous research (Ekberg et al., 2019) by exploring practical ways that therapists use physical objects to engage young children via the particular telehealth medium of videoconferencing.

Data and Methods

This chapter reports additional analysis of data that were used for a study that has been published elsewhere (Ekberg et al., 2019). The previous study explored interactional differences between telehealth and physically co-present therapy sessions for young child clients. The analysis reported here focuses on data collected from the two youngest telehealth clients who participated in the study. Three thirty-minute sessions were recorded for each client. Each client's sessions were with the same therapist (although each client had a different therapist) from the same child development service in Brisbane, Australia. A parent was present for each of the sessions but was not necessarily sitting with the client and regularly contributing to the progress of the therapy session. The clients accessed therapy via using the videoconferencing software *Skype*. Each therapist and client used a webcam that mostly focused on their faces, although therapists often toggled between this webcam and a document camera that displayed materials such as word cards (see Figure 10.1). Therapists had a range of toys and activities positioned beside the computer for use throughout the session. These resources were used to support play-based therapeutic activities, which are typical for therapeutic interventions with young children (Freckmann et al., 2017; Roulstone et al., 2004; Tykkyläinen, 2009; Sharp and Hillenbrand, 2008; Iacono, 1999). Although clients could not physically manipulate these objects, the therapist could show these objects using either the webcam or the document camera.

This study uses conversation analysis methods (Drew et al., 2001), which have been adopted to facilitate detailed exploration of the ways in which therapy sessions are organised by therapists, clients and family members, with a particular focus on interactional practices involving objects (Hutchby, 2001; Rosenbaun and Licoppe, 2017; Fasulo et al., 2017; Nevile et al., 2014). Conversation analysis is underpinned by an assumption that

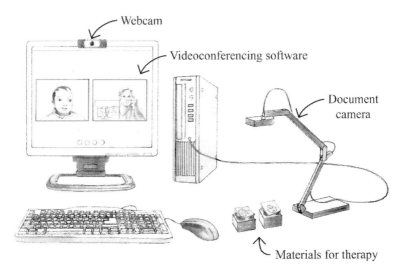

FIGURE 10.1
Telehealth setup comprised of a computer, webcam and document camera.

social interaction might exhibit 'order at all points', and therefore involves fine-grained analysis to identify ways in which the parties to an interaction attend to this potential orderliness (Sacks, 1984). The analysis that is reported in this chapter demonstrates how the fine-grained details of this orderliness can be consequential for the delivery of speech and language therapy via videoconferencing. This analysis is reported by considering several fragments of data that represent some of the diversity of the phenomenon of interest. This use of fragments is the standard way of reporting conversation analytic research, as it allows readers to critically appraise analytic claims against the materials upon which they are based (Peräkylä, 1997). Participant names have been replaced with pseudonyms in the transcripts.

To facilitate fine-grained analysis, detailed transcription conventions are employed within conversation analytic research (Hepburn and Bolden, 2013; Mondada, 2018). In addition to understanding what is said, these conventions enable an exploration of the ways in which something is said (e.g. its prosody), as well as aspects of non-vocal conduct (e.g. gestures). These conventions are used to transcribe the data fragments reported in this chapter. Although these transcripts may, at least initially, appear inaccessible to readers who are unfamiliar with the transcription conventions, these details are included to provide information for critically appraising the empirical basis for analytical claims (Peräkylä, 1997). Please refer to Table 10.1 for an abridged list of key transcription conventions. Explanations of transcription conventions not explained here are available in published material about transcription practices for conversation analytic research (Hepburn and Bolden, 2013; Mondada, 2018), as well as a previous study of the same data considered here (Ekberg et al., 2019).

TABLE 10.1

Key Transcription Conventions Employed in this Chapter

Speaker Labels	
CLI	Labels in upper case indicate lines that transcribe verbal conduct
cli	Labels in lower case indicate lines that transcribe embodied conduct
Temporal Dimensions	
Wo[rd]	Square brackets mark speaker overlap, with left square brackets
[Wo]rd	indicating overlap onset and right square brackets indicating overlap offset
Word (0.4) word	A number within parentheses refers to silence, measured to the nearest tenth of a second. A full stop within parentheses indicates a micropause of less than two-tenths of a second
Vocal Conduct	
Word.	A full stop indicates falling intonation at the end of a unit of talk
Word,	A comma indicates slightly rising intonation
Word¿	An inverted question mark indicates moderately rising intonation
Word?	A question mark indicates rising intonation
Word_	An underscore symbol indicates level intonation
Word!	An exclamation mark indicates animated tone
<u>Word</u>	Underlining indicates that emphasis on the underlined sounds
Wo:::rd	Colons indicates the stretching of the immediately preceding sound, with multiple colons representing prolonged stretching
£Word£	Pound signs encase utterances produce with smile voice
.hhh	A full stop followed by the letter 'h' indicates audible inhalation
(Word)	Words encased within single parentheses indicate an utterance that was unclear to the transcriptionist
Embodied Conduct	
ΔactionΔ ⌂action⌂	Triangles or house symbols encase descriptions of embodied actions by therapists
action ●action●	Asterisks or bullet points encase descriptions of embodied actions by clients
+action+	Plus signs encase descriptions of embodied actions by parents
Δ--> -->Δ	An arrow indicates an action continues across subsequent lines, until a corresponding arrow is reached
Δ-->3.15	An arrow followed by numbers is used when an embodied action continues for an extended period. The number before the full stop indicates the line where the action commences and the number following the full stop indicates the line where the action ends
. . . .	Full stops indicate the preparation of an action
- - - -	Dashes indicate the maintenance of an action
, , , ,	Commas indicate the retraction of an action
ca: /y/	The abbreviation 'ca' refers to a 'cued articulation' gesture. The sound being gestured follows.

Analysis

When speech and language therapy is conducted via contemporary video-conferencing software such as *Skype*, the therapist and client do not share access that enables them to mutually manipulate objects, even virtual ones (Ekberg et al., 2019). This is a challenge for therapeutic interventions with young clients, as therapists routinely use objects in playful ways to support therapeutic activities. Analysis of the data collected for this study indicates that therapists address this challenge in one of two ways. First, therapists made use of the physical objects that were in their own possession. Therapists tended to show these objects to clients, using either their webcam or document camera. A second approach was for therapists to use the same object that a client also had in their possession. This enabled both parties to engage with the physical object contemporaneously. Through both strategies, therapists sought to incorporate these objects into the therapeutic process. The remainder of the analysis section uses fragments taken from the collected data to explore these strategies in detail.

Using Objects Solely in a Therapist's Possession

Fragment 1 is taken from a speech therapy session involving a therapist and a 6-year-old client diagnosed with global developmental delay. The current therapeutic goal for the client was to produce 50 clear and meaningful words that he could use in his everyday interactions with others. To achieve this goal, the current focus was to target the early sounds of speech production and foster the client's engagement during therapy sessions. In the following fragment, the therapist works to achieve this goal with a set of large blocks and a set of cards containing images that illustrate the client's 50 target words.

As shown in Figure 10.2, the therapist places two cards on top of two blocks, with all these under the document camera (which is displayed on the bottom left-hand corner of the video transmitted from the therapist's computer). One card displays the image of a bottle and glass of milk, while another depicts a face with a 'yucky' expression. The client's task is to verbalise one of the two words that are illustrated: 'milk' or 'yucky'. If the young client does this to the therapist's satisfaction, the therapist removes the block underneath the corresponding card. Releasing the block then facilitates the playful element of the activity that follows. The therapist adds the block to a tower that she is progressively building. Once the tower reaches a particular height, the client is invited to instruct the therapist to knock over the tower. In order for this playful component to be realised, the client is required to practise his pronunciation of words contained on his target word list.

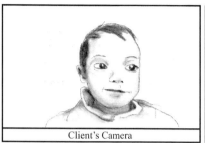
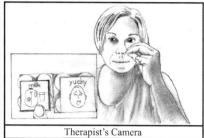

| Client's Camera | Therapist's Camera |

FIGURE 10.2
The therapist points to the 'milk' card while making the cued articulation gesture for /m/.

Fragment 1: C04/2015-03-05/11:35-12:15

```
01 THE:      Do you want the Δ*m:::::Δ:::milk?Δ
                             Δpoints-Δca: /m/-Δ
   cli:                     *drinking-->
02           (1.8)
03 THE:      ΔOr theΔ y:::Δucky one.Δ*
             Δpoints Δ.....Δca: /y/--Δ
   cli:                    -->*
04           (1.6)
05 CLI:      Ma:h?
06           (0.4)
07 THE:      Δ>Milk,<Δ=
   the:      Δpoints-Δ
08 CLI:      =(Yah?)
09           (0.2)
10 THE:      Or Δyu:kkyΔ block.
   the:         Δpoints Δ
11           (0.6)*(0.4)*(1.2)
   cli:           *.....*points-->
12 THE:      ΔI can't ↑see↑ >you're gonna have to< tELL me:_Δ
             Δopen palms, raised upwards-------------------Δ
13           (0.5)
14 THE:      Δ>Do you< want Δthe m::Δ::ΔΔ:::ΔΔmiΔlkΔ
             Δ.............Δ---1---Δ..Δ.Δ--2-Δ,,,Δ
                                     Δ....Δ--3--Δ
                            1 = left hand (LH) touching nose
                            2 = LH pointing to picture
                            3 = right hand (RH) ca: /m/
15           (0.7)
16 THE:      ΔOr the Δy[:::::::]ukky.Δ
17 CLI:                [(huhn¿)]
   the:      Δ.......Δca: /y/-------Δ
18           (1.7)
19 CLI:      (Huhn¿)
```

```
20              (1.5)*(1.4)
    cli:              *raises arm
21 CLI:         *Ya-°k°
                *points-->
22              (0.4)
23 THE:         YUCKY!
24              (.)
25 THE:         Δ↓Al*right,Δ ↑let's >here we go<¿ .hhh=
                Δ..........Δblock in RH and tower in LH-->
    cli:          -->*
26 THE:         =↑>We're gunna< put itΔ on: top?
                                -->Δplacing block on tower-->
27              (0.3)
28 THE:         .hhΔhpt!
                -->Δ
29              (0.4)
30 THE:         There: it go:es Δ↑we're building it up↑Δ
                           -->Δlowering RH----------Δ
31              Δ↓so::::big¿Δ
                Δ-----4-----Δ
                     4 = picks up new card with RH
32              (0.2)
33 THE:         ΔAre you ready let's get ano:ther Δblock from
                Δleans down---------------------Δstraightens-->

34 THE:         Δdown here.Δ
                Δmoving block-->>
                     -->Δ
```

This fragment illustrates how objects in a therapist's possession become a central aspect of therapeutic activity. Here, the therapist creates a context in which the client must select between, and then verbalise, one of two target words. To achieve this outcome, the therapist exploits a range of affordances that are available to her via the videoconferencing medium that she is using to interact with the client. For instance, she uses the audio channel to ask a question (lines 1–3) that restricts relevant responses from the client to two options: the target words 'milk' and 'yucky'. Reflecting the current focus on promoting the early sounds of speech production, the therapist elongates her pronunciation of the initial sound of each target word. The therapist also uses the video channel to support this activity, pointing to each card that displays the image of the target words and using cued articulation gestures to highlight the first sound of each word (see Figure 10.2). By making use of both audio and video streams, the therapist provides a rich multimodal indication of what the client should do next.

The therapist's repeat of some of these verbal and non-verbal behaviours across lines 7–10 indicates that the client's initial responses, at lines 5 and 8, are in some way inadequate. The client then produces a different response, pointing towards his screen (line 11). Although this response is appropriate insofar as it selects one of the two options made relevant by the therapist's earlier question, it does not align with a therapeutic goal of promoting the early sounds of speech production. By reporting that she cannot see where the client is pointing (line 12), she creates a warrant for indicating to the client that a verbal response is necessary. The therapist thus exploits another affordance of this telehealth medium to help realise her therapeutic objective.

The therapist continues to indicate an expectation of a verbal response by progressively upgrading the emphasis on the verbal and visual cues (lines 14–17). The therapist verbally elongates her pronunciation of the initial sound of each target word and maintains her cued articulation gestures and pointing to the sound cards for a longer time than she previously did at lines 1–3. These multimodal strategies are carefully coordinated to model the correct articulation and provide a visual cue for the client relating to the two possibilities afforded by the alternative question.

The therapist's ongoing pursuit of her question eventually results in a response from the client (line 21) that the therapist accepts (lines 23–25). Her conduct that follows shows that the progression of their activity was contingent upon the client producing one of the target words to the therapist's satisfaction. Having achieved this outcome, the therapist commences the playful part of the activity, which is to add the block to a tower that she is building on the client's behalf (lines 25–31). The therapist displays a sense of playfulness, excitement and joy about this part of the activity by audibly inhaling with an animated tone (line 28) and builds anticipation by slowly placing the block on top of the tower (lines 25–28), which she holds in a position that can be recorded by her webcam. The therapist proceeds to move the block tower to the side, highlighting that together they are building the tower so 'big' (line 31), deferring (but not ending) the tower-building activity until the client produces another target sound. This instance shows how objects that are routinely used in physically co-present therapy can also be used to support play-based therapy via telehealth. Nevertheless, therapists must identify creative solutions to some of the differences between therapies conducted across these different settings.

The second fragment is drawn from a session with a 4-year-old boy diagnosed with autism spectrum disorder. As in Fragment 1, the therapy session is conducted via videoconferencing. In contrast to Fragment 1, where the client's mother was present but off-screen, in Fragment 2 the client is seated on his mother's lap. Moreover, the mother is actively involved in the interaction. The therapeutic goal for this client is spontaneous word production. To support achievement of this goal, the therapist implements activities that target word elicitation. The session involves the use of a game that the therapist has opened on a tablet computer that is within her possession. She makes this game visible to the client via her document camera. The activity requires the client to verbally label items of clothing, which are then dragged by the therapist and placed on the character Mr Potato Head. As physical access to the tablet is only available to the therapist, the client must produce words verbally to 'play' the game.

Unlike Fragment 1, where the therapist displayed a composite image of
her head and torso from her webcam overlaid with a view from her document camera, in this fragment the therapist only transmits video from her
document camera. Compared to Fragment 1, this means that there are fewer
options available for the therapist to use multimodal interactional practices
such as gestures, although she does use her right hand to cover some objects
displayed on the tablet. With restricted multimodal means of interaction,
vocal expression may be relatively more important to promote and sustain
the client's engagement in this activity. In contrast to Fragment 1, the client's
mother is involved in this spate of interaction.

Fragment 2: C2/2015-02-19/17:00-17:13

```
01 THE:      >What do I need< first ↑Heath¿
02           (0.7)
03 CLI:      Luh-
04           *(1.2)
             *Leans toward screen-->
05 CLI:      *H:a:* (°t°)
             *--1-*,,,,,,-->
                1 = points at screen
06 MUM:      *Hat* >good boy_<
   cli:   -->*,,,*
07 THE:      Uh h:A::t o↑kayΔ (0.4) Δ*£>he:re comes< ↑the
                           Δ.......Δdrags hat on tablet-->
   cli:                          *eyes follow hat-->
08 THE:      ha↑::t_£*
                  -->*
09 THE:      Δ(0.8)Δ
   the:   -->Δ,,,,,Δ
10 THE:      .hhhhpt!
11           (0.4)
12 THE:      £What's ne::xt,£
13           (2.0)
14 CLI:      °A°* shew::↓oo::.=
                *leans toward screen, pointing?-->
```

The activity seems to be familiar to the client as there was no evidence of the
therapist explaining how to play the game. Rather, she initiates the activity by
asking the client which item of clothing she should select first to place onto Mr
Potato Head (line 1). This question supports the therapeutic goal by making
word production a relevant next action. The client's first response (line 3) is not
responded to by the therapist and is followed by another response comprised
of an utterance and gesture (line 5). The verbal response is repeated and treated
as adequate by the client's mother (line 6) and then the therapist (line 7).

As in Fragment 1, the client's production of some target utterance to the
satisfaction of the therapist (and, in this case, his mother) facilitates progression to the playful component of this activity. Also as in Fragment 1, the

therapist displays a sense of joy about this part of the activity, using smile voice (lines 7–8) and animated inhalation (line 10). Moreover, she elongates the pronunciation of her words to match the time it takes to drag and drop the hat onto Mr Potato Head (lines 7–8).

There are many differences between Fragments 1 and 2, only some of which are highlighted here. First, the therapist uses physical objects in Fragment 1 and digital objects in Fragment 2. Second, the therapist in Fragment 1 displays a composite image comprised of her webcam and document camera whereas the therapist in Fragment 2 only displays video from her document camera. Third, the client's mother is an active participant in Fragment 2. Notwithstanding these differences, there are important similarities across the two fragments. In both, the therapist finds ways to promote the client's engagement with objects that they cannot themselves manipulate. The therapists exploit both the audio and visual channels of the videoconferencing medium, closely coordinating their vocal and non-vocal conduct to indicate to clients what is required in a current activity. When therapists use objects in their own possession to support play-based therapy conducted via videoconferencing, this highlights the importance of exploiting the affordances of a particular telehealth medium to maximise the playfulness of an activity.

Using Identical Objects in Both a Therapist's and Client's Possession

In addition to occasions where therapists used objects that were solely in their possession, there were also instances where the therapist and the client each possessed the same physical object and they could therefore simultaneously use these identical objects within the therapeutic activity. For example, the therapist and one client each possessed the same set of toy jumping frogs, enabling both the therapist and client to 'jump' the frog following the client's successful production of some target utterance.

The following fragment comes from the same session as Fragment 1. Both the therapist and child client possess the same set of Miccio Character Cards (Miccio and Elbert, 1996). The goal of this activity is to encourage the production of speech sounds and receptive matching. Rather than displaying these cards underneath her document camera, the therapist holds these cards up so they are shown, along with her head and torso, via her webcam. Please note that there is audio feedback in parts of this fragment, which is transcribed with the speaker label 'COM' (for 'computer').

```
Fragment 3: C4/2015-03-05/05:41-06:18

01 THE:      *Δ>Can you<Δ find this one_
   cli:      *>>holding newt picture-->
   the:       Δ.........ΔLH: holds up bear picture-->01.22
02             *Δ(2.2)
   cli:    -->*showing newt picture-->02.17
   the:       ΔRH: writing-->
```

```
03 THE:      Ba::by, ↑bea:r,
04           (1.2)
05 CLI:      (>Ave ah,< roo:k)Δ
   the:                   -->Δ
06           (0.4)
07 THE:      Ba::by bear,=Δ↑>Where's you:r< baby bea:r.↑
                           Δopen palms, raised upwards-->
08           (1.1)
09 CLI:      ↑Noh:.↑
10           ●(0.4)
   cli:      ●gazing away-->10.18
11 THE:      ΔN↑o:↑?Δ
             Δ--1---Δ
               1 = shakes head
12           (0.4)
13 COM:      N↑o:↑?
14 THE:      £>Where is<£ he.
15           (.)
16 COM:      (>£>Where is<£ he.<)
17           (1.0)*(0.8)*(3.8)*
   cli:          -->*,,,,,*--2--*
                         2 = searching?
18 CLI:      ●(Ah *buh!)
   cli:    -->●    *--holding bear card-->
19             (0.6)
   cli:
20 THE:      Ah Δ>Bah- bah-Δ Δbah- for< ba:by Δbear?=
             Δca:/b/ /b/Δ              Δ......-->
21           =Δ£↑HighΔ fi::ve ↓>little< man.   ↑good
             -->Δ......ΔRH palm open towards screen-->
22           *jo↑::*↓::Δ::b.*Δ=Great wo::rk.
                 -->Δ   -->Δ
   cli:      *.....*---3----*
                     3 = RH palm open to screen
23 THE:      .hhhh ΔWhere's Δour .hhh puh- puh- pig¿
             Δ........Δshows card-->>
```

Prior to the beginning of this fragment, the client had been holding a card displaying an image of a newt. At line 1, the therapist holds up a card displaying the image of a bear dressed as a baby and asks him if he can find the same card in his own set. Instead, however, the client rotates the newt card that he is holding so it becomes visible to the therapist (line 2). From the outset, then it becomes apparent that a challenge with using an object that is also in the possession of the client, is that the client may seek to engage with these objects with a different intention to that of the therapist. Here, the therapist addresses this matter by verbally indicating the card that she wants the client to find (line 3) and continues to pursue this over time (at lines 7 and 14). Eventually, the client both identifies the matching card and vocalises the name of the image displayed on the card (line 18).

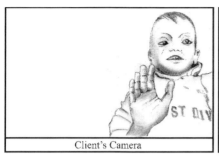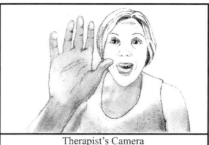

Client's Camera | Therapist's Camera

FIGURE 10.3
The therapist invites, and the client moves to reciprocate, a 'high five'.

As in Fragments 1 and 2, the therapist in Fragment 3 treats the client's response as adequate by producing a response that displays her joy and excitement. She repeats the sound that the client has just produced (line 20), and then displays how to use this sound to produce the full name of the card (line 20). Next, she recruits the client to 'high five' by placing their hands together, holding up one of her own hands to the screen (line 21), an action that is reciprocated by the client (line 21; see Figure 10.3). This emulates, in a virtual manner, the sort of physical contact that would be possible to 'high five' in contexts where therapists and clients are physically co-present with each other.

The use of objects in both the possession of a therapist and a client can create challenges for therapeutic activities. As seen in Fragment 3, a client may not, at least initially, engage with the objects in the way that a therapist might intend. Nevertheless, managing this challenge affords therapeutic opportunities that might not be easily realised with objects that are only in the possession of the therapist. In this fragment, for instance, it enables the client to practise his receptive language skills by following the therapist's instruction to match a specific card from his set with the identical card from her set. This approach highlights that carefully considering the design of activities can support particular therapeutic objectives, such as developing receptive language skills, as well as ensuring that an activity is suitable for the medium through which therapy is conducted.

Discussion

Everyday technologies, such as videoconferencing, are a widely available resource that can enhance access to specialist speech and language therapy services. The current study suggests that the success of therapy delivered across telehealth media such as videoconferencing depends upon a therapist's ability to adapt activities to suit a telehealth setting. This is especially the case for therapeutic interventions with young children, which tend to be play based. Physically co-present settings enable therapists and child clients to share access to physical objects such as toys. This shared access enables such objects to be used in particular ways that support therapeutic objectives. This shared access to physical objects is not afforded by contemporary videoconferencing technologies such as Skype (Ekberg et al., 2019). Therapists seeking to deliver play-based therapy to young children via such media must therefore identify ways of creatively adapting therapeutic activities to suit the affordances and constraints of a particular telehealth medium.

The analysis reported in this chapter identifies two major ways in which therapists can incorporate objects into therapy sessions conducted via videoconferencing. On some occasions, an object that was solely in the therapist's possession was used. These objects often were the same as those also used in the physically co-present therapy sessions conducted at the child language development service. Nevertheless, analysis highlighted how therapists used these objects in ways that suited a telehealth context in which clients could not physically manipulate the objects in therapists' possession. In particular, therapists used both the audio and visual channels of the videoconferencing medium, closely coordinating their vocal and non-vocal conduct to indicate to clients what is required in the current therapeutic activity. On some occasions, an adult who was physically present with a child client supported the therapist in the facilitation of therapeutic activities.

An alternative approach to incorporating objects into videoconferenced therapy involved the use of an identical object in the possession of both the therapist and their child client (e.g. the same set of Miccio Character Cards, as in Fragment 3). Although many of the same practices used by therapists for objects in their sole possession also were used when identical objects were in the possession of both the therapist and client, the client's possession of an object afforded different possibilities. For example, Fragment 3 demonstrates how the therapist used identical objects in her own and her client's possession to invite the client to practise his receptive language skills by matching a specific card from his set with the identical card from the therapist's set.

A third possible approach, which was not present in the available data, might be for therapists to use objects solely in a client's possession to facilitate therapeutic activities. For example, a therapist could invite the client to engage in 'show and tell' activities that promote their use of expressive language. This could be the subject of future research.

The findings of the current study highlight a number of practical aspects that warrant consideration by healthcare professionals who are contemplating or already using everyday technologies such as videoconferencing to support play-based interventions with young children:

- Identify basic equipment (e.g. a document camera) that can be used to enhance the delivery of therapy.

- Consider, in advance, ways in which the use of an object might be modified to suit the affordances and constraints of a particular telehealth medium (e.g. the audio and visual streams of videoconferencing).
- Ensure a range of diverse objects is available in case a particular object fails to facilitate an adequate level of engagement by a client.
- Determine whether specific therapeutic activities would be best supported by using objects in the possession of the therapist, the client or both parties.
- Where possible, ask an adult (e.g. a parent or teacher) to sit with a client and support the therapist by undertaking physical actions on their behalf.

This study reveals some practical ways in which telehealth technologies can affect the moment-by-moment delivery of healthcare. Considering the ways in which a particular telehealth medium might affect the delivery of speech and language therapy shows that there are unique aspects to the delivery, but they should not be seen as insurmountable obstacles for using telehealth with young children. As this study suggests, creative adaptations make possible the use of everyday technologies to facilitate healthcare interactions between professionals and clients without them necessarily needing participants to be in the same room.

Acknowledgement

The illustrations in this chapter were made by Genevieve Loy Callaghan and are reproduced here with permission.

Funding

This chapter is based upon a study funded by a Queensland University of Technology (QUT) Engagement Innovation Grant (EIG).

References

Campbell, F., Conti, G., Heckman, J. J., Moon, S. H., Pinto, R., Pungello, E. & Pan, Y. 2014. Early childhood investments substantially boost adult health. Science, 343, 1478–1485.

Conti-Ramsden, G., Durkin, K., Toseeb, U., Botting, N. & Pickles, A. 2018. Education and employment outcomes of young adults with a history of developmental language disorder. International Journal of Language and Communication Disorders, 53, 237–255.

Cronin, P., Reeve, R., McCabe, P., Viney, R. & Goodall, S. 2017. The impact of childhood language difficulties on healthcare costs from 4 to 13 years: Australian longitudinal study. International Journal of Speech-Language Pathology, 19, 381–391.

Doyle, O., Harmon, C. P., Heckman, J. J. & Tremblay, R. E. 2009. Investing in early human development: Timing and economic efficiency. Economics and Human Biology, 7, 1–6.

Drew, P., Chatwin, J. & Collins, S. 2001. Conversation analysis: A method for research into interactions between patients and health-care professionals. Health Expectations, 4, 58–70.

Dunkley, C., Pattie, L., Wilson, L. & McAllister, L. 2010. A comparison of rural speech-language pathologists' and residents' access to and attitudes towards the use of technology for speech-language pathology service delivery. International Journal of Speech-Language Pathology, 12, 333–343.

Eadie, P., Conway, L., Hallenstein, B., Mensah, F., McKean, C. & Reilly, S. 2018. Quality of life in children with developmental language disorder. International Journal of Language and Communication Disorders, 53, 799–810.

Ekberg, S., Danby, S., Theobald, M., Fisher, B. & Wyeth, P. 2019. Using physical objects with young children in 'face-to-face' and telehealth speech and language therapy. Disability and Rehabilitation, 41, 1664–1675.

Fasulo, A., Shukla, J. & Bennett, S. 2017. Find the hidden object. Understanding play in psychological assessments. Frontiers in Psychology, 8, 323.

Freckmann, A., Hines, M. & Lincoln, M. 2017. Clinicians' perspectives of therapeutic alliance in face-to-face and telepractice speech-language pathology sessions. International Journal of Speech-Language Pathology, 19, 287–296.

Hepburn, A. & Bolden, G. B. 2013. The conversation analytic approach to transcription. In: Sidnell, J. & Stivers, T. (eds) *The Handbook of Conversation Analysis*. Chichester: Wiley-Blackwell, 57–76.

Hill, A. J. & Miller, L. E. 2012. A survey of the clinical use of telehealth in speech-language pathology across Australia. Journal of Clinical Practice in Speech-Language Pathology, 14, 110–117.

Hutchby, I. 2001. *Conversation and Technology: From the Telephone to the Internet*. Malden, MA: Polity Press.

Iacono, T. A. 1999. Language intervention in early childhood. International Journal of Disability, Development and Education, 46, 383–420.

Manzanares, B. & Kan, P. F. 2014. Assessing children's language skills at a distance: Does it work? Perspectives on Augmentative and Alternative Communication, 23, 34–41.

Mashima, P. A. & Doarn, C. R. 2008. Overview of telehealth activities in speech-language pathology. Telemedicine and e-Health, 14, 1101–1117.

McCormack, J., Harrison, L. J., McLeod, S. & McAllister, L. 2011. A nationally representative study of the association between communication impairment at 4–5 years and children's life activities at 7–9 years. Journal of Speech, Language, and Hearing Research, 54, 1328–1348.

McCormack, J., McLeod, S., McAllister, L. & Harrison, L. J. 2009. A systematic review of the association between childhood speech impairment and participation across the lifespan. International Journal of Speech-Language Pathology, 11, 155–170.

Miccio, A. W. & Elbert, M. 1996. Enhancing stimulability: A treatment program. Journal of Communication Disorders, 29, 335–351.

Mondada, L. 2018. Multiple temporalities of language and body in interaction: Challenges for transcribing multimodality. Research on Language and Social Interaction, 51, 85–106.

Nevile, M., Haddington, P., Heinemann, T. & Rauniomaa, M. 2014. On the interactional ecology of objects. In: Nevile, M., Haddington, P., Heinemann, T. & Rauniomaa, M. (eds) *Interacting with Objects: Language, Materiality, and Social Activity.* Amsterdam: John Benjamins Publishing Company, 3–26.

Norbury, C. F., Gooch, D., Wray, C., Baird, G., Charman, T., Simonoff, E., Vamvakas, G. & Pickles, A. 2016. The impact of nonverbal ability on prevalence and clinical presentation of language disorder: Evidence from a population study. Journal of Child Psychology and Psychiatry, 57, 1247–1257.

O'Callaghan, A. M., McAllister, L. & Wilson, L. 2005. Barriers to accessing rural paediatric speech pathology services: Health care consumers' perspectives. Australian Journal of Rural Health, 13, 162–171.

Overby, M. S. 2018. Stakeholders' qualitative perspectives of effective telepractice pedagogy in speech–language pathology. International Journal of Language and Communication Disorders, 53, 101–112.

Peräkylä, A. 1997. Reliability and validity in research based on tapes and transcripts. In: Silverman, D. (ed.) *Qualitative Research: Theory, Method and Practice.* London: SAGE Publications Ltd.

Rosenbaun, L. & Licoppe, C. 2017. Showing 'digital' objects in web-based video chats as a collaborative achievement. Pragmatics, 27, 419–446.

Roulstone, S., Glogowska, M., Peters, T. J. & Enderby, P. 2004. Building good practice: Lessons from a multimethod study of speech and language therapy. International Journal of Therapy and Rehabilitation, 11, 199–205.

Sacks, H. 1984. Notes on methodology. In: Atkinson, J. M. & Heritage, J. (eds.) *Structures of Social Action: Studies in Conversation Analysis.* Cambridge: Cambridge University Press, 21–27.

Sharp, H. M. & Hillenbrand, K. 2008. Speech and language development and disorders in children. Pediatric Clinics of North America, 55, 1159–1173.

Suchman, L. 2005. Affiliative objects. Organization, 12, 379–399.

Sutherland, R., Trembath, D., Hodge, A., Drevensek, S., Lee, S., Silove, N. & Roberts, J. 2016. Telehealth language assessments using consumer grade equipment in rural and urban settings: Feasible, reliable and well tolerated. Journal of Telemedicine and Telecare, 23, 106–115.

Theodoros, D. G. 2008. Telerehabilitation for service delivery in speech-language pathology. Journal of Telemedicine and Telecare, 14, 221–224.

Tykkyläinen, T. 2009. Task-setting at home and in speech and language therapy. Child Language Teaching and Therapy, 25, 319–340.

van den Bedem, N. P., Dockrell, J. E., van Alphen, P. M., de Rooij, M., Samson, A. C., Harjunen, E. L. & Rieffe, C. 2018. Depressive symptoms and emotion regulation strategies in children with and without developmental language disorder: A longitudinal study. International Journal of Language and Communication Disorders, 53, 1110–1123.

Waite, M. C., Theodoros, D. G., Russell, T. G. & Cahill, L. M. 2010a. Assessment of children's literacy via an Internet-based telehealth system. Telemedicine and e-Health, 16, 564–575.

Waite, M. C., Theodoros, D. G., Russell, T. G. & Cahill, L. M. 2010b. Internet-based telehealth assessment of language using the CELF-4. Language, Speech, and Hearing Services in Schools, 41, 445–458.

Waite, M. C., Theodoros, D. G., Russell, T. G. & Cahill, L. M. 2012. Assessing children's speech intelligibility and oral structures, and functions via an Internet-based telehealth system. Journal of Telemedicine and Telecare, 18, 198–203.

Wales, D., Skinner, L. & Hayman, M. 2018. The efficacy of telehealth-delivered speech and language intervention for primary school-age children: A systematic review. International Journal of Telerehabilitation, 9, 55–70.

Wilson, L., Lincoln, M. & Onslow, M. 2002. Availability, access, and quality of care: Inequities in rural speech pathology services for children and a model for redress. Advances in Speech Language Pathology, 4, 9–22.

11

Digital Communication and Social Media for People with Communicative and Cognitive Disabilities

Margret Buchholz
University of Gothenburg
Sahlgrenska University Hospital

Ulrika Ferm
Sahlgrenska University Hospital

Kristina Holmgren
University of Gothenburg

CONTENTS

Introduction 194
Three Perspectives on Remote Communication for People with
Communicative and Cognitive Disabilities 196
    Professionals' Views on Texting with Pictures and Speech 196
    Experiences of and Views on Remote Communication by
    People with Communicative and Cognitive Disability 197
    Support Persons' Views on Remote Communication for the
    Target Group 198
Discussion 200
    Self-Determination and Participation... 200
    Safety and Security.. 202
    Access to Technology 203
    Access to Support.. 205
Methodological Considerations... 205
Summary 206
References 207

Introduction

Remote communication means communication between people who are not physically in the same place. For instance, using everyday technology like smartphones, tablets and computers, including services for calls (e.g. WhatsApp), messaging (e.g. Messenger), video calls (e.g. Skype) and social media are common means of communication in contemporary society (Statista, 2018; Zhou, 2017). Communication through digital channels is increasing as a required means of communication for interactions for daily activities, like contact with healthcare, insurance or banks and, therefore, has become a prerequisite for participation in society. Remote communication is used for social interactions with friends and groups and finding or signing up to participate in leisure activities that are commonly advertised through social media. It is also used to book activities, like haircuts, restaurant reservations or sport club sessions. Citizens are expected to have access to the Internet and digital devices for taking care of one's health by booking healthcare appointments, handling medication prescriptions and having contact with healthcare insurance providers. E-health is a relatively recent healthcare practice supported by electronic communication, and it is developing rapidly (WHO, 2018). Physical, more old-fashioned means (e.g. tellers and reception desks) of contact are being shut down, making access to remote communication a must in order to handle essential daily life activities.

Despite this common use of the Internet and social media, several groups of people do not have Internet access or other means of remote communication at present due to older age or disability (Jaeger, 2012). Using remote communication has been shown to reduce isolation while enhancing social contact, independence and participation (Raghavendra et al., 2015; Caron and Light, 2017). Being able to use common forms of remote communication require functional speech (phone calls and video calls) and the ability to read and write (texting, e-mailing or chatting). There are several medical conditions, such as congenital, acquired and progressive disorders that can affect communication abilities. People with a combination of communicative and cognitive disabilities may have limited speech and comprehension abilities as well as restricted reading and writing skills, which means that both their spoken and written communication are affected. Those who lack access to remote communication will most likely end up on the wrong side of the digital divide and become excluded from the digitalised world of today (Jaeger, 2012; Light and McNaughton, 2014).

Freedom of speech is a fundamental human right described by the United Nations (UN) in the Universal Declaration of Human Rights (1948). The right to communicate is described by the American Speech-Language-Hearing Association (2018) and in the UN-Convention on the Rights of Persons with Disabilities (2007). Disability occurs in the context of both personal and environmental factors, which influence how disability and subsequently participation are experienced by the individual (WHO, 2001). Disability affecting the ability to communicate can affect self-determination because it decreases opportunities to initiate contact, engage in conversation and plan and participate in activities in the same way as others (Wehmeyer, 2005). Participation is a common goal for communication interventions and an important outcome measure in research (Lund and Light, 2006; McNaughton and Bryen, 2007).

People who have a restricted ability to communicate can use augmentative and alternative communication (AAC; i.e. methods to compensate for restrictions in their ability to produce and/or comprehend spoken and written communication). An AAC system involves assistive technology that is adjusted to the individual's communication needs (Beukelman and Mirenda, 2013). People who have difficulties communicating may also have cognitive problems and difficulties reading and writing. For them, AAC can include graphic symbols and text-to-speech for assisted reading (Beukelman and Mirenda, 2013; Light and McNaughton, 2012). Assistive technology means products, environmental modifications, services and processes that enable occupation and participation for people with disabilities (Cook and Polgar, 2015). This includes mainstream, off-the shelf technology and specialised devices. Assistive technology can, to some extent, connect to and be used for remote communication. Remote communication to a large degree depends on access to mainstream technology and services. Having access to mainstream technology and services is, therefore, vital for communication and, as such, should be deemed a human right (McEwin and Santow, 2018).

For a person with disability, remote communication, including social media, may facilitate societal relationships, self-determination and participation (Caron and Light, 2016, 2017; Raghavendra et al., 2015; Hamm and Mirenda, 2006; Hemsley et al., 2015; Hynan et al., 2015). People who have difficulties with oral communication in combination with reading and writing problems tend to find it hard to handle mainstream communication technology, but research has shown that they may benefit from specialised software or well-designed mainstream technology (Stock et al., 2008; Wennberg and Kjellberg, 2010). Remote communication based on speech, such as phone calls or video calls, can be hard to manage. Remote communication involving writing, such as e-mail, chat, social media or texting, is also difficult (Light and McNaughton, 2014).

Communicative and cognitive disabilities can result in decreased interaction with other people, self-determination and participation in society. To further complicate matters, technology that could enable remote communication is often not designed for people with these disabilities. The research described in this chapter aimed to explore and describe remote communication for people with communicative and cognitive disabilities who have limited reading and writing abilities. This research explored remote communication in relation to self-determination and participation from the perspectives of professionals (occupational therapists and speech language pathologists), the people themselves and support persons.

Three Perspectives on Remote Communication for People with Communicative and Cognitive Disabilities

This chapter is based on four studies: three qualitative and a mixed method with qualitative focus. Data collection was carried out in a major city in Sweden (in cooperation with a regional centre for AAC and assistive technology). All qualitative data were recorded and transcribed verbatim.

Professionals' Views on Texting with Pictures and Speech

This study aimed to explore professionals' views on remote communication, including texting with picture symbols and speech synthesis for people with communicative and cognitive disabilities after an intervention period (Buchholz et al., 2013). The participants were seven professionals: four occupational therapists and three speech language pathologists who had participated in an intervention project to test text messaging with picture symbols and speech synthesis (TMSS) (Mattsson Müller et al., 2010). They had worked with seven people with communicative and cognitive disabilities who also participated in the project. The professionals were interviewed in semi-structured interviews that were analysed by content analysis (Graneheim and Lundman, 2004; Patton, 2015).

The findings from the interviews with professionals highlighted areas of importance to achieve user satisfaction with a smartphone and suggested that TMSS could increase independence and participation in people with cognitive and communicative disabilities from the professionals' point of view. There were three main areas of importance to achieve satisfaction with a smartphone for people with communicative and cognitive disabilities according to the professionals: *acceptance, functionality* and *usability* (Buchholz et al., 2013). *Acceptance*: In order for the users to accept the smartphone, it had to live up to the user's expectations; he or she had to feel comfortable in using it in social situations and accept it as a natural part of daily life activities. *Functionality*: Technology needed to be functional for the users. It was important that the devices were easy to handle and that the speech synthesis was intelligible. *Usability*: Usability concerned how the devices were perceived to have met the needs of the user and how the devices could be part of a meaningful activity. Learning to use the device was viewed as vital to be able to start using it, and this was an obstacle for some. Speech synthesis and functions for reading and writing support were indispensable features.

The professionals' views of the users' participation concerned two main areas: *independence* and *interaction with other people* (Buchholz et al., 2013). *Independence* was perceived to be related to the users making their own decisions and taking the initiative to participate through remote communication. When using remote communication, the users managed more things on their own. The professionals experienced that the users with cognitive and communicative disabilities felt safer in their daily life situations, which increased confidence and gradually led to more independence. *Interaction with other people* was important and was enabled by TMSS giving users sufficient time to express themselves. There were issues regarding the setup of the AAC system and findings described how using TMSS was an opportunity to practice other aspects of communication.

Experiences of and Views on Remote Communication by People with Communicative and Cognitive Disability

The aim of this second study was to explore the experiences of people with communicative and cognitive disabilities using remote communication (Buchholz et al., 2018b). The participants were 11 adolescents and adults who had communicative and cognitive disabilities, including limited abilities in reading and writing. In order for them to be able to give informed consent, participation in interviews and gathering as much data as possible, rigorous planning and interview adaptation were undertaken (Buchholz, 2016; Cameron and Murphy, 2007). Semi-structured interviews were combined with Talking Mats for communicative and cognitive support to enable their participation (Murphy et al., 2013). Talking Mats is a visual framework that allows individuals with communicative and cognitive disabilities to reflect upon and express their views on different issues. Talking Mats is used by placing a picture representing the conversational topic at the bottom of the mat, and then pictures representing an evaluation scale are placed on the top of the mat by the interviewer. A set of pictures, one for each question, relating to the topic are placed under the pictures of the evaluation scale by the respondent as answers to open questions (see Figure 11.1). The participants placed the picture accompanying each question under the scale step picture (good, bad or in-between good and bad) that best represented his or her opinion (see Figure 11.1). The participants were stimulated to complete their

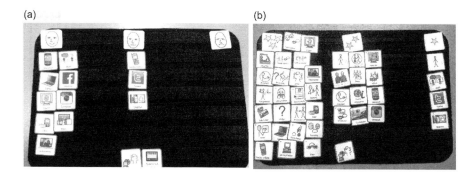

FIGURE 11.1
Example of Talking Mats in conversations about services, applications and devices (a) and the importance of the different activities, services and devices (b).

answers with their preferred means of communication (orally and/or by the use of AAC).

This study was a qualitatively driven mixed-method study (Schoonenboom and Johnson, 2017). The data collected by the placing of pictures with Talking Mats resulted in ordinal scales. The participants' views, as expressed orally and with body communication and aids, in parallel with the placement of the pictures on the mat, were analysed with systematic text condensation (Malterud, 2012).

Three main categories emerged from people with communicative and cognitive disabilities' experiences: *to get through in one's own way*, *own strategies to enable communication* and *technology not meeting needs*. These categories each consisted of three subcategories (Buchholz et al., 2018b). *To get through in one's own way*: Being able to make oneself understood and get through with a message was described as important but difficult. Usual means of communication did not work and participants described how they felt not being heard. Support from assistants was regarded as both wanted and unwanted depending on the situation, and the participants wished to be able to decide in which situations to get support. For instance, in communication situations where personal integrity was important to them, they did not want as much assistance to ensure they had some privacy. Decisions regarding means of communication and human support related to the concept of self-determination. *Own strategies to enable communication*: Participants described several of their own communication strategies to manage remote communication. This could be, for instance to adapt their communication to facilitate for the communication partner or prepare for future communication. For example, those who were able to use writing (e.g. chat or text messaging) as an alternative to problematic spoken remote communication (e.g. phone calls). *Technology not meeting needs*: There was a lack of access to useful technology and dependence on technology, meaning they were further vulnerable to changes in technology. Participants also expressed a need for training. Technology issues could lead to the abandonment of the technology altogether.

Support Persons' Views on Remote Communication for the Target Group

Two studies aimed to gather the views of support persons. The participants were 21 support persons to people with communicative and cognitive disabilities who were family members and/or staff who worked in sheltered housing, schools or as personal assistants. Data for the studies were collected through a series of focus groups that are characterised by group discussions where participants interact with one another in order to gather data on a certain topic (Krueger and Casey, 2015). Focus groups are a qualitative research method with its own methodological principles and research procedures including analysis (Dahlin Ivanoff and Hultberg, 2006).

The first of these two studies aimed to explore support persons' views on remote communication for people with communicative and cognitive disabilities and on factors that enabled their self-determination and participation (Buchholz et al., 2018a). The analysis of the focus groups resulted in three themes: *the right to communicate, increased control in life through access to remote communication* and *challenges in responsibilities of support persons*. The main themes each consisted of three to four subcategories (Buchholz et al., 2018a). *The right to communicate*: The support persons saw how the communicative rights of the users were not being met. Participants described a need for better access to technology and information. They wished for better competency concerning remote communication among staff for the users with cognitive and communicative disabilities and coordination in professional efforts and interventions. The users needed ongoing individual training on remote communication. *Increased control in life through access to remote communication*: The participants experienced how remote communication could enhance self-determination and participation, and how this was important for the safety and security of people with communicative and cognitive disabilities. *Challenges in responsibilities of support persons*: There were challenges in the responsibilities of the support persons. There were feelings of concern, insecurity, frustration and insufficiency. Perceived risks regarding online safety led to ethical dilemmas for the support persons.

The second focus group study aimed to describe support persons' views on varying aspects of and functions in technology for remote communication that enabled and stimulated independent communication, self-determination and participation for people with communicative and cognitive disabilities (Buchholz et al., 2018c). The analysis resulted in three themes: *use of standard technology, use of assistive technology* and *combining standard technology and assistive technology*, each of which encompassed categories describing aspects of technology that facilitated or impeded remote communication as well as suggestions for improvements. *Use of standard technology*: The findings described the support persons' views on the importance of being able to use standard technology for remote communication for people with communicative and cognitive disabilities. Some functions of standard technology could facilitate independent remote communication, like video calls and asynchronous communication. However, others could be challenging in terms of understandability, compatibility and Internet access. *Use of assistive technology*: Assistive technology was important in enabling remote communication through compensating functions, for instance, in reading and writing support, but certain issues restricted the opportunities. The participants discussed that there was a need to further develop assistive technology. *Combining standard technology and assistive technology*: The findings suggested an importance of being able to combine standard technology and assistive technology in order to have access to remote communication, but the results also highlighted that there were technical limitations and that information must be available online. They felt remote communication technology must be made more accessible and easier to use for both people with disabilities and people in their networks. The findings included a detailed list of required technology development (Buchholz et al., 2018c).

Discussion

The overall aim of this research was to explore and describe remote communication for people with communicative and cognitive disabilities with limited reading and writing abilities. Remote communication was explored from the perspectives of professionals, the people themselves and support persons (see Figure 11.2). The findings suggested how remote communication relates to self-determination and participation. The findings also highlighted needs in the areas of safety and security, access to technology and support.

Self-Determination and Participation

The findings of this research described how engaging in remote communication could result in increased control over one's own life because it allowed people to make their own decisions on how they interact with others and

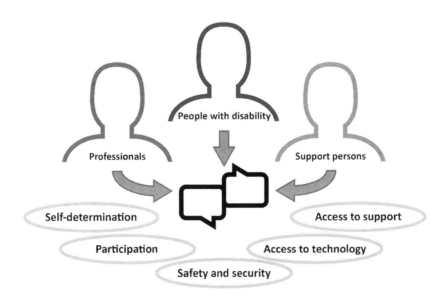

FIGURE 11.2
The figure shows the three different perspectives on remote communication for people with communicative and cognitive disabilities in this research project. Illustration by: Sofia Wallin.

have control over their own social network. Well-functioning remote communication was described to increase participation. Having access to remote communication could help people participate in social networks and engage in interests and meaningful activities.

Making one's own appointments was important and could be achieved in two manners: independently by using remote communication or by having assistance. According to the participants with disabilities, having control over the communication, especially in situations where personal integrity mattered, was vital for self-determination, which is in line with previous research (Hynan et al., 2015). This involved the user having a choice of whether to be independent or not in remote communication and determining how assistance was received. Having control over one's remote communication is a vital step in gaining confidence towards independence (Wennberg and Kjellberg, 2010). Remote communication was described to compensate for physical, cognitive and social limitations, for instance, by virtual meetings which is in line with other research (Sallafranque-St-Louis and Normand, 2017). However, research has highlighted how people with disabilities have structural barriers to healthcare due to problems in booking appointments and transportation (Henning-Smith et al., 2013; Morris et al., 2013).

Having a broader social network than only family was essential, and without this, participation in daily life and society was more limited. Caron (2016) has described the importance of being able to use social media to expand the amount of contact for people who use AAC.

According to our research, using mainstream technology could help users to expand their interests, blend in and also gain status for possessing and using popular technology. Access to remote communication seemed to enable participation on more equal terms. It was described as important to look or seem like everyone else by being able to use mainstream looking technology. The findings point at the importance of participating in online activities and choose one's own online persona, including deciding whether or not to reveal one's disability. Communication partners only saw the result (i.e. the final message) and not the process used to create it, and then the person with a disability could participate on his or her own terms.

Access to remote communication could enable participation in meaningful activities, for instance, engaging in gaming or social media, according to the findings of this research, which aligns with previous research (Caron and Light, 2015). From the perspectives of people with disability, professionals and support persons, there were descriptions of how it was not necessary that the activity be carried out independently to be meaningful. This was also found by Caron (2016) who described how only watching content on social media had benefits in participation and even despite minimal interaction, it allowed connection with the world for people experiencing online barriers.

Safety and Security

Remote communication could affect users' security in different ways as described in this research. On one hand, access to remote communication could increase safety and security by increasing the ability to contact someone when needing help or support. However, using the Internet and social media could also mean taking risks due to online safety issues.

From the perspectives of professionals and support persons, independent remote communication was perceived to enable users to manage more things independently in society or to stay home alone. Being able to call for assistance was described as increasing and developing the users' confidence and independence. Access to remote communication was also necessary to be able to make emergency calls in case of danger, which was not described as working well by the users themselves. Even if possible, it is doubtful that emergency personnel would know how to communicate with the person calling (RERC, 2018). Feeling safe is a basic need, which needs to be met for all citizens. It is essential that professionals acknowledge that if a person with a disability ever spends time on their own, it must be ensured that he or she can call for help independently to be safe, which is a basic human right (UN, 1948).

From the support persons' perspectives, the subject of safety had both advantages and disadvantages. Support persons described how they strived for increased self-determination and participation for their users and encouraged them to use different means of remote communication, but they experienced how using the Internet and social media could cause harm. Online safety is an issue for everyone today, and people with communicative and cognitive disabilities face risks when using remote communication on their own (Seale and Chadwick, 2017). Sorbring et al. (2017) have described how parents of intellectually challenged young people were worried that their children were in danger of unwelcome content and interactions on the Internet. However, research has shown that in spite of the online risks, the users gained increased self-determination and social contacts, maintained long-distance relationships and received social support through Internet use (Sallafranque-St-Louis and Normand, 2017). From the focus group discussion with support persons, it emerged how support persons who care for users could provide safety and help the users to identify online risks. The drawback is that support persons themselves can become a barrier to Internet access, self-determination and participation for the users when trying to protect them from any potential online risks (Hemsley et al., 2017). Research has described how people providing support to adolescents and adults with intellectual and developmental disabilities negotiated and handled risks online (Seale and Chadwick, 2017; Seale, 2014). They found that normal life means to be digitally included, which involves taking risks and exercising the same human rights as others and they proposed a framework of a positive risk-taking, involving support persons.

Access to Technology

An important, and perhaps not surprising, finding from our research was that access to technology was perceived as crucial for being able to use remote communication. The findings pointed out that communicational rights of people with communicative and cognitive disabilities were not met due to limitations in access to remote communication technology.

Findings of this research described how people with communicative and cognitive disabilities needed technology that is functional, useful, reliable and up to date. In the interview study with people with disability, a user said, when talking about smartphones and the need for alternative access to be able to use it: 'It will probably be like with everything else, a big damned thing that becomes difficult to bring with me, and then to hell with it!'. This is a colourful illustration of technology not meeting the users' needs and how that can lead to abandonment of assistive technology and subsequently decreased participation. Larsson Ranada and Lidström (2017) have highlighted the importance of a client-centred approach achieving the desired goals of participation in everyday activities in relation to satisfaction with assistive technology. People with communicative and cognitive disabilities needed individually assessed and adapted technology.

Cost can be a factor limiting access to remote communication if the user must purchase technology themselves as emerged from focus group discussions with support persons. Even with provided devices and applications, there were still costs for the Internet and mobile subscriptions. People with communicative and cognitive problems often have low or no income, which can inhibit access to remote communication for a group that already experiences obstacles in communication. These findings are in line with Jaeger's description of a digital divide for people with disabilities (2012). If the goal is equal access to communication for all, the issue of costs must be considered.

According to the findings of this research, technology must be easy to handle, and the findings from the perspectives of people with disability and support persons described how this was not the case. There were issues with handling touch screens and a lack of alternate access, leading to communication limitations. Technology was described as too complicated to use for both people with communicative and cognitive disabilities and support persons. When the supporters cannot help, what can the users do? Difficulties in handling remote communication technology have been described in other research (Caron and Light, 2017; McNaughton and Light, 2013; Raghavendra et al., 2012).

In daily remote communication, the common user switches between different devices, applications and services depending on which he or she wants to reach and preferred ways to communicate. People with disabilities may only have access to one specific device or software, limiting their choices and potentially excluding them from participating fully. If a person has difficulties texting with a smartphone but can have a conversation over

Messenger with assistive technology, he or she still has the possibility to participate with remote communication. The ability to use at least one mode of remote communication is vastly different compared to having no accessible devices, applications or services that he or she can use. The lack of interconnectivity described by support persons complicated the use of technology. Switching between applications and specific devices in the way that is necessary in mobile technology today was difficult for people with communicative and cognitive disabilities. The importance of interconnectivity has also been described in other research (Caron and Light, 2016; McNaughton and Bryen, 2007). It is of utmost importance to enable interconnectivity between technology for AAC and remote communication to make remote communication accessible for those who use AAC-technology.

Our research point at speech synthesis as a beneficial function. It was described as a major prerequisite for constructing and reading messages that should be available in all remote communication applications. This finding is in line with previous research (Mattsson Müller et al., 2010). Speech synthesis has gone from expensive assistive technology to a standard function in off-the-shelf devices, on webpages and in standard software and is today aiming for a more natural and personalised voice (Mills et al., 2014). Hopefully, this development can increase access to speech synthesis for those who need it.

From the perspective of support persons, another beneficial function was video calls. This was an example of easy to handle universal design that worked in favour of all users. The possibility of involving many visual means of AAC and body communication seemed to stimulate remote communication as others have found (Raghavendra et al., 2015). Even though video calls made it possible to incorporate means of AAC, it was not always easy to include communication boards or assistive devices or applications. Solutions for using different camera angles for AAC would be useful.

According to the findings of this research, there were also benefits in asynchronous communication in relation to the fact that producing messages using communication aids could be lengthy (Higginbotham et al., 2007). The person with a disability does not have to be fast to be listened to and the final message did not show the real amount of time and energy spent to produce it. In this way, communication with other people can be equalised.

An evaluation of Australian e-health service showed major limitations in access for people who could not read or write (Walsh et al., 2017). Based on our research, one can draw the conclusion that people with communicative and cognitive disabilities would have great difficulties in access to e-health, even if this was not evaluated in the four presented studies. There is a need for more knowledge concerning how people with disabilities could use remote communication to better interact with healthcare professionals (Henning-Smith et al., 2013; Morris et al., 2013; Paterson, 2017). Support for reading and writing must be included when developing platforms or systems aiming to be available for all. The advantages in speech synthesis, video calls and asynchronous communication should also be considered when aiming to include people with disabilities in digital communication.

Access to Support

Another important issue raised in the findings of our research was the need for support. It is essential for professionals to re-evaluate their responsibilities for support to users and their network. The professionals suggested that there should be improved teamwork between speech language pathologists and occupational therapists. The support persons pointed out that support to people with communicative and cognitive disabilities is a lifelong process. People with communicative and cognitive disabilities may hesitate to try new, unfamiliar technology and encouragement from their support network was central for them. This was also described by Raghavendra et al. (2012) who found that digital skills in family and friends influenced the users' online communication. It is necessary to approach and support users in their use of remote communication in a systematic way (Caron, 2016). Research has described that training and support to people with communicative and cognitive disabilities need to be individually adapted to the users' daily activities (Higginbotham et al., 2007). In an intervention study by Grace et al. (2014), youths with complex communication needs received training in using social media, and the findings describe how performance and satisfaction among the participants increased in terms of Internet use for social contacts. People with disabilities, as well as communication partners, need intensive support and technical assistance (Tegler et al., 2018). Findings from the perspective of support persons pointed to a lack of support from professionals and a non-existent coordination of services. Research has shown that a lack of support and insufficient training to those with cognitive and communicative difficulties led to the abandonment and/or underutilisation of assistive technology (Larsson Ranada and Lidström, 2017).

Methodological Considerations

This research is mainly based on qualitative studies, including a mixed-method study with a qualitative focus. The purpose of using a qualitative approach was to be able to explore a mostly unexplored research area and to find and describe its meaning. In qualitative research, one cannot argue for objectivity because every analysis and interpretation will have a trace of the paradigm of the researcher (Marshall and Rossman, 2011). Results cannot be generalised, thus the qualitative approach contributes an increased understanding and in-depth knowledge that is hard to research with a quantitative approach.

It is ethically questionable to draw conclusions about a group if efforts are not made in letting their voices be heard, but people with communicative and cognitive disabilities are often excluded from research (Lloyd et al., 2006; Paterson and Scott-Findlay, 2002). When designing studies, the researchers may not have the knowledge or necessary recourses to adapt the data collection to ensure the views of everyone in the target group get collected (Blackstone et al., 2007; Williams et al., 2008). In order to develop the understanding of remote communication for people with communicative and cognitive disabilities, obtaining the experiences from the target group themselves was the most crucial. To enable participation for people with communicative and cognitive difficulties, information must be understandable, and the researcher must take precautions to make sure that participants have understood and that their informed consent builds on their understanding (Buchholz, 2016; Cameron and Murphy, 2007). The participation of the target group themselves was very valuable. To enable participation of people who rarely participate in interview studies due to their communication challenges, ensuring comprehension and gathering as much data as possible, rigorous planning and interview adaptation were undertaken. Talking Mats was an important and reliable tool in order to gather the views of participants with communicative and cognitive disabilities as shown also in other research (Bunning et al., 2017; Murphy and Cameron, 2008; Stewart et al., 2018).

Summary

The overall aim of the research presented in this chapter was to explore and describe remote communication for people with communicative and cognitive disabilities with limited reading and writing abilities. It explored remote communication from the perspectives of the people themselves, professionals and support persons.

Access to remote communication is crucial for participation in today's society where an increasing part of human interaction is carried out through digital channels. Using remote communication can increase independence, self-determination and participation in daily life for people with communicative and cognitive disabilities. It can also increase safety.

Communication is a human right and must be available for all. There is a need for further technology development so that technology can be accessible for all. New development of technology used in society must also include people with communicative and cognitive disabilities, and there is a need for further studies involving this target group. People with disabilities and their network need improved support.

A health-related and low-researched topic is how it works to call for help in emergency situations for people with communicative and cognitive disabilities. What options are there, how are they used, and are there needs for development of technology and services? Another, also health-related, topic is how society can make sure that every citizen has access to the fast-developing e-health services that are projected to be a large part of the future health services. The findings of this research suggest that people with communicative and cognitive disabilities may encounter difficulties in accessing these services. Research working with this target group is very sparse, and studies are necessary to make sure that health services are available for everyone.

References

ASHA. (2018). Augmentative and Alternative Communication (AAC). American Speech-Language-Hearing Association. [Online] Available: www.asha.org/public/speech/disorders/AAC/ [Accessed June 19 2018].

Beukelman, D. R. & Mirenda, P. (2013). *Augmentative and Alternative Communication Processes*. Baltimore, MD: Paul H Brookes Publishing Co.

Blackstone, S. W., Williams, M. B. & Wilkins, D. P. (2007). Key principles underlying research and practice in AAC. *Augmentative and Alternative Communication*, 23, 191–203.

Buchholz, M., Ferm, U. & Holmgren, K. (2016). Including persons with complex communication needs in research – a methodology based on Talking Mats. ISAAC 2016 - Bringing Us Together, Toronto: ISAAC.

Buchholz, M., Ferm, U. & Holmgren, K. (2018a). Support persons' views on remote communication and social media for people with communicative and cognitive disabilities. *Disability and Rehabilitation*, 1–9. [Online] Available: www.tandfonline.com/doi/full/10.1080/09638288.2018.1529827.

Buchholz, M., Ferm, U. & Holmgren, K. (2018b). "That is how I speak nowadays" – experiences of remote communication among persons with communicative and cognitive disabilities. *Disability and Rehabilitation*, 40, 1468–1479.

Buchholz, M., Holmgren, K. & Ferm, U. (2018c). Remote communication for people with disabilities: Benefits, challenges and suggestions for technology development. In manuscript.

Buchholz, M., Mattsson Müller, I. & Ferm, U. (2013). Text messaging with pictures and speech synthesis for adolescents and adults with cognitive and communicative disabilities – professionals' views about user satisfaction and participation. *Technology and Disability*, 25, 87–98.

Bunning, K., Alder, R., Proudman, L. & Wyborn, H. (2017). Co-production and pilot of a structured interview using Talking Mats® to survey the television viewing habits and preferences of adults and young people with learning disabilities. *British Journal of Learning Disabilities*, 45, 1–11.

Cameron, L. & Murphy, J. (2007). Obtaining consent to participate in research: The issues involved in including people with a range of learning and communication disabilities. *British Journal of Learning Disabilities*, 35, 113–120.

Caron, J. (2016). Engagement in social media environments for individuals with who use augmentative and alternative communication. *NeuroRehabilitation*, 39, 499–506.

Caron, J. & Light, J. (2015). "My world has expanded even though I'm stuck at home": Experiences of individuals with amyotrophic lateral sclerosis who use augmentative and alternative communication and social media. *American Journal of Speech-Language Pathology*, 24, 680–695.

Caron, J. & Light, J. (2016). "Social media has opened a world of 'open communication": Experiences of adults with cerebral palsy who use augmentative and alternative communication and social media. *Augmentative and Alternative Communication*, 32, 25–40.

Caron, J. G. & Light, J. (2017). Social media experiences of adolescents and young adults with cerebral palsy who use augmentative and alternative communication. *International Journal of Speech-Language Pathology*, 19, 30–42.

Cook, A. M. & Polgar, J. M. (2015). *Assistive Technologies Principles and Practice*. Maryland Heights, MO: Mosby.

Dahlin Ivanoff, S. & Hultberg, J. (2006). Understanding the multiple realities of everyday life: Basic assumptions in focus-group methodology. *Scandinavian Journal of Occupational Therapy*, 13(2), 125–132.

Grace, E., Raghavendra, P., Newman, L., Wood, D. & Connell, T. (2014). Learning to use the Internet and online social media: What is the effectiveness of home-based intervention for youth with complex communication needs? *Child Language Teaching and Therapy*, 30, 141–157.

Graneheim, U. H. & Lundman, B. (2004). Qualitative content analysis in nursing research: Concepts, procedures and measures to achieve trustworthiness. *Nurse Education Today*, 24, 105–112.

Hamm, B. & Mirenda, P. (2006). Post-school quality of life for individuals with developmental disabilities who use AAC. *Augmentative and Alternative Communication*, 22, 134–147.

Hemsley, B., Balandin, S., Palmer, S. & Dann, S. (2017). A call for innovative social media research in the field of augmentative and alternative communication. *Augmentative and Alternative Communication*, 33, 14–22.

Hemsley, B., Dann, S., Palmer, S., Allan, M. & Balandin, S. (2015). "We definitely need an audience": Experiences of Twitter, Twitter networks and tweet content in adults with severe communication disabilities who use augmentative and alternative communication (AAC). *Disability and Rehabilitation*, 37, 1531–1542.

Henning-Smith, C., McAlpine, D., Shippee, T. & Priebe, M. (2013). Delayed and unmet need for medical care among publicly insured adults with disabilities. *Medical Care*, 51(11), 1015–1019. School of Public Health, Division of Health Policy and Management, University of Minnesota, Minneapolis, MN, VA Medical Center, Augusta, GA.

Higginbotham, D. J., Shane, H., Russell, S. & Caves, K. (2007). Access to AAC: Present, past, and future. *Augmentative and Alternative Communication*, 23, 243–257.

Hynan, A., Goldbart, J. & Murray, J. (2015). A grounded theory of Internet and social media use by young people who use augmentative and alternative communication (AAC). *Disability and Rehabilitation*, 37, 1559–1575.

Jaeger, P. T. (2012). *Disability and the Internet*. Boulder, CO: Lynne Rienner Publishers Inc.

Krueger, R. A. & Casey, M. A. (2015). *Focus Groups: A Practical Guide for Applied Research*. Thousand Oaks, CA: SAGE Publications, Inc.

Larsson Ranada, Å. & Lidström, H. (2019). Satisfaction with assistive technology device in relation to the service delivery process—A systematic review, *Assistive Technology*, 31:2, 82–97.

Light, J. & McNaughton, D. (2012). Supporting the communication, language, and literacy development of children with complex communication needs: State of the science and future research priorities. *Assistive Technology*, 24, 34–44.

Light, J. & McNaughton, D. (2014). Communicative competence for individuals who require augmentative and alternative communication: A new definition for a new era of communication? *Augmentative and Alternative Communication*, 30, 1–18.

Lloyd, V., Gatherer, A. & Kalsy, S. (2006). Conducting qualitative interview research with people with expressive language difficulties. *Qualitative Health Research*, 16, 1386–1404.

Lund, S. K. & Light, J. (2006). Long-term outcomes for individuals who use augmentative and alternative communication: Part I – what is a "good" outcome? *Augmentative and Alternative Communication*, 22, 284–299.

Malterud, K. (2012). Systematic text condensation: A strategy for qualitative analysis. *Scandinavian Journal of Public Health*, 40, 795–805.

Marshall, C. & Rossman, G. B. (2011). *Designing Qualitative Research*. Thousand Oaks, CA: SAGE Publications Inc.

Mattsson Müller, I., Buchholz, M. & Ferm, U. (2010). Text messaging with picture symbols – experiences of seven persons with cognitive and communicative disabilities. *Journal of Assistive Technologies*, 4, 11–23.

McEwin, A. & Santow, E. (2018). The importance of the human right to communication. *International Journal of Speech-Language Pathology*, 20, 1–2.

McNaughton, D. & Bryen, D. N. (2007). AAC technologies to enhance participation and access to meaningful societal roles for adolescents and adults with developmental disabilities who require AAC. *Augmentative and Alternative Communication*, 23, 217–229.

McNaughton, D. & Light, J. (2013). The iPad and mobile technology revolution: Benefits and challenges for individuals who require augmentative and alternative communication. *Augmentative and Alternative Communication*, 29, 107–116.

Mills, T., Bunnell, H. T. & Patel, R. (2014). Towards personalized speech synthesis for augmentative and alternative communication. *Augmentative and Alternative Communication*, 30, 226–236.

Morris, M. A., Dudgeon, B. J. & Yorkston, K. (2013). A qualitative study of adult AAC users' experiences communicating with medical providers. *Disability and Rehabilitation: Assistive Technology*, 8, 472–481.

Murphy, J. & Cameron, L. (2008). The effectiveness of Talking Mats with people with intellectual disability. *British Journal of Learning Disabilities*, 36, 232–241.

Murphy, J., Cameron, L. & Boa, S. (2013). *Talking Mats - A Resource to Enhance Communication*. Stirling, Scotland: Talking Mats Ltd.

Paterson, H. L. (2017). The use of social media by adults with acquired conditions who use AAC: Current gaps and considerations in research. *Augmentative and Alternative Communication*, 33, 23–31.

Paterson, B. & Scott-Findlay, S. (2002). Critical issues in interviewing people with traumatic brain injury. *Qualitative Health Research*, 12, 399–409.

Patton, M. Q. (ed.) (2015). *Qualitative Research and Evaluation Methods*. Thousand Oaks, CA: Sage Publications Inc.

Raghavendra, P., Newman, L., Grace, E. & Wood, D. (2015). Enhancing social participation in young people with communication disabilities living in rural Australia: Outcomes of a home-based intervention for using social media. *Disability and Rehabilitation*, 37, 1576–1590.

Raghavendra, P., Wood, D., Newman, L. & Lawry, J. (2012). Why aren't you on Facebook? Patterns and experiences of using the Internet among young people with physical disabilities. *Technology and Disability*, 24, 149–162.

RERC. (2018). The RERC on communication enhancement - emergency communication. The Rehabilitation Engineering Research Center on Communication Enhancement. [Online] Available: http://aac-rerc.psu.edu/index.php/pages/show/id/18 [Accessed November 9 2018].

Sallafranque-St-Louis, F. & Normand, C. L. (2017). From solitude to solicitation: How people with intellectual disability or autism spectrum disorder use the Internet. *Cyberpsychology: Journal of Psychosocial Research on Cyberspace*, 11. [Online] Available: https://cyberpsychology.eu/article/view/6757/6215.

Schoonenboom, J. & Johnson, R. B. (2017). How to construct a mixed methods research design. *Kölner Zeitschrift für Soziologie und Sozialpsychologie*, 69, 107–131.

Seale, J. (2014). The role of supporters in facilitating the use of technologies by adolescents and adults with learning disabilities: A place for positive risk-taking? *European Journal of Special Needs Education*, 29, 220–236.

Seale, J. & Chadwick, D. (2017). How does risk mediate the ability of adolescents and adults with intellectual and developmental disabilities to live a normal life by using the Internet? *Cyberpsychology: Journal of Psychosocial Research on Cyberspace*, 11. [Online] Available: https://cyberpsychology.eu/article/view/6764/6238.

Sorbring, E., Molin, M. & Löfgren-Mårtenson, L. (2017). "I'm a mother, but I'm also a facilitator in her every-day life": Parents' voices about barriers and support for Internet participation among young people with intellectual disabilities. *Cyberpsychology: Journal of Psychosocial Research on Cyberspace*, 11. [Online] Available: https://cyberpsychology.eu/article/view/6758/6218.

Statista. (2018). Social media & user-generated content. Statista. [Online] Available: www.statista.com/markets/424/topic/540/social-media-user-generated-content/ [Accessed November 28 2018].

Stewart, K., Bradshaw, J. & Beadle-Brown, J. (2018). Evaluating service users' experiences using Talking Mats®. *Tizard Learning Disability Review*, 23, 78–86.

Stock, S. E., Davies, D. K., Wehmeyer, M. L. & Palmer, S. B. (2008). Evaluation of cognitively accessible software to increase independent access to cellphone technology for people with intellectual disability. *Journal of Intellectual Disability Research*, 52, 1155–1164.

Tegler, H., Pless, M., Blom Johansson, M. & Sonnander, K. (2018). Speech and language pathologists' perceptions and practises of communication partner training to support children's communication with high-tech speech generating devices. *Disability and Rehabilitation: Assistive Technology*, 1–9. [Online] Available: www.tandfonline.com/doi/full/10.1080/17483107.2018.1475515.

United Nations. (1948). Universal declaration of human rights. United Nations.

United Nations. (2007). Convention on the rights of persons with disabilities United Nations.

Walsh, L., Hemsley, B., Allan, M., Adams, N., Balandin, S., Georgiou, A., Higgins, I., McCarthy, S. & Hill, S. (2017). The e-health literacy demands of Australia's My Health Record: A heuristic evaluation of usability. *Perspectives in Health Information Management*, 14, 1f.

Wehmeyer, M. L. (2005). Self-determination and individuals with severe disabilities: Re-examining meanings and misinterpretations. *Research and Practice for Persons with Severe Disabilities*, 30, 113–120.

Wennberg, B. & Kjellberg, A. (2010). Participation when using cognitive assistive devices - from the perspective of people with intellectual disabilities. *Occupational Therapy International*, 17, 168–176.

World Health Organization. (2001). International classification of functioning, disability and health. World Health Organization. [Online] Available: www.who.int/classifications/icf/en [Accessed November 13 2018].

World Health Organization. (2018). E-health. World Health Organization. [Online] Available: www.who.int/ehealth/en/ [Accessed November 13 2018].

Williams, M. B., Krezman, C. & McNaughton, D. (2008). "Reach for the stars": Five principles for the next 25 years of AAC. *Augmentative and Alternative Communication*, 24, 194–206.

Zhou, L. (2017). The world Internet project international report. In: Lebo, H. (ed.) 8th edn. Los Angeles, CA: USC Annenberg School Center for the Digital Future.

12

Mobile Technology to Facilitate Self-Management and Independence among Adolescents and Young Adults with Disabilities – Best Practices and the State of the Science[1]

Michelle A. Meade
University of Michigan

Marisa J. Perera
University of Miami

CONTENTS

Background 214
Engagement and Tailoring 215
Innovation 216
    Involvement of Stakeholders 217
    Context of Use 217
    Interdisciplinary Collaboration 218
Research: Its Role and Recommendations as Related to mHealth
Interventions 219
    Adoption of Community Participatory Research 220
    Integrate Theory into Design 220
    Identify and Apply Appropriate Methodological Approaches with
    Sufficient Rigor to Advance Understanding 220
    Create Consensus and Standardize Assessment Measures and
    Practices 221
    Engage Participants to Appropriately Power Studies 222
Integrating Technology into HealthCare, Rehabilitation and
Independent Living 222

---

[1] This chapter was written by Dr Michelle A. Meade and Ms. Marisa Perera on behalf of the Panellists and Discussants at the TIKTOC RERC State of Science Conference, which occurred between 19th and 20th October 2017. The TIKTOC RERC SOS Workgroup comprised of collaborating investigators for the TIKTOC RERC, participants of the five panels presenting at the conference, and identified discussants participating in the conference.

Learning Health Systems 223
Support of Key Stakeholders 224
Sustainability and Technology Transfer: Models and Best Practices 225
Transferring Technology 226
Licensees 227
Partnerships 228
Platforms and App Stores 229
Open Source 229
In Summary 230
References 230

Background

Adolescents and young adults (AYAs) with disabilities represent a diverse and often underserved group with unique needs, strengths, challenges, experiences and skills. Mobile technology – including sensors, apps, games and other innovations – represents an opportunity to include and engage AYAs and their family so as to better address their needs and support their transitions to health self-management and independence. The potential benefits associated with mobile technology, though, are likely to be lost if development and innovation do not occur in a space where there is an opportunity for shared understanding and discussion. The processes of development and innovation cannot occur in silos; they must be informed by the knowledge and expertise of individuals with disabilities and their families. Mobile technologies are utilized in different environments including healthcare, education and employment settings, each of which has inherent challenges and potential supports.

This chapter provides guidance and recommendations that should be considered when developing new mobile health (mHealth) technologies to support the self-management and transition of AYAs with disabilities to independence. While not exhaustive, this discussion is relevant to many of the key stakeholders who are likely to be involved in this process. We provide recommendations identified by panellists and participants at the October 2017 State of the Science conference conducted by the *Technology Increasing Knowledge: Technology Optimizing Choice* (TIKTOC) *Rehabilitation Engineering Research Center* (RERC). Funding for the conference was provided by the National Institute of Disability, Independent Living and Rehabilitation Research (NIDILRR), Administration on Community Living (ACL) in the Department of Health and Human Services (HHS; #90RE5012). The present chapter discusses key issues and recommendations related to engagement and tailoring, innovation, research, integration and sustainability.

Engagement and Tailoring

If mHealth is going to be utilized by AYAs with disabilities, it must be usable, useful and engaging (Warschausky et al., 2017a). Patterns of use of mobile technology vary by target population and individual; therefore, mHealth development must consider the user's specific patterns and needs. AYAs with disabilities have unique needs due to undergoing significant developmental, social, emotional, physical and cognitive changes in their transition to emerging adulthood (Sawyer et al., 2007). In contrast to adults, responsibility for an AYA with disabilities' health management is typically negotiated with caregivers and healthcare professionals. As AYAs with disabilities mature, they are expected to take on increased responsibility in managing their health, dealing not only with all the challenges of normal development, but also the tasks and behaviours specific to managing their condition or impairment while still participating in family, peer, educational, employment and/or community activities. To successfully engage these groups/populations, mHealth must consider their unique circumstances.

An important initial consideration in fostering engagement is the end user's motivation to manage his/her personal health (Warschausky et al., 2017b). Among AYAs with disabilities and chronic health conditions, a common barrier to motivation for health self-management is feeling excluded and vulnerable in social situations (Hilli et al., 2018). A desire to fit in can have a negative effect on motivation and self-care (e.g. hiding a diabetes syringe when in public; poor body image due to insulin-related weight gain). To address this barrier and engage AYAs, mHealth can offer opportunities for AYAs to experience belongingness and connectedness to other AYAs with disabilities via mobile platforms. In addition, creating a more structured life during emerging adulthood and integrating disability self-management into routines can aid in enhancing motivation (Hilli et al., 2018). Moreover, mHealth gamification of routine self-care can promote self-management by providing rewards and incentives for completing routine self-management behaviours (Sattoe et al., 2015). For example, in the iMHere 2.0 app (Fairman, 2017; Parmanto et al., 2013), rewards and gamification are integrated with educational information and self-report functions to enhance engagement. Serious games can also be developed as tailored approaches to teach self-management skills and either to model recommended behaviours or demonstrate consequences of poor behavioural compliance (Baranowski, 2017). For example, in the mobile game *SCI Hard*, which was designed for AYAs with spinal cord injuries (SCI) and dysfunction, the player's character must figure out how to get around with SCI, manage their health and engage in activities to save the world, receiving either rewards or negative consequences as a result of their choices as they progress through the game (Meade & Maslowski, 2018).

Mastery motivation, the psychological force that drives a person to persist in attempting to master challenging tasks, is associated with a person's health self-management skills (Hauser-Cram et al, 2014). AYAs with disabilities are at risk for lower mastery motivation levels than typically developing peers (Majnemer et al., 2010). The relation between mastery motivation and health self-management is mediated by executive functioning, suggesting that, despite being motivated to care for oneself and one's health, the individual must possess certain capabilities or have supports for those capabilities to engage in goal-directed, self-care behaviours (Warschausky et al., 2017c). *Executive dysfunction*, or deficits in inhibitory control, working memory or flexible thinking, persist over time and affect the ability to self-manage disability.

During adolescence and young adulthood, executive problems have been speculated to become more problematic (Heffelfinger et al., 2008) and performance of self-management behaviours is low (Psihogios et al., 2015). mHealth must be built to be engaging while also considering and compensating for potential executive deficits. For AYAs with disabilities and executive dysfunction, it is important to assess AYA's capabilities and executive skills over time to ensure that they can adopt and utilize the technology (Jacobson, 2017).

In addition to enhancing motivation, it is important to tailor the presenting problems (i.e. executive dysfunction, sensory/physical impairment) and solutions to the target user community in order to promote effective engagement (Warschausky et al., 2017a). To do so, it is important to draw upon a wide range of expertise while designing the technology. This expertise includes direct involvement of individuals who will use the technology in various environments (e.g. health, educational, employment) as well as programmers and researchers to ensure that the technology can be implemented and sustained. Obtaining information on the users' ability to successfully utilize the technology is imperative to sustain the use of the technology. An *iterative design process* of consistent testing and retesting to track usage patterns over time is critical to ensure that the technology helps the user manage the disability in the longer term. Technology that is scalable and insensitive to time (i.e. independent of proprietary software or hardware that can become inaccessible to users) is imperative for continued engagement with the technology.

Innovation

The vanguard of technology is a dynamic target. At the time this chapter was written, current innovative technical trends that may be incorporated into mHealth approaches included sensing and context awareness, personal informatics, social computing, augmentative and alternative communication (AAC) technologies, artificial intelligence, virtual and augmented reality, virtual personal assistants, robotics and support for DIY practices such as 3D printing. On the other hand, stable factors that foster innovation of mobile technology for self-management and independence among AYAs with disabilities include developing platforms and processes for strong interdisciplinary interaction, attending to the context of technology use, and involving end users throughout development.

Involvement of Stakeholders

Successful innovation in mHealth for AYAs with disabilities requires involvement of the multiple stakeholders. Caregivers (i.e. parents) and health professionals play significant roles in promoting the development of AYA's skills to self-manage health and disability. Involvement, engagement and participation of AYAs and their families in the planning and development of mHealth is likely to contribute to accepted and understood interventions among AYAs (McDonagh & Bateman, 2012). Participatory design allows developers to engage with potential users as data sources and as designers by having them not just provide data about what would work and not work, but actually having them participate in generating ideas for the design itself. Similarly, citizen science allows contributions from individuals with different perspectives in order to reach a specific objective (Newman et al., 2012). One such citizen science organization is Nightscout, an app developed by parents of children with type 1 diabetes to facilitate access to data collected using a glucose monitor via remote monitoring (Lee et al., 2016). Parents voluntarily enter a child's data to a cloud-based shared repository that serves as a resource for both parents and researchers. Building research infrastructure (registry; application) that connects people who want to participate in research with researchers and developers can foster innovative production of technology.

If the goal is to embed the mHealth system into clinical practice, healthcare providers and the healthcare team are critical stakeholders in the participatory design process (Aldiss et al., 2010). Despite technical advances and innovation, care via mHealth is unlikely to advance without engagement of the clinical providers. An example of one such app is GeoPain, which was designed in collaboration with clinicians to allow patients to model and track their pain experience (Maslowski et al., 2014).

Context of Use

When developing apps, interventions or tools to facilitate behaviour change, it is critical to consider the social-environmental pressures around the AYAs with the disability and the context in which the mHealth technology is meant to be used. Only when all phases of development are considered in parallel with the people, organizations and environments that surround the user will the technology be implemented and sustained.

In the face of exponential data growth and tools such as ecological momentary assessment (Rofey et al., 2010; Runyan et al., 2013), the availability of large and precise data sets can aid the innovation process. Specifically, through self-monitoring and availability of big data, AYA users can configure their own patterns and contexts of use. However, big data presents challenges that must be addressed, including protection of privacy of data and time constraints to thoughtfully review large quantities of data.

In addition, there is a need to bridge research prototype efforts with the context of mHealth use by identifying mechanisms that will lead to an efficient and sustainable production system for the technology. Individuals motivated to create prototypes may not be motivated to invest the effort required to move the product into the real world for mass distribution. It is imperative to identify individuals who will bridge the gap from research prototype to sustained production system. A requisite of this process of bridging is consideration of real-world constraints, such as realistic expectations for clinicians and limitations of electronic health records (EHRs; i.e. privacy, security and data ownership).

Interdisciplinary Collaboration

Identification of shared publication venues and priorities across disciplines and across research and applied contexts is important to provide a space for continued innovation. Different research traditions exist and are likely to arise when working across disciplines. For instance, the engineer may consider testing a methodology from the perspective of the usability of a product. Meanwhile, a different and more subjective approach is evaluating whether the methodology improves community living. In either case, it is fundamental to build knowledge that has an inarguable statistical outcome and can be communicated to the appropriate audience. However, if the outcome pertains to how people interact with a computer, pure statistics may not suffice. Rather, qualitative and behavioural knowledge related to the human interaction must be built.

Perhaps more importantly, it is critical to recognize the types of results, outputs and outcomes that are valued by various partners in an interdisciplinary collaboration (Durfee et al., 2017). Within academic environments, for example, many medical researchers may look for partners in schools/departments of engineering, computer science or information with the idea that those individuals would be able and interested in doing the actual development of the mHealth application. However, PhDs who teach in these departments (and their associated graduate students) may be interested and possibly even required to develop unique contributions to the field and to the science. So while computer and information scientists have much to add to an mHealth programme, particularly if the collaboration will be developing something that may be relevant 5 years into the future, they are not contractors or craftsman whose involvement should be expected to be limited to implementing the ideas of others (Durfee et al., 2017).

Research: Its Role and Recommendations as Related to mHealth Interventions

mHealth interventions and approaches have the potential to fit the 'triple aim' paradigm of biomedical research of (1) improving the experience of care and health of populations while also (2) reducing per capita costs and (3) offering opportunities to add significant value to payers and patients by providing low-cost, scalable interventions (Berwick et al., 2008; Wegener, 2017). To achieve such a paradigm, the methodological foundation must be strengthened, the evidence base expanded and the connection between industry development and academic research enhanced. The technology industry has developed thousands of apps to assist individuals with chronic conditions and disabilities in managing their health; however, most include minimal involvement of key stakeholders (including users, clinicians and healthcare providers) and have not been tested for efficacy in a standard process. Simultaneously, academia is developing new technologies and testing for efficacy; however, these apps are generally not available in the marketplace (Kitsiou, 2017). Moreover, because technology is changing so rapidly, few academic institutions can afford to regularly update their apps.

As of the writing of this chapter, research on mHealth for the self-management of AYAs with disabilities was in early stages, with most research in the proof-of-concept phase with few participants (Jones et al., 2018). The high degree of variability between studies limits the ability to identify effective approaches and interventions. Specifically, there is variability in the ways interventions are developed and described, how target populations are identified and defined and the assessment measures used to determine intermediate and long-term outcomes (Zwerink et al. 2014). Gaps in research include lack of evidence for determination of timing and techniques for each group of subjects, inadequate power to detect differences in behaviours and lack of tools to study behavioural change, inconsistent use of theory-based approaches and poor understanding of mechanisms of change. A foundation of evidence must be created, providing evidence on reliability, device validity and efficacy of mHealth for supporting the self-management and independence of AYAs with disabilities. For this to occur, the current status of the research must be recognized in order for proactive steps to be taken to improve its future status.

Adoption of Community Participatory Research

As previously discussed, a keystone to ensure that mHealth approaches improve the experience of care for AYAs with disabilities and other patients is participatory action research that involves stakeholders early in the design phase as well as in setting the agenda, designing the study, implementing the plan, disseminating the study results and sustaining the clinical services and programmes (Ehde et al., 2013). mHealth research for AYAs with disabilities should focus on the adolescent transition to independent living, with attention to the role of caregivers/parents and others (i.e. peers) during this process. Community participatory research can also aid researchers in understanding the perspectives of AYAs with disabilities, as well as their support structures and systems, because the use and integration of mHealth technology most often occurs within a social context.

Integrate Theory into Design

There is a general need to integrate theory and research into design, development and evaluation assessments of the technology (Kitsiou et al., 2017; Meade et al., 2017; Riley et al., 2011). An underlying theoretical basis can inform effective design and content decisions, especially when end user views contradict due to inherent individual differences. For example, mHealth programmes and apps based on principles of cognitive behavioural therapy (CBT) would be expected to promote enhanced health by increasing knowledge, awareness and positive attitudes about specific health issues, with the expectation that positive, congruent behaviours would follow. Assessing effectiveness, then, should include assessments of the degree of change in knowledge and self-efficacy as well as behaviours and health outcomes. Similarly, mHealth interventions based on the theory of planned behaviour would be designed to facilitate goal planning and be evaluated on the extent to which components of this process changed in response to using the app.

Identify and Apply Appropriate Methodological Approaches with Sufficient Rigor to Advance Understanding

The type of research and quality of metrics must be considered given that the individuals who develop and evaluate mHealth technology come from diverse fields and may have different standards, approaches and priorities. Within the health sciences, the general hierarchy of evidence starts with expert opinion, moves on to case studies and cohort studies and advances to randomized controlled trials (RCTs). When designing and evaluating the efficacy of mHealth technology for low-frequency populations, such as individuals with SCI or spina bifida, RCTs involve both time and resources that may be prohibitive in most cases; that is, involving the number of sites to recruit adequate participants may be cost prohibitive or take too long to be relevant for informing technological development. As a result, those RCTs with AYAs with disabilities that are conducted are likely to either be underpowered or inappropriately use broad criteria for inclusion in an attempt to obtain a sufficient sample size. It is critical to be able to conduct the research with the rigor needed to conduct valid results; a well-designed single-subject study may provide richer information than a poorly executed clinical trial (Wills, 2017).

The research pyramid, however, may not be fitting for mHealth as the development of apps is not concerned with proving a concept but rather with working within a business model to reach an effective product. For example, RCTs demand a level of evidence based on standards of statistical significance (i.e. $p < 0.05$) while mHealth demands evidence that some people find the technology helpful. Moreover, mHealth technology and development of apps is advancing faster than the science, and technology can be outdated by the time proof of concept is available. Thus, adopting a business model approach should significantly improve the app technology development process rather than adopting the typical health science approach.

Given the diversity of the audiences and applications, success (acceptance) of the mHealth app or technology itself is going to be defined in a variety of ways that will then be confirmed by the actions of end users. For some it would be reliable employment, and for others it might be just being able to live at home and take meds on time. End users will not rely on the results of an RCT or a review in the medical literature. The end user will try the app and ask if it helps, or ask friends whether it works or not, or is the cost acceptable. Although patients and families make decisions based on those criteria, adoption by clinicians or healthcare systems will be based on scientific evidence as well as the impact of the app on workflow and cost. Thus, it will be important to demonstrate successful outcomes for end users who have different needs and capabilities in defined contexts.

Create Consensus and Standardize Assessment Measures and Practices

Measures and assessment strategies need to be developed and perhaps even mandated to ensure methodological rigor and allow for pooling of data and comparison of outcomes across studies. Assessment strategies may need to consider mediating factors that affect self-efficacy, measurement of change in knowledge base and factors that affect sustainability, including planning for next-generation technology. Consensus standards and recommendations may be developed in collaboration with funding agencies to foster their adoption. It may also be appropriate to bring together experts to develop recommendations to be built into requests for proposals (RFPs). Similar efforts have been successful in promoting international standards and assessments for implementation and reporting of behavioural interventions (Davidson et al., 2003).

Moreover, mHealth usually allows for the capture of data on log-ins, time spent in the app and on what the time is spent. Such usage data should regularly collected for analysis and reported in a standardized manner. Additionally, standardization of terms and the aspects of data that are reported can help to build national networks to promote engagement and recruitment of participants. It is also important to standardize the decision-making process for mHealth development and ensure it is iterative.

Finally, when conducting research on and with AYAs with disabilities, there is a benefit in developing mHealth technology as well as data collection procedures and methodologies that are aimed at the environment and not dependent on individual action. This implies using technology (such as sensors) which can be integrated into the environment and capturing information either on an ongoing or event-specific basis.

Engage Participants to Appropriately Power Studies

As previously stated, most research on mHealth for the self-management of AYAs with disabilities is in the proof-of-concept phase with relatively few participants (Jones et al., 2018). Studies are typically underpowered, have small sample sizes and reliability and validity of data are low due to heterogeneity of assessment measures (Meade et al., 2017). Researchers and funding organizations can address this issue through the creation of national networks to partner with disability organizations and promote participant engagement and recruitment. Alternatively, Centers for Knowledge Translation, such the NIDILRR-funded Center for Knowledge Translation on Technology Transfer (KT4TT) (Buffalo, 2018), may contribute by assessing mediating and moderating factors of core mHealth components to improve methodology and study design. Other methods to engage participants may include being active on social media, reaching out to minority communities and partnering with technology companies to evaluate apps as they are released. Alternatively, it may be possible to partner with various stakeholders to obtain data that is collected on an ongoing basis. Specifically, similar to how insurance claims data can be accessed and analysed by researchers with specific hypotheses, it may be possible to partner with technology companies, insurers or others interested in understanding the cost-effectiveness of a product to access and analyse data from mHealth applications.

Integrating Technology into HealthCare, Rehabilitation and Independent Living

When developing mHealth and other technology to support the self-management and independence of AYAs, three considerations are critical:

(1) how data enters and is used or applied within systems; (2) the social-ecological context of healthcare; and (3) how mobile technology data is incorporated into personal, clinical and employment decisions (Farris et al., 2017). To varying degrees, each of these factors are influenced by *EHRs*, the value placed on creating *learning health systems* (AHRQ, 2018), and the priorities and ability of key stakeholders to use mHealth technologies to enhance existing workflows.

EHRs were introduced in the early seventies, but were not widely adopted until the Health Information Technology for Economic and Clinical Health (HITECH) Act was passed in 2009 and federal funding became available to hospitals in 2011 to support their adoption and set standards for their maintenance (Mann, 2017; Washington et al., 2017). Later policies, including *Fast Healthcare Interoperability Resources (FHIR)* and *Meaningful Use II*, supported better health data transfer between various computers and apps and improved data transfer related to patient portals (HL7.org, 2018; Kitsiou et al., 2006). Today, EHRs are virtually universal, FHIR is improved, many patent portals and mobile health apps exist and smartphones are ubiquitous. Accessibility and engagement is increasing, and there is a flood of data being processed. These resources, however, are not available to all patients, and how to facilitate access to these technologies to allow for the most effective use of the data is not well developed. The future of integrating mHealth and EHRs is focused on improving clinical outcomes and delivering value. To do that, barriers for technical integration must be reduced or eliminated, which requires shared patient/clinician cooperative development that is agile and human centred. Moreover, policy must continue to support the development of accessible health records, patient portals and apps to promote their integration into the healthcare practice (Farris et al., 2017).

Learning Health Systems

The Institute of Medicine (now National Academy of Medicine) called for capturing data from the healthcare encounter and applying the data to improve practice (Academies, 2011; Butzer, 2017). Consistent with this goal, the focus of learning health systems are to systematically integrate internal data and experience with external evidence and then use that knowledge to provide higher quality, safer, and more efficient care (AHRQ, 2018; Academies, 2011). mHealth systems provide a potential mechanism for contributing to this process as information can be collected by individuals or tracked by sensors and sent to the clinician/ health system. There must, however, be a plan to identify the types of data and variables that are worth collecting and managing (Washington et al., 2017). Decisions about what data to collect as well as how to sort, analyse and create visualizations of the data should be based on the data's utility in informing clinical practice and the actions of the provider, patient or someone else in the healthcare system. Issues and ethics associated with privacy also needs to be discussed, as patients need to be able to make informed decisions about who will be able to review their health information and how this will be done (e.g. if the data will be examined individually or in aggregate) to improve processes.

Support of Key Stakeholders

The transition of AYAs with disabilities to independent living, including employment, involves receiving support from key stakeholders (Farris et al., 2017). Transition is not only moving from family-supported living at home to independent living alone – any change is a transition that must be managed. The aftermath of a traumatic injury is a sudden time of transition, but the normal ageing experience is a transition as well, although more gradual. Beyond the role of healthcare providers in transition, there is a less well-defined natural support system for individuals with disabilities that involves family, friends and paid and unpaid caregivers as well as vocational rehabilitation counsellors, therapists, teachers, social workers and others. Mobile technologies, therefore, may be used by (and should be designed with the input of) one or more members of these various groups in order to optimize desired outcomes. Developing based on the interest, motivation and use context of the identified user is therefore critical.

Apps and systems developed for use by clinicians and healthcare providers are often met with a lukewarm reception (Fairman, 2017). Clinicians are wary about additional burdens on their time and can have barriers that prevent adoption. In contrast, reception by AYAs with disabilities and their family members is often more enthusiastic, as they welcome the opportunity to test any tools that may promote better outcomes. Contextual factors such as organizational mandates or peer pressure that may support or hinder the use of technology in general or specific apps should be considered.

Given these considerations, five key recommendations for the integration of apps and mHealth into systems to support AYAs with disabilities are:

1. mHealth development should be based on strong methodology while remaining agile and adaptable. Both development and evaluation should be iterative, which may not be easy for those who are accustomed to the RCT environment. Funding agencies should consider encouraging partnerships for each project that include health systems, research organizations and academia as well as industry. Such partners should value the combination of implementation science and innovative development, and work with one another and end users.

2. Develop a prototype as economically as possible, make the prototype available in the marketplace, obtain funding to support development and evaluation within the marketplace and in the health system, the education system and wherever else the technology most appropriately fits.

3. Conduct a literature review concomitantly with a user review. Funders may require this to answer the question of who will use the app, and whether it has a clear usefulness.

4. Incorporate case examples when describing and conducting outreach associated with mHealth technologies to encourage focus on the objective and to improve the chances of successful adoption and integration. It is critical that the data generated from the app is useful to the physicians or other clinicians, and it must be available promptly, preferably while the user is also immediately available, and it must be easy to understand (perhaps visually). The data must also be accepted and supported by leaders of the organization who own the data.

5. Finally, big data is becoming more important, especially to the research agencies (NIH, CDC, HRSA, etc.), and it should be considered in the context of health in general, mHealth, individualized education plans (IEPs) and employment data. It is particularly critical to remember that the original purpose and intent of many of the codes being analysed, that is, diagnostic codes, measures of functional independence (i.e., FIM scores) and other codes were developed, at least in part, to allow for billing of services. Each entity using the data will submit it and manage it in a way that provides the greatest benefit or, in other words, a way that gets the most money. Clearly, there are incentives, and therefore potential biases, in a system that uses codes tied to payments. A specific example discussed earlier was the different use of the functional independence measure (FIM), which may be calculated one way to show a rapid recovery (which financially benefits the hospital) or another way to show a need for a longer rehabilitation (which financially benefits the rehabilitation facility).

Sustainability and Technology Transfer: Models and Best Practices

Mobile technology requires regular review and maintenance for its continued use and sustainability. Apps, sensors and other mHealth require updates, bug fixes and associated programming every time there is an update of operating systems – whether on mobile phones or computers (for web-based technologies). It is critical that developers plan early for sustainability and technology transfer (Bennett et al., 2017).

Within the context of mHealth, *sustainability* refers to the ability to maintain a usable app, system or product. While funds may be available to create or build a product, finding money to sustain it can be a challenge. Ensuring the longevity of an app or other mHealth technology requires a commitment of time, effort and often money by someone. While the funding source does not have to be the developer/creator of the technology, the developer should expect to provide at least a degree of ongoing effort to facilitate the transition of the product either to another entity or into the open-source community. Without the ongoing expertise and vision of the development team, the transfer process is likely to consist of an idea or model rather than sustainability of the actual product. The more a developer can connect with the variety of groups who may be involved in adopting, sustaining or licencing the product, the more likely it will be sustained.

It is beneficial to the transfer process to spend time at the very beginning of product development to first develop a clear concept of the product before beginning to write code. Without a specific proposal for the app, those persons writing the code may have problems manifesting the idea. The tools and resources available to help developers work out their ideas are better and cheaper now, making it possible to define the product before code needs to be written.

Technical obsolescence also needs to be considered, as it affects most types of mHealth, including apps. Within 5 years, the programs and technology created by the developer may be completely surpassed by either existing options or alternatives that have not yet been envisioned. The research community has a lot to offer on an ongoing basis with respect to the current state of the art as well as the ongoing research of the original development team, offering up new thoughts and options for the future. For this reason, it is important that the project does not end when the research stops. The research community could stay involved at a different level after the app moves to the market, providing their input, advice and guidance for its use, placement, next generations and ongoing development. To continue to maintain awareness of the impact through various phases of the project makes it easier to engage with appropriate partners and to keep options open.

Transferring Technology

Tech transfer involves a diverse ecosystem with varied perspectives and motivations. The genesis of the present technology transfer process began with the Bayh-Dole Act in 1980. Prior to that year, when the federal government funded research, the rights to the intellectual property (IP) stayed with the government. There was little incentive for universities to become involved. The Act allowed universities to become licenced agents for the technology and move it into the marketplace. For those in university or academic settings, Offices of Technology Transfer can both assist with IP protection as well with planning for commercialization. Their primary priority is commercialization and dissemination so as to transfer innovation outside of the university in a good fit with the potential opportunity to have a big impact. The personnel who work in University Tech Transfer Offices are a mix of people with expertise in contract law, sales, marketing, fund development (venture), business operations and relationship building.

The ecosystem of technology transfer involves (1) the researcher and their team, (2) the customer, (3) the public, (4) investors, (5) the licensee, (6) the market and (7) any partners that may exist. It is critical that research and the development team who create the product communicate their vision to their technology transfer office; the sooner this conversation happens, the sooner both parties can identify potential targets to pick up the technology. Many of the activities conducted through Offices of Technology Transfer are about eliminating friction and connecting that fabric between potential endpoints and the people inside in that process. Great partnerships between developers, technology transfer offices and companies start with building a trusting relationship in the space, a common purpose and clear expectations about the objectives which in turn influence contractual milestones.

It is important to remember that the assistive technology space is relationship driven. To give relationships the best chance to survive, there are several key aspects juxtaposed with as many barriers. First, long-term vision must be paired with short-term evaluation and the celebration of small achievements. Another key is maximizing strengths and encouraging partners to share their unique talent and/or understanding of the product's functionality. Similarly, sharing research, development and marketing experience can allow more effective use of intellectual resources in these areas. However, because this is a relationship-based enterprise, failing to build a foundation of trust can be a huge obstacle to success. Avoiding poor communication with peers and partners requires clearly identifying points of contact and ensuring accountability is understood. This should extend to organizational leadership where mutual trust can accelerate the process. There should also be an organizational commitment to the product or process as a defined and unified commitment to success can avoid missteps. Similarly, there must be buy-in at all organizational levels, from the leadership of the organization to the hands-on staff. Some projects fall short, perhaps because the great idea that was developed did not really meet a need, or because an improvement to a technology overcomplicated an aspect of use that users wanted simplified. One outcome of all the effort has been that the research and development processes must be informed by and developed in harmony with the sales and marketing processes.

In the mHealth/mobile technology space, there are four major tech transfer approaches: (1) licensee (traditional) relationships, (2) partnerships, (3) platforms and (4) open source (Bennett, 2017).

Licensees

In the licensee relationship, the researcher/developer owns the product and the university may write the license and find another party, often a commercial entity (or a non-profit), to shepherd the product to market. In this case, the technology transfer process is based on developing partnerships between the individuals, groups or organizations that create the technology and the organization that licences and sustains it. The licencing process does not add value to the product, but it is an activity that must be done in order to attain rights.

In traditional license arrangements, the developers themselves pick up the licence and potentially form a start-up company. The start-up space is highly competitive, and there are significant risks, especially when the start-up is small, thus it is sensible to establish protections. Protections in the 1980s were trademarks and patents, and it was initially believed that all aspects of a start-up needed protection to provide a sufficient period of time to initiate the business and grow. However, building restrictions around the IP and product had limitations. For example, while protective, a non-disclosure agreement (NDA) requires much time and effort and thus may not fit the company's needs.

Finally, the possibility of tiered licencing exists – each person does not have to pay the same amount. Those who can pay should do so, whereas those who cannot pay should consider not doing so. Free versions for people who are in a need-based situation or resource constrained, non-profit-level pricing and commercial pricing are viable options when introducing technology into the marketplace since each individual may not want to use the technology in the same way. However, while freeware may be a helpful option, it does not relieve the licenser of the long-term challenge of supporting the application through programming updates, 'bug fixes' and other activities.

Risk considerations must be assessed when investors join because investors are particularly sensitive to risks that may threaten their investment. Owning a patent has positives and negatives: positives include exclusive control of the product and negatives can result because patents must be defended and litigation is expensive, especially for a small start-up. A start-up needs the right infrastructure to support protections.

In brief, developers need to identify the right partners and, if there is proprietary IP, to determine if protections are needed and develop a clear rationale for establishing them.

Partnerships

The next approach to technology transfer is partnerships. There are three primary types of partnership-based activity: (1) cause based, (2) professional based and (3) community based. These partnerships occur when an academic institution partners with an organization with a higher purpose than just profit. The challenge in a cause-based activity with a higher social obligation commitment is balancing the pros and cons. On the positive side, the enterprise is dedicated and usually market driven; the cons are that it involves managing costs, harmonizing expectations of the various players (product promotion for the benefit of the market or a simple profit objective), measuring progress and gauging the market. As such, it is worthwhile to have discussions with professional and non-profit organizations (particularly those associated with the specific population the mHealth is designed for) that might be willing to adopt, sustain and steward the application for a period of time.

Platforms and App Stores

As of the writing of this chapter, the iTunes store is at its 10-year anniversary. When the store launched, it had 500 apps; today there are approximately 2.2 million apps with approximately 1,300 new apps added each day. Each person utilizing these platforms still have the same challenges of addressing marketing, awareness and community building to promote accessibility and use of the product. As such, as the product is being built, it is worth considering creating a component rather than a stand-alone app; sometimes you do not have to build the house, you only have to build the living room. There are a number of online marketplaces in the algorithm space, including Algorithmia, Apervita and Alteryx, that can be investigated to get a better perspective of what may be involved. In particular, if you have something that you do not necessarily believe needs to be taken the last mile, you may be able to make it available to the public through such methods.

Open Source

Open source refers to freely available code that can be used without (many) restrictions (https://opensource.org/osd). Providing open access can foster growth and flexibility, allowing the technology to develop in ways driven by a user community with both time and resources. At its core, though, open source is a licencing approach and a distribution technique that does not take away the need for potential users to learn about your product or the potential the product may have for their own work and objectives. As such, the impact of the product will be a function of one's ability to build a community around it and to deal with ancillary issues such as identifying and addressing problems and keeping track of versions. The large volume of content available through open-source platform should also be considered as it heightens the importance of having a product that is attention grabbing. Examples of communities and projects that have been built around open-source content include Project Possibility (out of UCLA), FEVA (out of the University of Michigan) and OpenAPS. Project Possibility, in particular, includes many people with disabilities developing and sharing code freely.

In Summary

mHealth development requires more than simply developing a product and releasing it to the public. Even mHealth applications that are created using evidence-based processes and shown to enhance outcomes are likely to be left behind unless there is a clear process for both integrating them into existing systems and ensuring their sustainability. For this reason, it is critical that would-be developers (particularly those in academia) familiarize themselves with the entire process required for an mHealth application to reach a potential user's hands not just now, but also 5 years from now. They need to get a sense of their own time, interests and limitations within this process, and develop relationships with people and organizations who may share at least some of their interests in the identified outcomes. Moreover, as scientists, they should identify existing standards and best practices, document the steps and processes they engage in and share the outcomes that they experience, whether positive or negative, so the researchers who follow them can build on their work.

References

AHRQ. (2018). Learning health systems. From www.ahrq.gov/professionals/systems/learning-health-systems/index.html.

Aldiss, S., Taylor, R. M., Soanes, L., Maguire, R., Sage, M., Kearney, N., & Gibson, F. (2010). Working in collaboration with young people and health professionals. A staged approach to the implementation of a randomised controlled trial. *J Res Nurs*, 16(6), 561–576. doi: 10.1177/1744987110380803.

Baranowski, T. (2017, October 19, 2017). Online and mobile games. *Paper Presented at the TIKTOC RERC State of the Science*, Arlington, VA.

Bennett, D. (2017). Sustainability: Creative solutions to project longevity. *Paper Presented at the TIKTOC RERC State of the Science*, Arlington, VA.

Bennett, D., Herold, R., Maslowski, E., & Parmanto, B. (2017). Sustainability and technology transfer - models and best practices. *Paper Presented at the TIKTOC RERC State of the Science*, Arlington, VA.

Berwick, D. M., Nolan, T. W., & Whittington, J. (2008). The triple aim: Care, health, and cost. *Health Aff*, 27(3), 759–769. doi: 10.1377/hlthaff.27.3.759.

Buffalo, U. O. (2018). Center for Knowledge Translation on Technology Transfer (KTT4TT). From http://sphhp.buffalo.edu/cat/kt4tt.html.

Butzer, J. (2017). Learning health systems: Improving practice via health encounter data. *Paper Presented at the TIKTOC RERC State of the Science*, Arlington, VA.

Davidson, K. W., Goldstein, M., Kaplan, R. M., Kaufmann, P. G., Knatterud, G. L., Orleans, C. Tracy, Spring, B., Trudeau, K. J., & Whitlock, E. P. (2003). Evidence-based behavioral medicine: What is it and how do we achieve it? *Ann Behav Med*, 26(1), 161–171. doi: 10.1207/S15324796ABM2603_01.

Durfee, E., Newman, M., Ackerman, M., Cutrell, E., Ding, D., & Hurst, A. (2017). Innovation in the development of mobile apps. *Paper Presented at the TIKTOC RERC State of the Science*, Arlington, VA.

Ehde, D. M., Wegener, S. T., Williams, R. M., Ephraim, P. L., Stevenson, J. E., Isenberg, P. J., & MacKenzie, E. J. (2013). Developing, testing, and sustaining rehabilitation interventions via participatory action research. *Arch Phys Med Rehabil*, 94(1 Suppl), S30–S42. doi: 10.1016/j.apmr.2012.10.025.

Fairman, A. (2017). Integrating technology into health care, rehabilitation, and independent living. *Paper Presented at the TIKTOC RERC State of the Science*, Arlington, VA.

Farris, K., Butzer, J., Fairman, A., Lord, S., & Mann, D. (2017). Integrating technology into health care, rehabilitation, and independent living. *Paper Presented at the TIKTOC RERC State of the Science*, Arlington, VA.

Hauser-Cram, P., Woodman, A. C., & Heyman, M. (2014). Early mastery motivation as a predictor of executive function in young adults with developmental disabilities. *Am J Intellect Dev Disabil*, 119(6), 536–551. doi: 10.1352/1944-7588-119.6.536.

Heffelfinger, A. K., Koop, J. I., Fastenau, P. S., Brei, T. J., Conant, L., Katzenstein, J., & Sawin, K. J. (2008). The relationship of neuropsychological functioning to adaptation outcome in adolescents with spina bifida. *J Int Neuropsychol Soc*, 14(5), 793–804. doi: 10.1017/S1355617708081022.

Hilli, Y., Lööf, H., Malmberg, J., & Hess, D. (2018). Young and motivated for self-care? An interview study with young adults suffering from type 1 diabetes. *Clin Nurs Stud*, 6(4), 36. doi: 10.5430/cns.v6n4p36.

HL7.org. (2018). FHIR overview. From www.hl7.org/fhir/overview.html.

Institute of Medicine (IOM) of the National Academices. (2011). The learning health system and its innovation collaboratives: Update report. IOMOTN Academies. From www.nationalacademies.org/hmd/Activities/Quality/~/media/Files/Activity%20Files/Quality/VSRT/Core%20Documents/ForEDistrib.pdf.

Jacobson, L. (2017). Considerations for tailoring technology: Executive function. *Paper Presented at the TIKTOC RERC State of the Science*, Arlington, VA.

Jones, M., Morris, J., & Deruyter, F. (2018). Mobile healthcare and people with disabilities: Current state and future needs. *Int J Environ Res Public Health*, 15(3), 515. doi: 10.3390/ijerph15030515.

Kitsiou, S. (2017, October 19, 2017). Mobile apps and connected health devices for self-management of physical, cognitive, and developmental disabilities. *Paper Presented at the TIKTOC RERC State of the Science*, Arlington, VA.

Kitsiou, S., Manthou, V., & Vlachopoulou, M. (2006). Framework for the evaluation of integration technology approaches to healthcare. From http://medlab.cc.uoi.gr/itab2006/proceedings/eHealth/106.pdf.

Kitsiou, S., Pare, G., Jaana, M., & Gerber, B. (2017). Effectiveness of mHealth interventions for patients with diabetes: An overview of systematic reviews. *PLoS One*, 12(3), e0173160. doi: 10.1371.journal.pone.0173160.

Lee, J. M., Hirschfeld, E., & Wedding, J. (2016). A patient-designed do-it-yourself mobile technology system for diabetes promise and challenges for a new Era in medicine. *JAMA*, 315(14), 1447–1448. doi: 10.1001/jama.2016.1903.

Majnemer, A., Shevell, M., Law, M., Poulin, C., & Rosenbaum, P. (2010). Level of motivation in mastering challenging tasks in children with cerebral palsy. *Dev Med Child Neurol*, 52(12), 1120–1126. doi: 10.1111/j.1469-8749.2010.03732.x.

Mann, D. (2017). Integrating technology into healthcare and the EHR. *Paper Presented at the TIKTOC RERC State of the Science*, Arlington, VA.

Maslowski, E., DaSilva, A., Petty, S., & Sheehan, S. (2014). U. O. Michigan. www.geopain.com/ by Moxytech, Inc., Accessed June 12, 2019.

McDonagh, J. E. & Bateman, B. (2012). 'Nothing about us without us': Considerations for research involving young people. *Arch Dis Child Educ Pract Ed*, 97(2), 55–60. doi: 10.1136/adc.2010.197947.

Meade, M., Baranowski, T., Houlihan, B., Kitsiou, S., Wegener, S., & Wills, H. (2017). What does the research say? Evaluation and efficacy of programs and technology for adolescents and young adults. *Paper Presented at the TIKTOC RERC State of the Science*, Arlington, VA.

Meade, M. & Maslowski, E. (2018). Development of a serious gaming app for individuals with spinal cord injury. *J Technol Pers Disabil*, 6, 162–180.

Newman, G., Wiggins, A., Crall, A., Graham, E., Newman, S., & Crowston, K. (2012). The future of citizen science: Emerging technologies and shifting paradigms. *Front Ecol Environ*, 10(6), 298–304. doi: 10.1890/110294.

Parmanto, B., Pramana, G., Yu, D. X., Fairman, A. D., Dicianno, B. E., & McCue, M. P. (2013). iMHere: A novel mHealth system for supporting self-care in management of complex and chronic conditions. *JMIR mHealth uHealth*, 1(2), e10. doi: 10.2196/mhealth.2391.

Psihogios, A. M., Kolbuck, V., & Holmbeck, G. N. (2015). Condition self-management in pediatric spina bifida: A longitudinal investigation of medical adherence, responsibility-sharing, and independence skills. *J Pediatr Psychol*, 40(8), 790–803. doi: 10.1093/jpepsy/jsv044.

Riley, W., Rivera, D., Atienza, A., Nilsen, W., Allison, S., & Mermelstein, R. (2011). Health behavior models in the age of mobile interventions: Are our theories up to the task? *Transl Behav Med*, 1(1), 53–71.

Rofey, D. L., Hull, E. E., Phillips, J., Vogt, K., Silk, J. S., & Dahl, R. E. (2010). Utilizing ecological momentary assessment in pediatric obesity to quantify behavior, emotion, and sleep. *Obesity (Silver Spring)*, 18(6), 1270–1272. doi: 10.1038/oby.2009.483.

Runyan, J. D., Steenbergh, T. A., Bainbridge, C., Daugherty, D. A., Oke, L., & Fry, B. N. (2013). A smartphone ecological momentary assessment/intervention "app" for collecting real-time data and promoting self-awareness. *PLoS One*, 8(8), e71325. doi: 10.1371/journal.pone.0071325.

Sattoe, J. N., Bal, M. I., Roelofs, P. D., Bal, R., Miedema, H. S., & van Staa, A. (2015). Self-management interventions for young people with chronic conditions: A systematic overview. *Patient Educ Couns*, 98(6), 704–715. doi: 10.1016/j.pec.2015.03.004.

Sawyer, S., Drew, S., & Duncan, R. (2007). Adolescents with chronic disease--the double whammy. *Aust Fam Physician*, 36(8), 622–627.

Warschausky, S., Jacobson, L., Joye, D., Maslowski, E., & Seel, R. (2017a). Engagement and tailoring of mobile apps. *Paper Presented at the TIKTOC RERC State of the Science*, Arlington, VA.

Warschausky, S., Jacobson, L., Seel, R., Joye, D., & Maslowski, E. (2017b). Engagement and tailoring of mobile technologies for health self-management. *Paper Presented at the TIKTOC RERC State of the Science*, Arlington, VA.

Warschausky, S., Kaufman, J. N., Evitts, M., Schutt, W., & Hurvitz, E. A. (2017c). Mastery motivation and executive functions as predictors of adaptive behavior in adolescents and young adults with cerebral palsy or myelomeningocele. *Rehabil Psychol, 62*(3), 258–267. doi: 10.1037/rep0000151.

Washington, V., DeSalvo, K., Mostashari, F., & Blumenthal, D. (2017). The HITECH Era and the path forward. *N Engl J Med, 377*(10), 904–906. doi: 10.1056/NEJMp1703370.

Wegener, S. (2017, October 19, 2017). Building an evidence base for mHealth applications: foundations and future. *Paper Presented at the TIKTOC RERC State of the Science*, Arlington, VA.

Wills, H. (2017, October 19, 2017). Technology-based self-monitoring: School, work, community. *Paper Presented at the TIKTOC RERC State of the Science*, Arlington, VA.

Zwerink, M., Brusse-Keizer, M., van der Valk, P. D., Zielhuis, G. A., Monninkhof, E. M., van der Palen, J., Frith, PA, & Effing, T. (2014). Self-management for patients with COPD. *Cochrane Database Syst Rev.* From http://airplusr.com/wordpress/wp-content/uploads/2017/07/Zwerink_et_al-2014-The_Cochrane_Library.pdf.

13

Principles and Practical Uses of Virtual Reality Games as a Physical Therapy Strategy

Lorena Cruz

Faculdades Integradas da União Educacional do Planalto Central (Faciplac)

Felipe Augusto dos Santos Mendes, Silvia Gonçalves
Ricci Neri, and Rodrigo Luiz Carregaro

Universidade de Brasília (UnB)

CONTENTS

Terminology, General Concepts and Distinctions 235
Possible Uses of VRGs in Physical Therapy Practice 237
Evidence of VRGs in the Physical Fitness Context 239
   Main Characteristics of VRG Interventions 240
   Effects of VRG Interventions 243
   Considerations 244
Evidence of VRGs in Rehabilitation: Emphasis on Parkinson's Disease 244
   Main Characteristics of VRG Interventions for PD 245
   Effects of VRG Interventions in PD 247
   Considerations 247
Clinical Case 248
Final Considerations 250
References 251

Terminology, General Concepts and Distinctions

According to Dempsey et al. (1996), 'a game is a set of activities involving one or more players. It has goals, constraints, payoffs, and consequences. A game is rule-guided and artificial in some respects. Finally, a game involves some aspect of competition, even if that competition is with oneself'. Some games do not require or improve skills used in other areas of activity, while others provide meaning and purpose outside the gaming context. The use of games with a focus beyond playfulness is known as gamification, a concept described by Deterding et al. (2011) as 'an umbrella term for the use of video game elements (rather than full-fledged games) to improve user experience and user engagement in non-game services and applications'.

Gamification provides interesting types of interventions, such as Edutainment games (EGs), which combine education and entertainment. In EGs, gaming elements can have a positive impact on attention and learning (Blumberg et al., 2013; Jarvin, 2015), as demonstrated by enhanced attention abilities in children after playing action video games (visual selective attention, attention time and faster accurate responses) (Qiu et al., 2018; Cardoso-Leite and Bavelier, 2014; Dye et al., 2009).

Serious Games (SGs) are an EG modality that presents an apparent contradiction because they combine educational contents and entertainment but with goals beyond playfulness. SGs aim to create instructionally sound and learning experiences for a wide variety of audiences (Charsky, 2010). 'Seriousness' can, for example, be used for health promotion and education by helping players to understand and improve the management of chronic conditions and to avoid risk factors such as tobacco and alcohol use, unhealthy diet and physical inactivity (Tolentino et al., 2015). This is an interesting application, given that the control of these factors has been shown to reduce the occurrence of morbidities such as obesity and hypertension (Prochaska and Prochaska, 2011). Changes in health-related behaviours were also found in children with cancer who played a game called Re-Mission© (HopeLab, 2004), in which a nanobot shoots cancer cells, overcomes bacterial infections and manages signs of nausea and constipation. This intervention succeeded in improving adherence to treatment, self-efficacy and cancer-related knowledge (Granic et al., 2014; Kato et al., 2008).

Active or interactive video games require players to be in constant movement in front of a screen as the player's body is the main game controller (avatar). When these games aim to provide some kind of enjoyable physical activity, they are called exergames (games to exercise). Such games can make use of immersion in augmented reality or just transfer the three-dimensional player's space into the two-dimensional game screen. This pervasive technology is an unexploited research field in the context of physical fitness. Exergames are motion based and the players have to move their body to complete challenges and attain goals. The energy expenditure can be twice as high as that of sedentary games (Lanningham-Foster et al., 2006). These applications focus mainly on improving the levels of physical activity and home-based exercise and rehabilitation (Choi et al., 2017; Dithmer et al., 2016) and are an effective way of promoting light- to moderate-intensity physical activity (Peng et al., 2011). In addition, exergames may help players to achieve the exercise levels recommended by the American College of Sports Medicine guidelines (Perrier-Melo et al., 2014), although they require keen visual–spatial skills, hand–eye or foot–eye coordination, divided attention and quick reaction time to operate and overcome the challenges. Thus, there are added benefits to the cognitive impact of exergames (Staiano and Calvert, 2011; Maillot et al., 2012).

In order to implement digital or virtual media elements as an intervention strategy, specific platforms or equipment can be adopted. Currently, mobile devices (e.g. smartphones, tablets and smartwatches), commercial consoles (e.g., Xbox, PlayStation and Nintendo) and desktop computers are widely available, and the choice may be influenced by several aspects. Smartphones and smartwatches are able to track daily activities and measure specific data such as level of physical activity, walking distance, heart rate and sleep quality, whereas consoles with motion sense technology can scan body movements to track their accuracy and motor skill levels. The use of computers and mobile devices are already blended within the real life and the 'virtual world', influenced by information and communication technologies in people's daily life. This interaction is called 'pervasive computing', 'everyware', or 'internet of things'. In this context, these games employ a so-called 'augmented reality', which combines virtual plots and characters with real places and objects to make the game as close to reality as possible. The contents and activities are located in real physical places, or demand actual physical activity, thus providing a feeling that the virtual reality can surpass the game itself (Waern et al., 2009). Some examples of games designed for mobile devices using GPS location-based augmented reality are Zombies, Run!© by Six To Start, SpecTrek© by Spectrekking, and, the most well-known, Pókemon Go© from Niantic Inc. The latter was able to increase the player's average physical activity by around 26% (Althoff et al., 2016). However, there are no follow-up studies, which examined the long-term effectiveness or sustainability, or even the accuracy of physical activity tracking (LeBlanc and Chaput, 2017).

Virtual reality games (VRGs) have a pervasive technology capable of creating an effect known as game transfer phenomena (GTP), described as altered sensory perception, mental process and behaviour transfer from the video-game 'world' to real life (Ortiz de Gortari et al., 2011). Possibly, due to an increased realism, the brain perceives virtual reality as an objective reality within optimal conditions (Dindar and Ortiz de Gortari, 2017). Players may experience altered visual, auditory and body perceptions, automated mental process and altered behaviours, usually occurring during daily activities. Also, memories from the games can even be as memorable as real-life ones (Dindar and Ortiz de Gortari, 2017; Ortiz de Gortari and Griffiths, 2016).

Possible Uses of VRGs in Physical Therapy Practice

VRGs are a promising healthcare tool (Tieri et al., 2018). Within the context of physical fitness and rehabilitation, VRGs are prescribed to encourage participation and to improve adherence to physical therapy (PT) interventions

(Warburton et al., 2007; Burke et al., 2009). This is particularly important, given that previous studies reported an association between high adherence and better results in functional outcomes (Lange et al., 2010; Campbell et al., 2005). VRGs can provide scenarios that successfully attract the players' attention. Additionally, simulated situations can be used to elicit a thrilling atmosphere, while the patient moves in a safe and controlled environment (Wüest et al., 2014). During gaming, players direct their attention to the experience rather than the physical impairment, which makes it enjoyable (Lange et al., 2010). Subsequently, patients are more likely to attend an adequate number of sessions, which will be a determining factor in increasing intervention frequency thus inducing neural plasticity and motor learning (Lange et al., 2010).

Rather than delivering motor and cognitive training in isolated sessions, VRGs also present an opportunity to combine physical activity and cognitively challenging tasks (Stanmore et al., 2017). The engagement of patients in virtual motor and cognitive activities, simultaneously, requires an integration of the movements and cognitive demands of these tasks (Mirelman et al., 2010). This means that VRGs could be explored as therapeutic tools to deliver meaningful and purposeful stimulation by means of motor-cognitive exercises in a quantifiable manner that allows real-time feedback and an enriched auditory and visual environment (Alves et al., 2018). That kind of training can promote neuroplasticity, stimulating motor learning and enhancing both cognitive and motor rehabilitation (Barry et al., 2014; Teo et al., 2016).

Another key feature of interventions using VRGs is the acquisition of skills in the context in which they need to be applied, resulting in more meaningful learning (Lange et al., 2010; Teo et al., 2016). By replicating real-life scenarios, VRGs provide greater potential for transference to activities of daily living (Dockx et al., 2016; Crocetta et al., 2017). In addition, VRGs offer two kinds of extrinsic and essential feedback for learning: knowledge of performance and knowledge of results. The former refers to information on movement performance (mainly given in the form of visual and audio feedback) and the latter refers to information on the outcome of the performance (mainly given in the form of scores during and at the end of the sessions) (Adamovich et al., 2009; van den Heuvel et al., 2013). It is important to highlight that this feedback is usually augmented compared to that of conventional interventions, and that visual feedback is more available than audio feedback. Another aspect of VRGs intervention is the enhancement of observational learning. The observation of goal-oriented movements activates parts of the brain involved with physical performance, allowing a motor programme to be developed, facilitating both motor planning and execution (Pelosin et al., 2010; Buccino et al., 2011).

Moreover, VRGs can be successfully implemented in a wide variety of settings (Levac et al., 2015), such as clinical environments (Howcroft et al., 2012; Shin et al., 2014) and at home (Schoene et al., 2013; Golomb et al., 2010). VRGs also have the potential for inclusion in a social context, where individuals can play with others or against each other in competitive circumstances. In addition, healthcare could shift from traditional approaches to more inclusive and innovative interventions. For instance, groups of participants could have the opportunity to play together, remotely, using the Internet (Skjæret et al., 2016).

Due to these possibilities, the use of VRGs is becoming increasingly popular. In Australia, approximately 76% of stroke rehabilitation units already have access to this tool (NSF, 2012). VRGs were also described as the most prevalent assistive technology used by physical therapists in stroke rehabilitation in the United Kingdom (Demain et al., 2013). In the United States, occupational and physical therapists were surveyed on their opinion on VRGs use during rehabilitation of patients with neurological conditions and the majority of the therapists found VRGs easy to operate, safe to use and, in their opinion, they should be used as a complementary tool during inpatient and outpatient care (Fung et al., 2010).

The competencies required by physical therapists to implement VRGs into their practice are similar to those required during conventional approaches. However, in order to include VRGs into clinical practice, some specific skills and basic knowledge should be addressed. First, basic training on how to use the technology (e.g. mobile, consoles or desktop) is necessary. Secondly, it is essential to learn how to link and/or choose the nature/types of VRGs (e.g. immersive) and their expected effects based on the primary and secondary outcomes. Finally, therapists need to be aware of the benefits and challenges provided by each tool/game and be able to monitor the rehabilitation progress and document whether outcomes are being achieved (Levac and Galvin, 2013).

Because an unskilled physical therapist can hinder the potential of the tool, or even render it dangerous, resources are emerging to support such clinical reasoning (Levac et al., 2015; Anderson et al., 2015; Galvin and Levac, 2011). For instance, Anderson et al. (2015) developed a practical guide on the use of VRGs to promote movement recovery in stroke rehabilitation, describing the characteristics of the patients and how the games could be beneficial. The authors also describe commonly available gaming systems that could be integrated into PT practice and compile examples of games that incorporate useful movements for rehabilitation (Anderson et al., 2015). Thus, we recommend a critical reading of these emerging resources as a guide to clinical decision-making.

Evidence of VRGs in the Physical Fitness Context

There is a range of effects attributed to VRGs that could be useful for improving physical function, such as dual-task training (de Bruin et al., 2010; Shubert, 2011) and the possibility of a self-paced experience (Kueider et al.,

2012). Older individuals can be one of the most benefited by VRGs given that this population is exposed to numerous risk factors, many influenced by physiological adaptations of the ageing process, causing an increase in physical deficits such as muscle weakness and balance problems (Nawaz et al., 2016; van Diest et al., 2013). These problems can lead to the occurrence of falls, one of the leading causes of impairment and accidental death (Nevitt et al., 1991). The annual prevalence of falling events varies from 30% to 50% in older individuals aged 65 years and older (Shubert, 2011). In this context, the use of VRGs as an intervention focused on the improvement of functional capacity can be useful (van Diest et al., 2013).

This section aims to present the use of VRGs as an intervention strategy for physical therapists and to summarize the applicability and scientific evidence. The main question is: Can the use of VRGs in individuals without dysfunction be a viable strategy to improve physical-related outcomes such as muscle strength, balance and mobility? For this purpose, studies with community-dwelling older adults without dysfunction will be explored.

Main Characteristics of VRG Interventions

The purpose of VRG interventions varies according to the population and the clinical condition. In older individuals without dysfunction, the objectives are mainly focused on the prevention of injuries/impairments and the improvement of outcomes related to physical function (Tripette et al., 2017). The most common outcome in VRG interventions is postural balance (Hsieh et al., 2014; Maillot et al., 2012, 2014; Bieryla and Dold, 2013; Lai et al., 2013; Schoene et al., 2013; Rendon et al., 2012; Singh et al., 2013; Duque et al., 2013; Franco et al., 2012; Pluchino et al., 2012; Toulotte et al., 2012; Szturm et al., 2011; Jorgensen et al., 2012; Tripette et al., 2017). Other outcomes of interest are lower-limb strength (Maillot et al., 2012, 2014; Daniel, 2012; Jorgensen et al., 2012), reaction time (Schoene et al., 2013; Maillot et al., 2012; Singh et al., 2013; Lee et al., 2011), mobility (Schoene et al., 2013; Singh et al., 2013; Szturm et al., 2011), energy expenditure, heart rate and oxygen consumption (Peng et al., 2011).

The intervention programme needs to be properly designed and well structured (e.g. weekly frequency and duration). Table 13.1[1] provides examples of different characteristics and protocols of VRG intervention. For instance, studies that used VRGs focusing on the improvement of physical fitness have adopted protocols lasting 2 to 20 weeks (Toulotte et al., 2012; Kubicki et al., 2011). Nonetheless, as an overall recommendation, the effects seem to be more evident when interventions at least 3–4 weeks in length are adopted. Regarding frequency, interventions may vary from 1 to 5 days a

---

[1] The table is merely descriptive and cannot be used as a definitive guide for choosing protocols. We recommend a critical reading and the analysis of the reviews cited in this chapter before clinical decision-making.

week (Toulotte et al., 2012; Hsieh et al., 2014), with sessions lasting 15–70 min (Toulotte et al., 2012; Pluchino et al., 2012; Maillot et al., 2012, 2014; Pichierri et al., 2012a, Schoene et al., 2013). Unfortunately, there is great heterogeneity in intervention protocols. To date, there are no standardized protocols for improving physical fitness and health-related outcomes in healthy older adults (Neri et al., 2017; Molina et al., 2014; Tripette et al., 2017).

TABLE 13.1

Examples of VRG Protocols and Intervention Effects

Authors	Participants	VRGs Description	Outcomes	Effects
Bieryla and Dold (2013)	Community-dwelling older adults	**Console:** Nintendo Wii (Wii Fit and Wii Balance Board). **Games:** Yoga (half-moon, chair, warrior), Aerobic (torso twists) and Balance (soccer heading, ski jump). **Description:** two sets for each game. **Protocol:** Session: 30 min Frequency: 3×/week Duration: 3 weeks (plus 1-month follow-up) Supervised	Balance (BBS), Mobility (TUG)	VRGs: Improved balance measurements (three points on the BBS) after 1-month follow-up. Mobility (TUG) was not different between pre- versus post-intervention
Maillot et al. (2014)	Community-dwelling older adults	**Console:** Nintendo Wii (Wii Remote, the Nunchuk and the Wii Balance Board) **Games:** Wii Tennis, Wii Boxing, Wii Soccer Headers, Wii Ski Jump, Hula Hoop and Wii Marbles **Description:** Each session divided into segments: (1) Playing Wii Tennis or Wii Boxing in pairs and (2) Playing in the Balance Board (Wii Soccer Headers, Wii Ski Jump, Hula Hoop and Wii Marbles) alone. **Protocol:** Session: 60 min Frequency: 2×/week Duration: 12 weeks No description whether supervised or not	Lower-limb strength (CS test), Cardiovascular fitness (6MWT)	VRGs: Pre- versus Post-intervention improvement of 26 chair stands on CS test and 55 m in the 6MWT

(Continued)

TABLE 13.1 (*Continued*)

Examples of VRG Protocols and Intervention Effects

Authors	Participants	VRGs Description	Outcomes	Effects
Jorgensen et al. (2012)	Community-dwelling older adults	**Console:** Nintendo Wii **Games:** Table tilt, slalom ski, perfect 10, tight rope tension, penguin slide **Description:** Each session included an initial balance exercise (games; two-thirds duration of the session) followed by a muscle conditioning exercise (standing rowing squat; one-third duration of the session). **Protocol:** Session: approximately 70 min Frequency: 2×/week Duration: 10 weeks Supervised	Mobility (TUG), Lower-limb strength (Leg Press MIVC)	VRGs: Mobility and strength were improved (250 N in the leg press MVIC and 1.3 s in the TUG)

6MWT: 6-m walking test; BBS, Berg balance scale; MVIC, maximum voluntary isometric contraction; TUG, Timed Up and Go test.

Commercial video game consoles such as Nintendo Wii or Microsoft Xbox are the most frequently used (Cho et al., 2014; Hsieh et al., 2014; Maillot et al., 2012, 2014; Bieryla and Dold, 2013; Singh et al., 2012, 2013; Franco et al., 2012; Pluchino et al., 2012; Toulotte et al., 2012; Jorgensen et al., 2012; Lai et al., 2013; Pichierri et al., 2012b; Tripette et al., 2017). From a practical standpoint, commercial gaming consoles and off-the-shelf games are cheaper and provide many options and variations, which may facilitate the implementation of VRGs in clinical practice. However, the selection of games available on these consoles should be based on the purposes of the intervention (and outcomes). For instance, Maillot et al. (2014) presented a structured programme focused on improving lower-limb strength, postural balance and cardiovascular fitness. Accordingly, the authors selected games characterized by wide movements that involved cardiorespiratory activity, muscle resistance (e.g. tennis and boxing), weight transfer and body weight resistance, all of which proved to be useful and sensitive to their purposes. Therefore, the properties of the games are an important step towards the benefits of VRG interventions. At the end of this chapter, we present a clinical case that illustrates the process of selecting a game and structuring the intervention.

VRGs usability is an interesting issue to be considered in the design of interventions. Nawaz et al. (2016) defined usability as 'the extent to which a product can be used by specified users to achieve specified goals with effectiveness, efficiency, and satisfaction'. Therefore, some aspects of VRGs should be considered, as they may help to improve adherence and motivation:

- Immediate and positive feedback (use of scores and audiovisual feedback);
- Competition (e.g. comparison of scores and adherence between or within participants);
- Social interaction between participants;
- Presence of challenge (e.g. game stages);
- Group play.

Effects of VRG Interventions

Balance is one of the most common outcomes in VRG interventions (Miller et al., 2014; Neri et al., 2017). According to van Diest et al. (2013), proper postural control requires several motor skills and is a prerequisite for daily life activities. Studies demonstrated that VRGs had significant and positive effects on balance in healthy older adults (Cho et al., 2014; Hsieh et al., 2014; Maillot et al., 2012, 2014; Bieryla and Dold, 2013; Lai et al., 2013; Schoene et al., 2013; Kubicki et al., 2011; Rendon et al., 2012; Lee et al., 2011; Jorgensen et al., 2012; Duque et al., 2013; Szturm et al., 2011). Moreover, the adoption of balance board and weight shift accessories seems to be an important strategy towards the improvement of balance (van Diest et al., 2013; Miller et al., 2014).

Miller et al. (2014) showed that balance improvements (measured by the Berg balance scale (BBS) and Single Leg Stance Time) were associated with sessions lasting 20–40 min, two to three times a week, for at least 6 weeks. Neri et al. (2017) showed that VRGs improved balance when compared to no treatment and conventional interventions. They found significant improvements of 2.99 points (95% CI: 1.80–4.18) in the BBS in favour of VRGs (versus no treatment) after training sessions lasting 30 min, three to five times a week, for 3–6 weeks. However, these findings should be interpreted with caution due to the high risk of bias of the studies.

Mobility is an important outcome commonly assessed by the Timed Up and Go (TUG) test (Molina et al., 2014). Previous systematic reviews showed improvements in TUG after VRG interventions (Neri et al., 2017; Molina et al., 2014). Neri et al. (2017) showed that VRGs led to significant improvement in the TUG test after 3–6 weeks (–1.2 s) and 8–12 weeks (–0.8 s) compared with no treatment. Overall, effects were attained by interventions composed of sessions lasting 30 min, three to five times a week (3- to 6-week duration) and 15–60 min, two to three times a week (8- to 12-week duration). However, the reviews show that even though VRGs may have positive effects on mobility, there are still many inconsistencies in the studies (Miller et al., 2014), in part due to the high risk of bias (Neri et al., 2017) and heterogeneity of the protocols (Molina et al., 2014).

Muscle strength is also benefited by VRGs (Rodrigues et al., 2018; Neri et al., 2017). Neri et al. (2017) showed increases in lower-limb strength attributed to VRGs and superiority of this intervention over no treatment and conventional treatment (such as usual care). Other studies demonstrated that the chair-stands test (CST) and maximum voluntary isometric contraction (MVIC), measured on the leg press, had improved after 10–12 weeks compared to a placebo intervention and no treatment, respectively (Maillot et al., 2014; Jorgensen et al., 2012) (See Table 13.1). Yet another study demonstrated that VRG dance training for 40 min per session, three times a week, for 12 weeks, increased the eccentric peak torque of the quadriceps muscle by 8.5% (Rodrigues et al., 2018); however, there are still some issues regarding this outcome. Molina et al. (2014) address guidelines showing that a minimum required amount of strengthening exercises, twice a week or more, is recommended for older adults. Their findings demonstrated that a combined intervention (e.g. VRGs and resistance and balance exercises) are more adequate and may provide greater gains in functionality. Conversely, the dosage and effects of VRG interventions alone on muscle strength are still unclear.

Considerations

Current evidence suggests that VRGs are a viable intervention tool for physical therapists seeking to improve fitness-related outcomes. VRGs may be successfully implemented in healthy populations (e.g. community-dwelling older adults). Accordingly, it is expected that outcomes such as balance, mobility and muscle strength improve after interventions that include VRGs, with a duration of at least 3–4 weeks. Nevertheless, there is no consensus regarding the most suitable protocol for attaining those effects due to the lack of standardization in the intervention protocols.

Evidence of VRGs in Rehabilitation: Emphasis on Parkinson's Disease

VRGs have been widely used in neurorehabilitation as they have been shown to be suitable and to provide skill re-learning and retention. Moreover, VRG interventions are deemed to induce motor and cognitive recovery for people with motor and/or mental health dysfunctions such as cerebral palsy, Parkinson's Disease (PD), traumatic brain injury, stroke and anxiety disorders (Teo et al., 2016; Alves et al., 2018). It is not surprising that VRGs have been suggested as a tool to engage patients with PD in long-term interventions, given that, first, PD is one of the most common neurodegenerative disorders worldwide; secondly, PD leads to motor and cognitive impairments;

thirdly, sustained exercise is considered essential to obtain optimal performance and maintain independence in daily life activities in these patients; and finally, people with PD are known to use visual and/or auditory cues to improve physical performance.

Recent reviews (Mirelman et al., 2010; Barry et al., 2014; Dockx et al., 2016; Harris et al., 2015; Stanmore et al., 2017; Cano Porras et al., 2018) showed positive effects of VRGs in patients with PD (mainly in gait, balance and cognitive tests) when compared to control interventions. Studies included in those reviews also demonstrated that VRGs are a viable option for these patients as they showed improved gameplay (dos Santos Mendes et al., 2012; Pompeu et al., 2012). However, VRGs need to be tailored towards specific disease features, taking into account safety and feasibility (dos Santos Mendes et al., 2012; Yang et al., 2016; Gandolfi et al., 2017). In addition, VRGs may be more useful for PD as an adjunct to conventional treatment rather than as a standalone intervention (Barry et al., 2014; Teo et al., 2016).

In this section, we discuss VRGs as an intervention strategy for patients with PD and summarize the applicability and scientific evidence. The main question is: Can the use of VRGs in patients with PD be a viable strategy to improve motor and cognitive outcomes? For this purpose, studies involving patients with PD will be explored.

Main Characteristics of VRG Interventions for PD

The current lack of standardization of tools, systems and dosage limit the evidence on VRGs (Mirelman et al., 2013). Moreover, the efficacy of VRGs cannot be determined for people with PD (Harris et al., 2015) as the evidence is still lacking regarding safety and effectiveness (Cano Porras et al., 2018). Nevertheless, VRGs can be a feasible intervention to minimize motor and cognitive impairments in people with PD (Mirelman et al., 2013; Barry et al., 2014; Dockx et al., 2016; Cano Porras et al., 2018).

Even though the results are inconclusive, VRG training is as effective as conventional therapies for PD (Dockx et al., 2016). The combination of VRGs and conventional interventions was considered safe and more effective compared to conventional or VRG interventions alone (Barry et al., 2014). While VRGs may complement exercise therapy, the use of commercial consoles may be too complex (Barry et al., 2014). Despite the common use of commercial VRGs systems, it is not known whether they are appropriate for all patients, given that they were developed for entertainment purposes (dos Santos Mendes et al., 2012; Teo et al., 2016).

To support the reader regarding the different characteristics and protocols used in some VRG interventions in PD studies, data from six recent reviews on the topic are described in Table 13.2.[1] The data extracted from these reviews provide information on important aspects that may help readers to design interventions. The interventions explored in these studies are mainly focused on the improvement of balance and gait. Data from two

TABLE 13.2

Main Characteristics of VRGs Interventions in PD Studies

Authors	Studies Included	Outcomes	Average Number of Sessions	Average Session Duration (min)	Average Sessions/ Week	Average Total Duration of Intervention (h)	Association with Conventional Therapy (%)	VRG Systems Used
Mirelman et al. (2013)	5	Gait and balance	15	33	2,4	8,5	60	60% used Nintendo Wii 40% used customized
Barry et al. (2014)	7	Gait and balance	14	50	2,5	13	NI	85% used Nintendo Wii 15% used Playstation
Harris et al. (2015)	2	Balance	13	45	2	10	100	50% used Nintendo Wii 50% used customized
Dockx et al. (2016)	8	Gait, balance and quality of life	16	38	2,5	9	50	38% used Nintendo Wii 62% used customized
Cano Porras et al. (2018)	18	Gait and balance	15	50	2,5	12,5	NI	NI
Stanmore et al. (2017)	3	Cognition	14	38	NI	9	33	66% used Nintendo Wii 34% used customized

NI, not informed.

reviews, however, also included quality of life (Dockx et al., 2016) and cognition (Stanmore et al., 2017).

Regarding the number of sessions, there were variations between 13 and 16 sessions, with duration between 33 and 50 min each, over a period of two to two-and-a-half weeks. Mirelman et al. (2013) established that a dosing effect associated with more-intense training leads to greater improvements, mainly in gait parameters. Overall, the studies combined VRGs with conventional interventions, and the majority of these studies used Nintendo Wii or customized virtual reality systems. Interestingly, studies adopting the Xbox Kinect were not included in these reviews, even though some studies adopted this system for individuals with PD (Galna et al., 2014; Pompeu et al., 2014).

Effects of VRG Interventions in PD

VRGs provide not only a useful alternative to conventional interventions for improvement in gait, but also other benefits when combined with a range of interventions. These additional benefits seem to rely on the capability of VRGs to explore task variation and repetition, multisensory feedback and motivation (Cano Porras et al., 2018). Studies demonstrated positive effects after VRG interventions in step and stride length (Liao et al., 2015; Shen and Mak, 2014, 2015), gait speed (Zettergren et al., 2011; Shen and Mak, 2014, 2015; Esculier et al., 2012), obstacle negotiation (Mirelman et al., 2011; Liao et al., 2015) and freezing of gait (Killane et al., 2015). Some studies also demonstrated improvement in dual-task performance during gait after interventions using the Nintendo Wii balance board (Killane et al., 2015; Alves et al., 2018) and treadmill training with virtual obstacles (Mirelman et al., 2010).

The efficacy of VRGs for improving balance cannot be determined for people with PD. However, some studies reported equivalent balance improvements comparing VRG interventions to conventional balance exercises (Harris et al., 2015). Balance has been measured more often by clinical tests such as the Berg balance scale and the TUG test. Furthermore, VRG interventions in PD have presented moderate to large effects on global cognition compared to active control groups (Stanmore et al., 2017). Studies have shown benefits of VRGs for domain-specific tasks of executive functions, such as inhibitory control and cognitive flexibility, and for visuospatial skills, attention and processing speed (Pompeu et al., 2012; Zimmermann et al., 2014), memory, attention and reversibility (Alves et al., 2018).

Considerations

The current evidence demonstrates potential applications of VRG interventions for people with PD, mainly in gait and balance impairments. However, relevant issues need to be addressed in the near future, such

as the risk of bias in PD clinical trials. Future research should standardize the outcome measures and implement adequate follow-up assessments
to examine the long-term effects of VRGs. Finally, empirical evidence is
required to provide well-substantiated recommendations regarding the
frequency, duration and content of VRG interventions. Further research
should attempt to differentiate clinically oriented VRG interventions performed with commercial consoles to establish whether any positive outcomes would imply real-world improvement (Cano Porras et al., 2018).
Additionally, VRGs specifically tailored for PD symptoms may help to
improve participant enjoyment, motivation and effectiveness (Barry et al.,
2014).

Clinical Case

In 2015, P.R., a 65-year-old retired male with 8 years of formal education, was
diagnosed with PD and classified as stage 2 on the Hoehn and Yahr scale.
He presented a Mini-Mental State Examination score of 24 and a score of 4
on the Geriatric Depression Scale. In addition, he was prescribed 100 mg of
levodopa divided into three daily doses.

   Although P.R. had good visual and auditory acuity, he had difficulty walking in crowded places or on unstable surfaces and reported a fall episode
during a cell phone call. As a result, he was referred to a PT clinic where
VRGs were used. The physical therapist in charge completed an assessment
and verified poor performance in the 10-m walk test, Berg balance scale, uni-
pedal stance test, cognitive TUG test and cognitive tests of executive functions. The goals established by the physical therapist were improvement in
gait velocity and its management in the dual-task condition and enhancement in static and dynamic balance and cognitive function, more specifically
executive function.

   After analysing the available VRG systems, the physical therapist, along
with the neuropsychologist of the multi-professional team, chose the
Nintendo Wii and a few off-the-shelf games (Wii Fit Plus package). All
selected games presented motor and cognitive demands that met the anticipated goals. The games and their main motor and cognitive demands are
presented in Table 13.3.

   The intervention was composed of 14 VRG sessions of 40 min each, twice
a week, under the supervision of a physical therapist during the 'on' phase
of the dopaminergic medication. To maximize the effects, the intervention
was designed to combine virtual training and conventional gait and balance
training. The conventional training was performed during the first 20 min
of each session. A rest period was allowed between exercises or games

TABLE 13.3

Main Tasks and Demands of Interest to Attain the VRG Intervention's Goals

Nintendo Wii Games	Tasks	Main Motor Demands	Main Cognitive Demands
Obstacle course	Walk as fast as possible on a course, avoiding obstacles	Fast stationary walk avoiding obstacles	Response inhibition and planning to avoid obstacles
Basic step	Alternate steps according to the game's music rhythm and visual stimuli	Alternate steps according to rhythm determined by game	Sustained attention and visuospatial capacity to follow visual and auditory cues which direct foot movements
Rhythm parade	Marching in place to the sound of a beat while moving arms according to the visual stimuli	Alternate steps while moving arms	Divided attention between alternating steps and moving both arms
Tightrope walk	Keep balance while walking on a tightrope and avoid obstacles	Shift centre of gravity latero-laterally	Sustained attention and decision-making on shifting direction

Source: Adapted from Alves et al. (2018).

according to the patient's needs. The game was projected onto a screen positioned 2 m in front of the patient (Figure 13.1).

P.R. played each game three times during each session. Before the start of the first VRG session, the physical therapist explained the goals and performed a familiarization trial. For clinical safety, heart rate and blood pressure were monitored in all sessions.

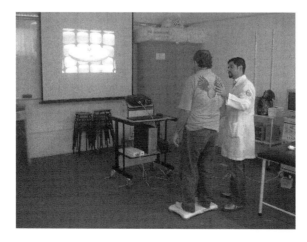

FIGURE 13.1
Training setup.

Final Considerations

It is worth noting that most VRG studies have recurrent biases, which weakens the scientific evidence (Miller et al., 2014; Neri et al., 2017). Bias can lead to overestimation of the true intervention effect (Gluud, 2006), and it compromises clinical recommendations. The systematic review by Neri et al. (2017) showed that the majority of studies using VRGs have not reported a proper description of randomization and allocation concealment. The purpose of randomization is to eliminate systematic biases that can influence the allocation of treatment groups (i.e. subjects should have the same chance of receiving any intervention) (Altman, 1991). Allocation concealment 'shields' researchers from knowing the upcoming assignments and, without it, the randomization is compromised and readers cannot rely on the results (Schulz and Grimes, 2002).

The heterogeneity of intervention protocols affects research replication, thus making it difficult to summarize the clinical evidence. Thus, professionals should consider their clinical reasoning in the selection of the best VRGs protocol. As time allows, physical therapists are encouraged to compile studies of interest (preferably systematic reviews, if any) to support the design and the characteristics of the intervention, integrating clinical experience and client/patient preferences and specificities (e.g. clinical condition, availability for training, outcomes of interest and personal demands).

Another aspect to be considered is the number of individuals who dislike VRGs and, consequently, will not attend the interventions. This is surprising, as it appears that part of the older population prefers paper-based instructions for self-regulated conventional exercise rather than computer-based exergames (Oesch et al., 2017).

Even though bias is a warning to researchers, the current body of knowledge and the weak evidence allow, to some extent, the implementation of VRGs in clinical practice. However, we agree that implementation is possible as long as it is done with caution. Professionals who choose to use VRGs should seek a standardized protocol and exercise prudence when designing an intervention (as discussed in this chapter). Professionals should also pay attention to the opinion and objectives of the client/patient. Another important aspect is that, depending on the outcome of interest (e.g. muscle strength, socialization/community interaction, increase in physical activity), professionals must be aware of the most consolidated interventions based on the strongest evidence available before deciding to adopt VRGs. However, if the main objective is the combination of effects on physical variables with cognitive outcomes, VRGs can provide positive effects with good applicability due to better adherence and motivation when compared to conventional interventions.

References

Adamovich, S. V., Fluet, G. G., Tunik, E. & Merians, A. S. 2009. Sensorimotor training in virtual reality: A review. *NeuroRehabilitation*, 25, 29–44.

Althoff, T., White, R. W. & Horvitz, E. 2016. Influence of Pokemon go on physical activity: Study and implications. *Journal of Medical Internet Research*, 18, e315.

Altman, D. 1991. Randomisation. Essential for reducing bias. *British Medical Journal*, 302, 1481–1482.

Alves, M. L. M., Mesquita, B. S., Morais, W. S., Leal, J. C., Satler, C. E. & Dos Santos Mendes, F. A. 2018. Nintendo Wii versus Xbox kinect for assisting people with Parkinson's disease. *Percept Mot Skills*, 125, 546–565.

Anderson, K. R., Woodbury, M. L., Phillips, K. & Gauthier, L. V. 2015. Virtual reality video games to promote movement recovery in stroke rehabilitation: A guide for clinicians. *Archives of Physical Medicine and Rehabilitation*, 96, 973–976.

Barry, G., Galna, B. & Rochester, L. 2014. The role of exergaming in Parkinson's disease rehabilitation: A systematic review of the evidence. *Journal of NeuroEngineering and Rehabilitation*, 11, 33.

Bieryla, K. A. & Dold, N. M. 2013. Feasibility of Wii Fit training to improve clinical measures of balance in older adults. *Clinical Interventions in Aging*, 8, 775–781.

Blumberg, F. C., Altschuler, E. A., Almonte, D. E. & Mileaf, M. I. 2013. The impact of recreational video game play on children's and adolescents' cognition. *New Directions for Child and Adolescent Development*, 2013, 41–50.

Buccino, G., Gatti, R., Giusti, M. C., Negrotti, A., Rossi, A., Calzetti, S. & Cappa, S. F. 2011. Action observation treatment improves autonomy in daily activities in Parkinson's disease patients: Results from a pilot study. *Movement Disorders*, 26, 1963–1964.

Burke, J. W., McNeill, M., Charles, D. K., Morrow, P. J., Crosbie, J. H. & McDonough, S. M. 2009. Optimising engagement for stroke rehabilitation using serious games. *The Visual Computer*, 25, 1085.

Campbell, A. J., Robertson, M. C., La Grow, S. J., Kerse, N. M., Sanderson, G. F., Jacobs, R. J., Sharp, D. M. & Hale, L. A. 2005. Randomised controlled trial of prevention of falls in people aged ≥75 with severe visual impairment: The VIP trial. *BMJ*, 331, 817.

Cano Porras, D., Siemonsma, P., Inzelberg, R., Zeilig, G. & Plotnik, M. 2018. Advantages of virtual reality in the rehabilitation of balance and gait: Systematic review. *Neurology*, 90, 1017–1025.

Cardoso-Leite, P. & Bavelier, D. 2014. Video game play, attention, and learning: How to shape the development of attention and influence learning? *Current Opinion in Neurology*, 27, 185–191.

Charsky, D. 2010. From edutainment to serious games: A change in the use of game characteristics. *Games and Culture*, 5, 177–198.

Cho, G. H., Hwangbo, G. & Shin, H. S. 2014. The effects of virtual reality-based balance training on balance of the elderly. *Journal of Physical Therapy Science*, 26, 615–617.

Choi, S. D., Guo, L., Kang, D. & Xiong, S. 2017. Exergame technology and interactive interventions for elderly fall prevention: A systematic literature review. *Applied Ergonomics*, 65, 570–581.

Crocetta, T. B., de Araújo, L. V., Guarnieri, R., Massetti, T., Ferreira, F. H. I. B., de Abreu, L. C. & de Mello Monteiro, C. B. 2017. Virtual reality software package for implementing motor learning and rehabilitation experiments. *Virtual Reality*, 1–11.

Daniel, K. 2012. Wii-hab for pre-frail older adults. *Rehabilitation Nursing*, 37, 195–201.

de Bruin, E. D., Schoene, D., Pichierri, G. & Smith, S. T. 2010. Use of virtual reality technique for the training of motor control in the elderly. Some theoretical considerations. *Zeitschrift für Gerontologie und Geriatrie*, 43, 229–234.

Demain, S., Burridge, J., Ellis-Hill, C., Hughes, A.-M., Yardley, L., Tedesco-Triccas, L. & Swain, I. 2013. Assistive technologies after stroke: Self-management or fending for yourself? A focus group study. *BMC Health Services Research*, 13, 334.

Dempsey, J. V., Lucassen, B. A., Haynes, L. L. & Casey, M. S. 1996. Instructional applications of computer games. *1996 Annual Meeting of the American Educational Research Association*, New York, USA.

Deterding, S., Dixon, D., Khaled, R. & Nacke, L. 2011. From game design elements to gamefulness: Defining "gamification". *Proceedings of the* 15th *International Academic MindTrek Conference: Envisioning Future Media Environments*, Tampere, Finland: ACM.

Dindar, M. & Ortiz de Gortari, A. B. 2017. Turkish validation of the Game Transfer Phenomena Scale (GTPS): Measuring altered perceptions, automatic mental processes and actions and behaviours associated with playing video games. *Telematics and Informatics*, 34, 1802–1813.

Dithmer, M., Rasmussen, J. O., Gronvall, E., Spindler, H., Hansen, J., Nielsen, G., Sorensen, S. B. & Dinesen, B. 2016. "The heart game": Using gamification as part of a telerehabilitation program for heart patients. *Games for Health Journal*, 5, 27–33.

Dockx, K., Bekkers, E. M., van den Bergh, V., Ginis, P., Rochester, L., Hausdorff, J. M., Mirelman, A. & Nieuwboer, A. 2016. Virtual reality for rehabilitation in Parkinson's disease. *The Cochrane Library*, 12, CD010760.

dos Santos Mendes, F. A., Pompeu, J. E., Modenesi Lobo, A., Guedes da Silva, K., Oliveira Tde, P., Peterson Zomignani, A. & Pimentel Piemonte, M. E. 2012. Motor learning, retention and transfer after virtual-reality-based training in Parkinson's disease--effect of motor and cognitive demands of games: A longitudinal, controlled clinical study. *Physiotherapy*, 98, 217–223.

Duque, G., Boersma, D., Loza-Diaz, G., Hassan, S., Suarez, H., Geisinger, D., Suriyaarachchi, P., Sharma, A. & Demontiero, O. 2013. Effects of balance training using a virtual-reality system in older fallers. *Clinical Interventions in Aging*, 8, 257–263.

Dye, M. W., Green, C. S. & Bavelier, D. 2009. The development of attention skills in action video game players. *Neuropsychologia*, 47, 1780–1789.

Esculier, J. F., Vaudrin, J., Beriault, P., Gagnon, K. & Tremblay, L. E. 2012. Home-based balance training programme using Wii Fit with balance board for Parkinsons's disease: A pilot study. *Journal of Rehabilitation Medicine*, 44, 144–150.

Franco, J. R., Jacobs, K., Inzerillo, C. & Kluzik, J. 2012. The effect of the Nintendo Wii Fit and exercise in improving balance and quality of life in community dwelling elders. *Technology and Health Care*, 20, 95–115.

Fung, V., So, K., Park, E., Ho, A., Shaffer, J., Chan, E. & Gomez, M. 2010. The utility of a video game system in rehabilitation of burn and nonburn patients: A survey among occupational therapy and physiotherapy practitioners. *Journal of Burn Care and Research*, 31, 768–775.

Galna, B., Barry, G., Jackson, D., Mhiripiri, D., Olivier, P. & Rochester, L. 2014. Accuracy of the Microsoft Kinect sensor for measuring movement in people with Parkinson's disease. *Gait Posture*, 39, 1062–1068.

Galvin, J. & Levac, D. 2011. Facilitating clinical decision-making about the use of virtual reality within paediatric motor rehabilitation: Describing and classifying virtual reality systems. *Developmental Neurorehabilitation*, 14, 112–122.

Gandolfi, M., Geroin, C., Dimitrova, E., Boldrini, P., Waldner, A., Bonadiman, S., Picelli, A., Regazzo, S., Stirbu, E., Primon, D., Bosello, C., Gravina, A. R., Peron, L., Trevisan, M., Garcia, A. C., Menel, A., Bloccari, L., Vale, N., Saltuari, L., Tinazzi, M. & Smania, N. 2017. Virtual reality telerehabilitation for postural instability in Parkinson's disease: A multicenter, single-blind, randomized, controlled trial. *BioMed Research International*, 2017, 7962826.

Gluud, L. L. 2006. Bias in clinical intervention research. *American Journal of Epidemiology*, 163, 493–501.

Golomb, M. R., McDonald, B. C., Warden, S. J., Yonkman, J., Saykin, A. J., Shirley, B., Huber, M., Rabin, B., Abdelbaky, M. & Nwosu, M. E. 2010. In-home virtual reality videogame telerehabilitation in adolescents with hemiplegic cerebral palsy. *Archives of Physical Medicine and Rehabilitation*, 91, 1.e1–8.e.1.

Granic, I., Lobel, A. & Engels, R. C. 2014. The benefits of playing video games. *American Psychologist*, 69, 66–78.

Harris, D. M., Rantalainen, T., Muthalib, M., Johnson, L. & Teo, W. P. 2015. Exergaming as a viable therapeutic tool to improve static and dynamic balance among older adults and people with idiopathic Parkinson's disease: A systematic review and meta-analysis. *Frontiers in Aging Neuroscience*, 7, 167.

Hopelab. 2004. *Re-Mission*. Palo Alto, CA: HopeLab.

Howcroft, J., Klejman, S., Fehlings, D., Wright, V., Zabjek, K., Andrysek, J. & Biddiss, E. 2012. Active video game play in children with cerebral palsy: Potential for physical activity promotion and rehabilitation therapies. *Archives of Physical Medicine and Rehabilitation*, 93, 1448–1456.

Hsieh, W.-M., Chen, C.-C., Wang, S.-C., Tan, S.-Y., Hwang, Y.-S., Chen, S.-C., Lai, J.-S. & Chen, Y.-L. 2014. Virtual reality system based on Kinect for the elderly in fall prevention. *Technology and Health Care*, 22, 27–36.

Jarvin, L. 2015. Edutainment, games, and the future of education in a digital world. *New Directions for Child and Adolescent Development*, 2015, 33–40.

Jorgensen, M. G., Laessoe, U., Hendriksen, C., Nielsen, O. B. F. & Aagaard, P. 2012. Efficacy of Nintendo Wii training on mechanical leg muscle function and postural balance in community-dwelling older adults: A randomized controlled trial. *The Journals of Gerontology Series A: Biological Sciences and Medical Sciences*, 68, 845–852.

Kato, P. M., Cole, S. W., Bradlyn, A. S. & Pollock, B. H. 2008. A video game improves behavioral outcomes in adolescents and young adults with cancer: A randomized trial. *Pediatrics*, 122, e305–e317.

Killane, I., Fearon, C., Newman, L., McDonnell, C., Waechter, S. M., Sons, K., Lynch, T. & Reilly, R. B. 2015. Dual motor-cognitive virtual reality training impacts dual-task performance in freezing of gait. *IEEE Journal of Biomedical and Health Informatics*, 19, 1855–1861.

Kubicki, A., Petrement, G., Bonnetblanc, F., Ballay, Y. & Mourey, F. 2011. Practice-related improvements in postural control during rapid arm movement in older adults: A preliminary study. *The Journals of Gerontology Series A: Biological Sciences and Medical Sciences*, 67, 196–203.

Kueider, A. M., Parisi, J. M., Gross, A. L. & Rebok, G. W. 2012. Computerized cognitive training with older adults: A systematic review. *PLoS One*, 7, e40588.

Lai, C.-H., Peng, C.-W., Chen, Y.-L., Huang, C.-P., Hsiao, Y.-L. & Chen, S.-C. 2013. Effects of interactive video-game based system exercise on the balance of the elderly. *Gait and Posture*, 37, 511–515.

Lange, B., Requejo, P., Flynn, S. M., Rizzo, A., Valero-Cuevas, F., Baker, L. & Winstein, C. 2010. The potential of virtual reality and gaming to assist successful aging with disability. *Physical Medicine and Rehabilitation Clinics*, 21, 339–356.

Lanningham-Foster, L., Jensen, T. B., Foster, R. C., Redmond, A. B., Walker, B. A., Heinz, D. & Levine, J. A. 2006. Energy expenditure of sedentary screen time compared with active screen time for children. *Pediatrics*, 118, e1831–e1835.

Leblanc, A. G. & Chaput, J. P. 2017. Pokemon Go: A game changer for the physical inactivity crisis? *Preventive Medicine*, 101, 235–237.

Lee, W.-H., Cho, K.-H., Kim, S.-H. & Lee, J.-H. 2011. The effect of a virtual reality-based exercise program using a video game on the balance, gait and fall prevention in the elderly women. *Journal of Sport and Leisure Studies*, 44, 605–614.

Levac, D., Espy, D., Fox, E., Pradhan, S. & Deutsch, J. E. 2015. "Kinect-ing" with clinicians: A knowledge translation resource to support decision making about video game use in rehabilitation. *Physical Therapy*, 95, 426–440.

Levac, D. E. & Galvin, J. 2013. When is virtual reality "therapy"? *Archives of Physical Medicine and Rehabilitation*, 94, 795–798.

Liao, Y. Y., Yang, Y. R., Cheng, S. J., Wu, Y. R., Fuh, J. L. & Wang, R. Y. 2015. Virtual reality-based training to improve obstacle-crossing performance and dynamic balance in patients with Parkinson's disease. *Neurorehabilitation and Neural Repair*, 29, 658–667.

Maillot, P., Perrot, A. & Hartley, A. 2012. Effects of interactive physical-activity video-game training on physical and cognitive function in older adults. *Psychology and Aging*, 27, 589–600.

Maillot, P., Perrot, A. & Hartley, A. 2014. The braking force in walking: Age-related differences and improvement in older adults with exergame training. *Journal of Aging and Physical Activity*, 22, 518–526.

Miller, K. J., Adair, B. S., Pearce, A. J., Said, C. M., Ozanne, E. & Morris, M. M. 2014. Effectiveness and feasibility of virtual reality and gaming system use at home by older adults for enabling physical activity to improve health-related domains: A systematic review. *Age and Ageing*, 43, 188–195.

Mirelman, A., Maidan, I. & Deutsch, J. E. 2013. Virtual reality and motor imagery: Promising tools for assessment and therapy in Parkinson's disease. *Movement Disorders*, 28, 1597–1608.

Mirelman, A., Maidan, I., Herman, T., Deutsch, J. E., Giladi, N. & Hausdorff, J. M. 2011. Virtual reality for gait training: Can it induce motor learning to enhance complex walking and reduce fall risk in patients with Parkinson's disease? *Journals of Gerontology, Series A: Biological Sciences and Medical Sciences*, 66, 234–240.

Mirelman, A., Maida, I., Jacobs, A., Mirelman, D., Giladi, N. & Hausdorff, J. 2010. Virtual reality for gait training in Parkinson's disease: A feasibility study. *Parkinsonism and Related Disorders*, 16, S83.

Molina, K. I., Ricci, N. A., de Moraes, S. A. & Perracini, M. R. 2014. Virtual reality using games for improving physical functioning in older adults: A systematic review. *Journal of Neuroengineering and Rehabilitation*, 11, 156.

Nawaz, A., Skjaeret, N., Helbostad, J. L., Vereijken, B., Boulton, E. & Svanaes, D. 2016. Usability and acceptability of balance exergames in older adults: A scoping review. *Health Informatics Journal*, 22, 911–931.

Neri, S. G., Cardoso, J. R., Cruz, L., Lima, R. M., de Oliveira, R. J., Iversen, M. D. & Carregaro, R. L. 2017. Do virtual reality games improve mobility skills and balance measurements in community-dwelling older adults? Systematic review and meta-analysis. *Clinical Rehabilitation*, 31, 1292–1304.

Nevitt, M. C., Cummings, S. R. & Hudes, E. S. 1991. Risk factors for injurious falls: A prospective study. *Journal of Gerontology*, 46, M164–M170.

NSF 2012. National Stroke Foundation. National stroke audit–rehabilitation services report. National Stroke Foundation Melbourne, Australia.

Oesch, P., Kool, J., Fernandez-Luque, L., Brox, E., Evertsen, G., Civit, A., Hilfiker, R. & Bachmann, S. 2017. Exergames versus self-regulated exercises with instruction leaflets to improve adherence during geriatric rehabilitation: A randomized controlled trial. *BMC Geriatrics*, 17, 77.

Ortiz de Gortari, A. B., Aronsson, K. & Griffiths, M. D. 2011. Game transfer phenomena in video game playing: A qualitative interview study. *International Journal of Cyber Behavior, Psychology and Learning*, 1, 15–33.

Ortiz de Gortari, A. B. & Griffiths, M. D. 2016. Prevalence and characteristics of game transfer phenomena: A descriptive survey study. *International Journal of Human–Computer Interaction*, 32, 470–480.

Pelosin, E., Avanzino, L., Bove, M., Stramesi, P., Nieuwboer, A. & Abbruzzese, G. 2010. Action observation improves freezing of gait in patients with Parkinson's disease. *Neurorehabilitation Neural Repair*, 24, 746–752.

Peng, W., Lin, J. H. & Crouse, J. 2011. Is playing exergames really exercising? A meta-analysis of energy expenditure in active video games. *Cyberpsychology, Behavior, and Social Networking*, 14, 681–688.

Perrier-Melo, R. J., Silva, T. C. D. A., Brito-Gomes, J. L., Oliveira, S. F. M. D. & Costa, M. D. C. 2014. Active video games, balance and energy expenditure in elderly: A systematic review. *ConScientiae Saúde*, 13, 289–297.

Pichierri, G., Coppe, A., Lorenzetti, S., Murer, K. & de Bruin, E. D. 2012a. The effect of a cognitive-motor intervention on voluntary step execution under single and dual task conditions in older adults: A randomized controlled pilot study. *Clinical Interventions in Aging*, 7, 175–184.

Pichierri, G., Murer, K. & de Bruin, E. D. 2012b. A cognitive-motor intervention using a dance video game to enhance foot placement accuracy and gait under dual task conditions in older adults: A randomized controlled trial. *BMC Geriatrics*, 12, 74.

Pluchino, A., Lee, S. Y., Asfour, S., Roos, B. A. & Signorile, J. F. 2012. Pilot study comparing changes in postural control after training using a video game balance board program and 2 standard activity-based balance intervention programs. *Archives of Physical Medicine and Rehabilitation*, 93, 1138–1146.

Pompeu, J. E., Arduini, L. A., Botelho, A. R., Fonseca, M. B., Pompeu, S. M., Torriani-Pasin, C. & Deutsch, J. E. 2014. Feasibility, safety and outcomes of playing kinect adventures! for people with Parkinson's disease: A pilot study. *Physiotherapy*, 100, 162–168.

Pompeu, J. E., Mendes, F. A., Silva, K. G., Lobo, A. M., Oliveira Tde, P., Zomignani, A. P. & Piemonte, M. E. 2012. Effect of Nintendo Wii-based motor and cognitive training on activities of daily living in patients with Parkinson's disease: A randomised clinical trial. *Physiotherapy*, 98, 196–204.

Prochaska, J. J. & Prochaska, J. O. 2011. A review of multiple health behavior change interventions for primary prevention. *American Journal of Lifestyle Medicine*, 5, 208–221.

Qiu, N., Ma, W., Fan, X., Zhang, Y., Li, Y., Yan, Y., Zhou, Z., Li, F., Gong, D. & Yao, D. 2018. Rapid improvement in visual selective attention related to action video gaming experience. *Frontiers in Human Neuroscience*, 12, 47.

Rendon, A. A., Lohman, E. B., Thorpe, D., Johnson, E. G., Medina, E. & Bradley, B. 2012. The effect of virtual reality gaming on dynamic balance in older adults. *Age and Ageing*, 41, 549–552.

Rodrigues, E. V., Guimarães, A. T. B., Gallo, L. H., Melo Filho, J., Pintarelli, V. L. & Gomes, A. R. S. 2018. Supervised dance intervention based on video game choreography increases quadriceps cross sectional area and peak of torque in community dwelling older women. *Motriz: Revista de Educação Física*, 24, e101868.

Schoene, D., Lord, S. R., Delbaere, K., Severino, C., Davies, T. A. & Smith, S. T. 2013. A randomized controlled pilot study of home-based step training in older people using videogame technology. *PLoS One*, 8, e57734.

Schulz, K. F. & Grimes, D. A. 2002. Allocation concealment in randomised trials: Defending against deciphering. *Lancet*, 359, 614–618.

Shen, X. & Mak, M. K. 2014. Balance and gait training with augmented feedback improves balance confidence in people with Parkinson's disease: A randomized controlled trial. *Neurorehabilitation and Neural Repair*, 28, 524–535.

Shen, X. & Mak, M. K. 2015. Technology-assisted balance and gait training reduces falls in patients with Parkinson's disease: A randomized controlled trial with 12-month follow-up. *Neurorehabilitation and Neural Repair*, 29, 103–111.

Shin, J.-H., Ryu, H. & Jang, S. H. 2014. A task-specific interactive game-based virtual reality rehabilitation system for patients with stroke: A usability test and two clinical experiments. *Journal of NeuroEngineering and Rehabilitation*, 11, 32.

Shubert, T. E. 2011. Evidence-based exercise prescription for balance and falls prevention: A current review of the literature. *Journal of Geriatric Physical Therapy*, 34, 100–108.

Singh, D., Rajaratnam, B., Palaniswamy, V., Raman, V., Bong, P. & Pearson, H. 2013. Effects of balance-focused interactive games compared to therapeutic balance classes for older women. *Climacteric*, 16, 141–146.

Singh, D. K., Rajaratnam, B. S., Palaniswamy, V., Pearson, H., Raman, V. P. & Bong, P. S. 2012. Participating in a virtual reality balance exercise program can reduce risk and fear of falls. *Maturitas*, 73, 239–243.

Skjæret, N., Nawaz, A., Morat, T., Schoene, D., Helbostad, J. L. & Vereijken, B. 2016. Exercise and rehabilitation delivered through exergames in older adults: An integrative review of technologies, safety and efficacy. *International Journal of Medical Informatics*, 85, 1–16.

Staiano, A. E. & Calvert, S. L. 2011. Exergames for physical education courses: Physical, social, and cognitive benefits. *Child Development Perspectives*, 5, 93–98.

Stanmore, E., Stubbs, B., Vancampfort, D., de Bruin, E. D. & Firth, J. 2017. The effect of active video games on cognitive functioning in clinical and non-clinical populations: A meta-analysis of randomized controlled trials. *Neuroscience and Biobehavioral Reviews*, 78, 34–43.

Szturm, T., Betker, A. L., Moussavi, Z., Desai, A. & Goodman, V. 2011. Effects of an interactive computer game exercise regimen on balance impairment in frail community-dwelling older adults: A randomized controlled trial. *Physical Therapy*, 91, 1449–1462.

Teo, W. P., Muthalib, M., Yamin, S., Hendy, A. M., Bramstedt, K., Kotsopoulos, E., Perrey, S. & Ayaz, H. 2016. Does a combination of virtual reality, neuromodulation and neuroimaging provide a comprehensive platform for neurorehabilitation? - A narrative review of the literature. *Frontiers in Human Neuroscience*, 10, 284.

Tieri, G., Morone, G., Paolucci, S. & Iosa, M. 2018. Virtual reality in cognitive and motor rehabilitation: Facts, fiction and fallacies. *Expert Review of Medical Devices*, 15, 107–117.

Tolentino, G., Ventura, A., Cruz, L., Vidal, S., Valeriano, R., Battaglini, C. & Oliveira, R. J. 2015. The serious games applied for health. In: Mehdi Khosrow-Pour, D. B. A. (ed.) *Encyclopedia of Information Science and Technology*, 3rd edn. Hershey, PA: IGI Global, 5641–5645.

Toulotte, C., Toursel, C. & Olivier, N. 2012. Wii Fit® training vs. Adapted physical activities: Which one is the most appropriate to improve the balance of independent senior subjects? A randomized controlled study. *Clinical Rehabilitation*, 26, 827–835.

Tripette, J., Murakami, H., Ryan, K. R., Ohta, Y. & Miyachi, M. 2017. The contribution of Nintendo Wii Fit series in the field of health: A systematic review and meta-analysis. *PeerJ*, 5, e3600.

van den Heuvel, M. R., van Wegen, E. E., de Goede, C. J., Burgers-Bots, I. A., Beek, P. J., Daffertshofer, A. & Kwakkel, G. 2013. The effects of augmented visual feedback during balance training in Parkinson's disease: Study design of a randomized clinical trial. *BMC Neurology*, 13, 137.

van Diest, M., Lamoth, C. J., Stegenga, J., Verkerke, G. J. & Postema, K. 2013. Exergaming for balance training of elderly: State of the art and future developments. *Journal of NeuroEngineering and Rehabilitation*, 10, 101.

Waern, A., Montola, M. & Stenros, J. 2009. The three-sixty illusion: Designing for immersion in pervasive games. *Proceedings of the SIGCHI Conference on Human Factors in Computing Systems*. Boston, MA: ACM.

Warburton, D. E., Bredin, S. S., Horita, L. T., Zbogar, D., Scott, J. M., Esch, B. T. & Rhodes, R. E. 2007. The health benefits of interactive video game exercise. *Applied Physiology, Nutrition, and Metabolism*, 32, 655–663.

Wüest, S., Langenberg, R. & Bruin, E. D. 2014. Design considerations for a theory-driven exergame-based rehabilitation program to improve walking of persons with stroke. *European Review of Aging and Physical Activity*, 11, 119.

Yang, W. C., Wang, H. K., Wu, R. M., Lo, C. S. & Lin, K. H. 2016. Home-based virtual reality balance training and conventional balance training in Parkinson's disease: A randomized controlled trial. *Journal of the Formosan Medical Association*, 115, 734–743.

Zettergren, K., Antune, S. M., Canhao, J. & Lavallee, C. 2011. The effects of Nintendo Wii Fit on gait speed, balance and functional mobility on idiopathic Parkinson's disease: A case study. *Gerontologist*, 51, 70.

Zimmermann, R., Gschwandtner, U., Benz, N., Hatz, F., Schindler, C., Taub, E. & Fuhr, P. 2014. Cognitive training in Parkinson disease: Cognition-specific vs nonspecific computer training. *Neurology*, 82, 1219–1226.

14

Project Career: The Matching Person and Technology Model and Everyday Technology in Action

Deborah Minton
Kent State University

Elaine Sampson
West Virginia University

Amanda Nardone
Boston University

Callista Stauffer
Kent State University

CONTENTS

Introduction 259
Traumatic Brain Injury 260
Project Career Overview 262
MPT Model and Data Collection 264
John's Experience 266
Project Career Outcomes 267
Summary 268
References 268

Introduction

Assistive Technology (AT) has the ability to change the lives of those who use it. As technology options and features have expanded, so has their use by individuals with disabilities. Expanded technology options have improved accommodation options. Unfortunately, the expanded technology choices and the multifaceted needs and expectations of the people using them require matching the person and the technology for the best fit for the individual (Scherer et al., 2005).

One model that has successfully interpreted the complex individualized issues with technology and those with disabilities using it is the Matching Person and Technology (MPT) model (Scherer, 1998). The MPT process centres on the individual's psychosocial characteristics, the personal myriad environmental elements that influence use and the desirable features of the most appropriate technologies for the individual's needs (Scherer, 2005). The MPT model is both personal and collaborative, as the service provider guides the individuals through the assessment process. In a recent federally funded demonstration grant, Project Career, the MPT model was used to provide 2- and 4-year college students with traumatic brain injury (TBI) assistance in identifying an individualized set of academic, vocational and personal applications (apps) used with an iPad.

Traumatic Brain Injury

To better understand the role of the MPT process, it is important to understand the impact of TBIs on the academic, vocational and psychosocial facets of an individual. Described as a global health emergency by the World Health Organization (WHO), TBIs are 'involved in nearly half of all traumatic deaths' (Basso et al., 2006). The WHO further reported that people with TBIs may require continuing assistance while adapting to the physical and cognitive impact of their injury as well as accompanying life changes that may include the loss of social networks and a lack of understanding in school and the workplace (Bootes & Chapparo, 2010; Leopold, 2018; National Association of State Head Injury Administrators (NASHIA), 2006; Wehman et al., 2005). The U.S. Centers for Disease Control and Prevention (CDC) determined that persons most likely to incur a TBI are between ages 15 and 24 and those ages 65 and older (CDC, 2011). The CDC also reported that the prevalence of TBIs occurring between ages 16 and 25 have increased by almost 60% between 2001 and 2015 with the majority of these injuries being recreational activity related (CDC, 2011). In addition, a record number of military service members have experienced a TBI during the past two decades. The Defense and Veterans Brain Injury Center reported in 2016 that more than 339,000 members of the U.S. armed services sustained TBIs between 2000 and the third quarter of 2015, many occurring in military combats (Defense and Veterans Brain Injury Center, 2016).

It is widely recognized that TBIs are underreported, and may have long-term implications and a permanent impact on functioning (Nardone et al., 2015; Basso et al., 2006; Bryan-Hancock & Harrison, 2010. Regardless of how mild or severe the injury, a TBI may not only influence a person's cognitive abilities but may also affect an individual's interlinked biopsychosocial functions (Toriello & Keferl, 2012). A 2008 study found that college students with mild TBIs reported fatigue, headaches and blurry vision, among other symptoms, at a higher rate than students without a TBI (Kennedy et al., 2008). A recent study examining the impact of repetitive TBIs on college students found that students with two or more TBIs reported more changes in cognitive functioning, worse executive functioning and more symptoms of depression. While impairments vary from person to person, most people who have sustained a TBI experience one or more of the following: impaired memory, inability to prioritize thoughts, difficulty concentrating; lack of awareness of impairments; accommodations needed for impairments; difficulty in problem-solving, decision-making, organizing and planning (Rumrill et al., 2019; Scherer, 2012). These key impaired skills are vital to succeeding in the classroom and in the workplace (NASHIA, 2006; Wehman, 2013). Students with TBI also reported changes in their emotional responses, including rapid or extreme mood changes, anger, anxiety and depression. These strong emotions may become barriers to their continued education and vocational goals (Bootes & Chapparo, 2010; NASHIA, 2006; TBI Model Systems, 2010; Todis et al., 2011).

Students with TBIs attending higher education institutions face many challenges that other students without TBIs may not face during the transition from high school or the military into academia and from academia to employment. The complications teens and young adults (ages 16–25) with TBI face include dealing with the impact of the injury at a time when they are starting to prepare for their future. This may include learning new skills, completing academic requirements and making career plans (Wehman, 2013; Wehman et al., 2014).Veterans with TBI experience similar challenges as they return to civilian life and return to academia to enhance their skills (Rumrill et al., 2016). Individuals with TBI who successfully transition to post-secondary education continue to deal with their injury and face more cognitive, emotional, psychological and social challenges than their uninjured counterparts; the culmination of these disparities include lower grades and higher dropout rates (NASHIA, 2006; Todis et al., 2011). In addition, research indicates that three-fourths of individuals returning to work after experiencing a TBI lose their job within 90 days due to insufficient or a lack of supports.

It is vital that individuals who have incurred a TBI receive appropriate accommodations to remove educational and vocational barriers. Research has long identified education as one a primary conduit to competitive employment and higher salaries. Accommodations enable students with TBI to manage and complete academic requirements, job tasks and engage as active and productive members of their community. Unfortunately, biased public perceptions and negative attitudes may affect accommodation requests. Many times, TBIs are an invisible disability forcing those who incurred one to challenge stigmas by providing information about their injury and its impact to receive accommodations (Bowen, 2008; Kelly et al., 2012). Others may attribute displays of behaviours such as disinhibition, aggression or excessive self-disclosure to one's personality instead of a brain injury, failing to acknowledge the inherent challenges of a TBI (Ruoff, 2008).

Few, if any, evidence-based practices supported the cognitive and service needs of individuals with TBIs seeking assistance in achieving academic and/or employment success. There was a lack of research on best practices to help individuals with TBI obtain skills and supports to adapt to changes in academic, employment and life situations for all levels of brain injury severity. Employment barriers during the job interview process and in the workplace include challenges with organizing, short-term memory problems and the inability to respond to and interact with co-workers and supervisors (Kennedy et al., 2008; Brainline.org, 2008).

One approach identified as lessening the impairments resulting from a TBI is the use of AT (e.g., Scherer, 2012). Leopold et al. (2015) completed an analysis of 28 studies published between 2000 and 2015 that used assistive technology for cognition (ATC) with individuals who had experienced a TBI. These authors found that ATCs could be used successfully by individuals who have a TBI to support various cognitive functions such as memory, processing and attention.

Project Career Overview

Project Career was designed to respond to the challenges experienced by individuals with TBI pursuing higher education and entering the workforce. Project Career, an interdisciplinary demonstration initiative, focused its objectives on improving the academic and employment successes of undergraduate veterans and civilians with a TBI attending colleges and universities.

Funded as a 5-year development grant (2013–2018) through the National Institute on Disability, Independent Living and Rehabilitation Research (NIDILRR) with the objective of demonstrating effective practices to address academic and employment success, Project Career aimed to improve the academic and long-term employment outcomes that presently affect post-secondary students with TBI. The programme operated at three programme sites: Boston University in Massachusetts, Kent State University in Ohio and West Virginia University. A technology and employment coordinator (TEC) was located at each site to supporting 50 individuals at each site. The multisite Project Career programme assisted participating students, but also identified best practices when working with other undergraduate students with TBI. Quantitative and qualitative evaluations completed by JBS International show that the programme's unique integrated components have provided positive results (Nardone et al., 2015).

In order to participate, the student had a documented TBI, experienced cognitive challenges due to the TBI and be enrolled in 2- or 4-year academic institution. Project Career students have consistently identified two barriers: limited access to individualized supports to accommodate cognitive and academic limitations and a lack of career-related services to prepare for and maintain employment.

Eligible students completed the MPT and other baseline assessments in order to determine next steps. The TECs provided comprehensive individualized services that included identifying and reviewing accommodations; articulating and advocating for himself/herself inside and outside of the classroom; information and referral; assessments; counselling and guidance; vocational training; support for technology selection and use; identifying school and community resources; job search, placement and coaching; assistance with developing and maintaining employer and co-worker relationships; as well as help with addressing job-related challenges. TECs followed up with students, often through technology-based communications - to support his/her technology use, stress management techniques, organization, time management strategies, exploring new opportunities, solving daily problems, addressing issues with various campus offices and responding to general life stressors.

TECs assist Project Career students with identifying and achieving career goals. They help students create and update their resumes, identify potential references and develop cover letters to obtain full- or part-time jobs or apply for internships. TECs connect students with campus accessibility services, commonly referred to as student accessibility services (SAS). It is critical for students with TBIs to work regularly with the campus SAS office, yet researchers have found that fewer than half of the students with TBI reported using this service. To receive an accommodation, college students must provide documentation to the SAS office regarding their disability. SAS staff then assists with obtaining needed accommodations and notifying students' professors (NASHIA, 2006; Todis et al., 2011; Wehman, 2013; Griffin & Stein, 2015).

In addition to the individualized vocational and academic case management assistance described, Project Career students used Cognitive Support Technology (CST) to assist cognitive functioning. Specifically, the iPads serve as the platform to provide CST in the form of applications (apps), as well as a virtual platform to provide coaching, education, counselling and career-mentoring services that maximize students' career readiness. Benefits of using iPad technology include that it is highly mobile, easy to use, has built-in accessibility features, connects easily to available wi-fi systems and does not stigmatize the user as a person with a disability as iPads are universally used. This CST improves functioning affected by TBIs through assisting with cognitive challenges including memory, attention, concentration and planning (Hendricks, 2015). Apps were selected specifically to support individual student needs. When the CST does not meet the student's functional needs, the student typically stops using the CST. One student reported that the TEC followed up to make sure they were able to use the technology.

Participating students also had the opportunity to work with a mentor. The project defined a mentor as a person who has knowledge about the academic experience and/or understands the student's chosen career field. A peer, faculty member or professional working in a student's field of interest may provide mentorship. Mentors serve as a career guide and provide support beyond that given by TECs. Students who have a mentor report that these relationships provide opportunities that may not otherwise have been available. Mentorship takes different forms depending on the venue and type of mentor. Some students were paired with their mentors by the TECs based on mutual interests, whereas others could independently select their mentors. This relationship is an important connection, providing support, encouragement, professional networking and assistance with identifying opportunities inside and outside the classroom (American Psychological Association, 2015).

The use of technology in combination with one-on-one assistance from the Project's TECs, academic/career mentors, as guided by results from the MPT process, has shown positive results. Students are completing academic pursuits, applying for and obtaining part-time and summer employment, obtaining experiential learning opportunities such as internships in their field of study, enhancing career readiness and attaining their career goals.

MPT Model and Data Collection

Project Career follows a formal protocol that began with an intake assessment, where the TECs noted basic demographic and medical documentation to determine if the individual qualifies for programme services. Eligible students complete a baseline assessment, which compiles employment-related attitudinal and behavioural measures that assess the student's employability, maturity, career decidedness, career self-efficacy, acceptance and perception of disability and employment history.

Each individual is given a MPT assessment, which measures attitudes and feelings towards technology, current supports and self-ratings of abilities in areas of reading skills, comprehension, hearing, seeing, schedule, time management, etc. (Scherer, 1998, 2012, 2016; Scherer et al., 2007). The MPT starts the conversation on the technology needs of students and the areas where the students feel they are experiencing the most challenges. As a self-reporting system, it provides the TECs with a glimpse into the thought process of the student and their attitude towards technology. Although we often think of the younger generation as the technology generation, it is important to remember that not all young people have had positive interactions with technology. The MPT helps the TECs to identify students who may be struggling with technology and its implementation. Since the assessment is self-report, it also makes students feel as if they are part of the process in determining what they need and choosing apps. Other vocational assessments may be completed based on the student's academic goals and needs.

While all Project Career students received the same base level of services, they were not all provided in the same manner, time frame or order. Each student's process was based on his or her specific needs and academic timeline. For example, a junior or a senior is encouraged to seek out or connect with a mentor faster than an incoming freshman. The student's academic timeline as well as his/her individual needs has a direct impact on the services timeline for that student. Just as no two TBIs are the same, no two personal experiences are the same in regards to how their TBI influences them, or the supports they may need. This disparity in experience impacted every aspect of the Project Career process. Some students will need only one training session on how to use apps, others could require several training sessions and supplemental materials to ensure they understand the app and all its functionality. Some students may benefit from a TEC attending class with them to understand how the technology is used in real time in the natural use environment. This is where the TECs use their experience and expertise to determine the best course of action for each student and implement the different training methods.

This customized approach does not end with app selection and training. The hallmark of Project Career is meeting students where they are, physically, emotionally, cognitively, academically and socially, and then taking that information and creating a one of a kind programme that meets the needs of both the student and the Project Career process. This combined individualized process and project foundation allow the student and the TEC to establish the best practices needed in overcoming the two most frequently reported challenges of not enough individualized supports and lack of career-related services. By meeting the students where they are, the TECs are able to adjust course and help the students overcome the barrier/s they are experiencing during that particular time. This may address the need for employment before finding a mentor, or addressing social issues above academic concerns. The timeline and process are directed by the student's needs and not a regimented schedule.

This personalization extended to the selection of apps and the different CST features used by the students. With assistance from the information gathered through the MPT process, the TECs are able to pinpoint the different challenges and strengths of the students and determine which challenges need the most support at any given time; App selection was based on that set of circumstances. For example, a student may need one set of apps during the academic year and a potentially different set during summer employment or an internship. The TECs assisted the students in identifying and determining which app was to be most beneficial during any given time in the student's academic or employment process. The MPT also aids the TECs in selecting apps from the myriad of apps available in the App Store. Using the information gained in the MPT, the TECs are able to specify if an app is going to meet the needs of the student. This information is invaluable in ensuring that the student continues to use the app.

For example, if a student is using a note-taking app and only types into the app because of hand tremors, there is no need to emphasize the handwriting capabilities of the app. Conversely, sharing the handwriting capabilities with a different student might open a new world of possibilities for him or her. This is where the individualized approach to the Project Career student comes into play. Through discussion, trial and error and time, the TEC is able to best determine not only the most suitable app, but also the preferred features of the apps thereby making the technology approachable and not overwhelming.

This individualized approach and the one-on-one nature of the process has led to higher retention and graduation rates among Project Career students than students with TBIs not participating in the programme. This approach has also led to a greater understanding of the individualized needs of the students and their particular objectives and goals.

John's Experience

John, a sophomore undergraduate premedical student, sought services from Project Career after having failed math, biology and chemistry. He stated that he wanted to study medicine 'to help people when they are at their worst'. John shared that he had incurred a severe TBI as the result of a car collision. John self-reported that he dealt with short-term memory loss, poor grip strength, leg weakness, difficulty walking, difficulty with speech, trouble focusing and poor decision-making skills. After administering the intake and the MPT protocol, John and the TEC focused on his challenges and how they influenced his ability to succeed in college and in his desired field of study, medicine.

As John and his TEC evaluated the MPT findings, the two discovered that in addition to the academic problems John was dealing with, he was also faced with physical challenges to becoming a physician. The MPT assessments revealed that in addition to having difficulties with grip strength, John had difficulty holding a pencil for more than 30 min, was prone to falling when walking, required at least 8 h of sleep every night and that he needed a regular meal schedule to avoid headaches. With this information, John and his TEC explored jobs in the medical field to determine if this was the right option for him. After accessing O*Net Online and reviewing the basic job skills and day-to-day requirements of people in the medical profession, after reviewing the information, John noted that between his physical and academic challenges, he may need to amend his vocational goals.

In addition to the vocational exploration, John fully implemented the technology provided through Project Career. John used his iPad and apps for note taking, recording his lectures, creating and checking off items on his to-do lists, studying Spanish with language learning apps, organizing his assignments and class schedule and managing weight to help with his mobility concerns.

With the assistance from his iPad, apps and information gained from the MPT assessments, John and his TEC explored other careers that would allow John to 'help people when they are at their worst'. John arrived at his answer when he shared, 'I remember the hospital Social Worker telling me it would all be okay [after the accident]. She really helped me when I needed it the most'. With that realization, John changed his major from pre-med to Social Work. Since changing his major and employing his individualized technology, successfully completed his programme, graduated, and was accepted into a Social Work Master's degree programme.

Project Career Outcomes

John's case is just one example of how Project Career combined technology and vocational rehabilitation's best practices to help students reach a positive outcome. As of spring 2018, 146 students participated in Project Career activities with 41 students graduating from their programme of study. Of these students, 27 were employed full-time, 6 part-time, and one individual provided unpaid family eldercare on a full-time basis. Seven graduates were not working, but were pursuing their education on a full-time basis as well as 10 of the 33 were employed graduates (Leopold, 2018; Rumrill et al., 2019).

In addition to the success of Project Career student participants, a compendium of technology application, guidelines, resources and training materials for professionals and consumers was created to provide information, assistance and resources to better assist students with TBIs in post-secondary settings. Divided into multiple categories, the Student, Technology, Accommodations, Resources (STAR) portal provides information for students, veterans, educators, employers and families to provide best practices regarding technology, academic success and long-term career assistance for persons with TBI. The STAR portal also includes information about the Project Career model, specific information about the

CST used in the project, app information and training materials. The portal can be accessed at http://www.projectcareertbi.org. (Rumrill et al., 2019).

Summary

College students with TBIs can experience challenges with executive functioning, attention and concentration, memory and many other areas of cognitive and mental functioning, which in turn impact the academic, vocational and psychosocial experiences of the individual. The students' academic and functional needs should be identified along with their goals, preferences and priorities. Project Career was funded by the U.S. government to develop and assess a process of service delivery modelled on the MPT model, academic and vocational support and case management. The approach has proven to be successful and resources have been developed so that it can be used and replicated more widely.

References

American Psychological Association. (2015). Disability mentoring program. Available at: www.apa.org/pi/disability/resources/ mentoring/ (Downloaded: 20 September 2018).

Basso, A., Previgliano, I., & Servadei, F. (2006). Section 3.10: Traumatic brain injury. In: *World Health Organization Neurological Disorders: Public Health Challenges* (pp. 164–175). Available at: www.who.int/mental health/neurology/neurological disorders report web.pdf?uu=1 (Downloaded: 22 September 2018).

Bootes, K. & Chapparo, C. (2010). Difficulties with multitasking on return to work after TBI: A critical case study, *Work*, 36, pp. 207–216.

Bowen, J.M. (2008). Classroom interventions for students with traumatic brain injuries. Available at: www.brainline.org/ content/2008/07/classroom-interventions-students-traumatic-brain-injuries pageall.html (Downloaded: 19 September 2018).

Brainline.org. (2008). TBI research review: Return to work after traumatic brain injury. Available at: www.brainline.org/content/2008/10/ tbi-research-review-return-work-after-traumatic-brain-injury pageall.html (Downloaded: 14 September 2018).

Bryan-Hancock, C., & Harrison, J. (2010). The global burden of traumatic brain injury: preliminary results from the Global Burden of Disease Project. *Injury Prevention*, 16(1), A17–A17.

Centers for Disease Control and Prevention. (2011). Nonfatal traumatic brain injuries related to sports and recreation activities among persons aged ≤ 19 years— United States, 2001–2009, *MMWR*, 60(39), pp. 1337–1342. Available at: www.cdc. gov/mmwr/ pdf/wk/mm6039.pdf (Downloaded: 18 September 2018).

Defense and Veterans Brain Injury Center. (2016). DoD worldwide numbers for TBI. Available at: http://dvbic.dcoe.mil/dod-worldwide-numbers-tbi (Downloaded: 14 September 2018).

Griffin, C. & Stein, M. (2015). Self-perception of disability and prospects for employment among U.S. veterans, *Work*, 50, pp. 49–58.

Hendricks, D., et al. (2015). Activities and interim outcomes of a multi-site development project to promote cognitive support technology use and employment success among postsecondary students with traumatic brain injuries, *NeuroRehabilitation*, 37, pp. 449–458.

Kelly, J., Amerson, E., & Barth, J. (2012). Mild traumatic brain injury: Lessons learned from clinical sports, and combat concussions, *Rehabilitation Research and Practices*. Available at: www.hindawi.com/journals/rerp/2012/37 1970/ (Downloaded: 22 September 2018).

Kennedy, M., Krause, M., & Turksta, L. (2008). An electronic survey about college experience after traumatic brain injury, *NeuroRehabilitation*, 23, pp. 511–520.

Leopold, A. (2018). *Project Career Data Report*. Bethesda, MD: JBS International.

Leopold, A., et al. (2015). The use of assistive technology for cognition to support the performance of daily activities for individuals with cognitive disabilities due to traumatic brain injury: The current state of the research. *NeuroRehabilitation*, 37(3), 359–378.

Nardone, A., et al. (2015). Project career: A qualitative examination of five college students with traumatic brain injuries, *Neurorehabilitation*, 37(3), 459–469.

National Association of State Head Injury Administrators (NASHIA). (2006). Traumatic brain injury facts: Vocational rehabilitation and employment services. Available at: www.nashia.org/ (Downloaded: 18 September 2018).

Rumrill Jr, P.D., et al. (2019). An Organizational Case Study of a 5-Year Development Project to Promote Cognitive Support Technology Use, Academic Success, and Competitive Employment Among Civilian and Veteran College Students With Traumatic Brain Injuries. *Journal of Applied Rehabilitation Counseling*, 50(1), 57–72.

Rumrill, P., et al. (2016). Promoting cognitive support technology use and employment success among postsecondary students with traumatic brain injuries, *Journal of Vocational Rehabilitation*, 45, pp. 53–61.

Ruoff, J. (2008). The student with a brain injury: Achieving goals for higher education. Available at: www.brainline. org/content/2008/10/student-brain-injury-achieving-goalshigher-education.html (Downloaded: 1 September 2018).

Scherer, M. (1998). *Matching Person and Technology*. Webster, NY: Institute for Matching Person & Technology.

Scherer, M., et al. (2005). Predictors of assistive technology use: The importance of personal and psychosocial factors, *Disability Rehabilitation*, 27(21), pp. 1321–1331.

Scherer, M., et al. (2007). A framework for modelling the selection of assistive technology devices (ATDs), *Disability and Rehabilitation: Assistive Technology*, 2(1), pp. 1–8.

Scherer, M. (2016). Matching person and technology: Purpose. Available at: www.matchingpersonandtechnology.com/purpose.html (Downloaded: 22 September 2018).

Scherer, M.J. (2012). *Assistive Technologies and other Supports for People with Brain Impairment*. New York: Springer Publishing Co.

TBI Model Systems. (2010). Emotional problems after traumatic brain injury. Available at: www.msktc.org/tbi/model-system-centers (Downloaded: 15 September 2018).

Todis, B., et al. (2011). Longitudinal investigation of the post-high school transition experiences of adolescents with traumatic brain injury, *Journal of Head Trauma Rehabilitation*, 26(2), pp. 138–149.

Toriello, P. & Keferl, J. (2012). A renaissance of consumer autonomy: Moving from self-determination theory to therapy. In: P.J. Toriello, M.L. Bishop, & P.D. Rumrill, editors. *New Directions in Rehabilitation Counseling: Creative Responses to Professional, Clinical, and Educational Challenges* (pp. 1–24). Linn Creek, MO: Aspen Professional Services.

Vynorius, K.C., Paquin, A.M., & Seichepine, D.R. (2016). Lifetime multiple mild traumatic brain injuries are associated with cognitive and mood symptoms in young healthy college students. *Frontiers in Neurology*, 7, 188.

Wehman, P. (2013). *Life Beyond the Classroom*, 5th edn. Baltimore, MD: Paul H. Brookes Publishing Company.

Wehman, P., et al. (2005). Productive work and employment for persons with traumatic brain injury: What have we learned after 20 years? *Journal of Head Trauma Rehabilitation*, 20(2), pp. 115–127.

Wehman, P., et al. (2014). Transition planning for youth with traumatic brain injury: Findings from the National Longitudinal Transition Survey-2, *NeuroRehabilitation*, 34(2), pp. 365–372.

15

Everyday Communication and Cognition Technologies

Jerry K. Hoepner
University of Wisconsin

Thomas W. Sather
University of Wisconsin and Mayo Clinic Health Systems

CONTENTS

Introduction 271
Technology Adoption and Self-Stigma 273
    Self-Stigma 274
Digital Participation 275
People with Disabilities Using Everyday Technologies 276
Self-Management Tools 278
    Assisted Prompting 279
    External Memory Aids 280
    Experience Sampling and Telehealth Monitoring 282
Potential Roles for the Clinician/Rehab Professional 284
Building the Support Cycle 285
Takeaways for the Rehabilitation Professional (or whomever) 286
References 287

Introduction

We live in an age of technology, where there is an app for just about anything and technologies to serve a wide-range of endeavours. As technology becomes increasingly ubiquitous, use of assistive technology and augmentative communication supports is no longer isolated to persons with cognitive or communication impairments. While persons with physical and cognitive-communication impairments may require specific adaptations to employ such supports, there is much potential value in the availability and normality of universally accessible, everyday technologies (Figure 15.1).

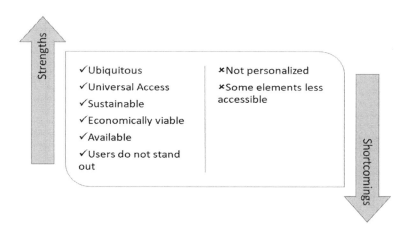

FIGURE 15.1
Considerations for repurposing versus developing individualized assistive technology supports.

Disruptions to cosmesis or perceptions of how others may see assistive technologies are an important element of the self-stigma that can arise from use of individualized assistive technologies. As the field of assistive technology and augmentative-alternative technologies has developed, more attention has been paid to these personal, human factors, as they have the potential to markedly influence implementation and use. Steps towards developing universal access have begun to address some of the factors that contribute to stigma and thus may impact implementation rates. Today's users of assistive technology have more options and potential to use ubiquitous and universal technologies to fill a very individualized cognitive-communication need. No one is likely to question use of a smartphone or tablet to access social media, calendar/reminder functions and a variety of other augmentative supports. Identifying the best fit for applications, technologies, training for implementation and providing ongoing technological supports is essential for ensuring implementation and sustainable use.

When I (first author) began working in the discipline of speech-language pathology, a device called the Liberator was used as an augmentative-alternative communication tool to support individuals with severe communication impairments. This device was about the size of a portable musical keyboard and instantly drew attention to the user. I distinctly recall having conversations wondering why it was not being used across contexts. Knowing what I learned throughout years of practice, it is obvious why adoption failed.

Persons with cognitive-communication impairments have identified a desire to use universal, as well as individualized assistive technologies, to augment their participation in life (Brown, Worrall, Davidson & Howe, 2010;

Buhr, Hoepner, Miller & Johnson, 2017; Miller, Buhr, Johnson & Hoepner, 2013; Worrall et al., 2011). They strongly desire to 'not stand out', a benefit that universal technologies may accomplish better than some individualized assistive technologies. It may help to operationalize what those individualized assistive technologies are, as compared to those that function on a universal platform like smart technologies. For simplicity and the purposes of this discussion, we will refer to those as dedicated devices. Dedicated devices and applications are designed for the purpose of addressing a specific set of cognitive-communication needs and may also serve to address physical or environmental access needs. In many cases, funding is linked to dedicated devices and/or available at a higher rate than everyday technologies, even though cost of everyday technologies are often substantially less. Further, the cosmesis related to universal appearance of those devices fall upon a continuum, with some *passing for* universal devices while others clearly stand out more as dedicated devices to support someone with physical, cognitive and communication impairments. The concept of *passing for* ordinary people or fitting in as ordinary people has been discussed in the context of assistive and augmentative/alternative technologies (Söderström & Ytterhus, 2010). Often assistive technologies that make individuals standout are rejected by the user, whenever possible (Söderström & Ytterhus, 2010; Kent & Smith, 2006). If given only the option of an overt assistive technology support, users who have some capacity to function without the device will often reject use in that context.

Technology Adoption and Self-Stigma

Younger people are particularly interested in using technology in their everyday lives (Buckingham, 2006; McMillan & Morrison, 2006). Information and communication technologies including Internet-based technologies, social media and mobile technologies are of particular value. Access to those technologies has become ubiquitous and modified access may be relatively easy in home or private contexts where other people will not see modifications. Acceptance and implementation may change when or if access modifications become more visible to others, making the user to stand out. In those cases, rejection of the modification is more likely. The Pew Research Center, a nonpartisan research think tank, tracks access and use rates of such technologies across age groups, geographical contexts and a variety of other factors. Pew data indicate widespread access and use by most age groups, with use lessening with older age groups. For specific information about age groups and geographical contexts pertinent to your work, we recommend examining those Pew data sets (www.pewresearch.org/). Particularly relevant to implementation of information and communication technologies and assistive technology are rates of use by persons with and without disabilities.

Of the 27% of adults in the United States living with a disability, most are significantly less likely to use online resources than their peers without disabilities (54% as opposed to 81% without a disability). Device owner-ship is also correlated with variables of age, income and education level. As of 2014 (Pew Research Center), 88% of American adults had a cell phone, 57% had a laptop, 19% owned an e-book reader and 19% owned a tablet device. Further, 63% of those individuals accessed Internet through those devices. Individuals with cognitive-communication and/or physical impair-ments face additional challenges to online access and social networking. Dobransky and Hargittai (2016) report that online access and experiences are heterogenous among individuals with disabilities, and that, while barriers to online access exist, there are unique opportunities online that may support participation and interaction beyond what may occur in an exclusionary, 'real-world' society. When controlling for demographic status including age and socioeconomic status, individuals with disabilities engage in primary online activities (downloading videos, gaming online, reviewing products, sharing content and posting to blogs) similarly to individuals without dis-abilities (Dobransky & Hargittai, 2016). However, because individuals with disabilities tend to be older and with lower socioeconomic status, there does continue to be a disproportionate reduction in Internet access and Internet skills among those with disabilities (Dobransky & Hargittai, 2016).

Self-Stigma

The user perception of universality and cosmesis (lack of standing out) appears central to adoption and use. This use or non-use, varying by con-text, appears dependent on stigmas and associations with those technolo-gies (Pape, Kim & Weiner, 2002; Parette & Scherer, 2004). Pape et al. (2002) found that people were more likely to abandon their assistive technology when it made them feel different from peers. Information and communi-cation technologies (aka everyday technologies) are associated with com-petence, independence and belonging to a social group. Conversely, use of assistive technology (especially when not disguised well or passing for universal technology) is associated with medically restricted, difference and dependency (Ravneberg, 2009; Wielandt et al., 2006). Therefore, mak-ing assistive technologies more aligned with, or combined with, universally designed information and communication technologies is central to increas-ing adoption/use across contexts. Söderström and Ytterhus (2010) identified factors that predict usability of assistive technologies, including a reduction in physical, cognitive and linguistic effort that promotes convenience, effi-ciency and productivity, while creating a positive impression by the user amongst pertinent peers. Unfortunately, there is typically a gap between release of mainstream technologies and assistive technologies. That gap may never be avoided, as individual needs are complex in spite of progress towards universal design. Universal design principles refer to a philosophy of designing products that are accessible to the widest range of capabilities, including those made accessible through assistive technologies (Section 3 of the Assistive Technology Act of 1998, U.S.C. § 3002). It is a mistake, however, to assume that universal design will replace assistive technology. Rose, Hasselbring, Stahl and Zabala (2005) identify universal design and assistive technology as two parallel interventions designed to reduce barriers. Universal design reduces barriers for everyone, while assistive technologies reduce barriers for persons with disabilities. Adjustments must often be made through individualized adaptations and training. Those adjustments extend beyond access modifications to address social acceptance. Some assistive technology users express a fear of looking incompetent while using their technologies (Shinohara & Wobbrock, 2011). They are more likely to use the technology in the midst of peers when they feel skilled and competent. This seems to emphasize the importance of effective training to mastery/level of confidence with the device or application. While technologies are constantly changing, principles of selecting, adapting and training use of assistive technologies in the form of everyday technologies are potentially more stable. As such, this chapter will attempt to examine some potential types of technologies and how they can be repurposed to support individuals with cognitive-communication impairments, rather than trying to address an exhaustive and ever-changing list of individualized supports and specific programmes. This fits well with principles of *mainstream accessibility* and *design for social acceptance* (Shinohara & Wobbrock, 2011). Table 15.1 includes a list of potential considerations for repurposing devices and applications.

Digital Participation

The Communications Consumer Panel (CCP) broadly defines digital participation as 'increasing the reach, breadth, and depth of digital technology use across all sections of society, to maximize digital participation and

TABLE 15.1

Considerations for Types of Cognitive-Communicative Needs that may be Met by Repurposing Universal Applications

Repurposing Applications
• Social media and peer networking
• Communication supports
• Self-management tools
• Assisted prompting
• External memory aids
• Video modelling
• Experience sampling
• Telehealth monitoring

the economic and social benefits it can bring' (Digital Britain Report, 2009; p. 4). While Internet usage continues to climb over the years, there remains a subset of individuals who are at higher risk of exclusion from such usage. While these factors for non-engagement are complex and go beyond one single factor, Helsper and Reisdorf (2013) suggest consideration of disengagement due to external and internal factors, including access, interest and self-preservation. The Consumer Framework for Digital Participation (CCPR, 2010) is a model developed through consumer input. As such, it provides a fairly tangible set of action steps for effective Internet engagement. Menger, Morris and Salis (2016) applied this framework to identify skills and factors relating to digital participation specifically among individuals with aphasia. The framework addresses interest, logistics of use, benefits of successful implementation and risk management.

People with Disabilities Using Everyday Technologies

The positive potential impact that social networks have on health and well-being is well documented (Umberson & Karas Montez, 2010; Smith & Christakis, 2008; Umberson, Crosnoe & Reczek, 2010). Social media, and subsequent everyday technologies that support social media access and use, may positively impact social networks. Although complex, there have been multiple implications (both positive and negative) for the role of social media and technology on both in-person and cyberspace social networks (Matsuba, 2006; Alloway, Runac, Qureshi & Kemp, 2014). Specific to individuals with cognitive-communication impairments, everyday technologies hold the potential to generate, enhance and maintain relationships with greater ease, efficiency and transparency than in the physical world. This may subsequently enhance one's social network and the potential advantages of a growing and robust social network.

People with communication impairments have identified a desire to use social networking technologies (Brown, Worrall, Davidson & Howe, 2010; Buhr, Hoepner, Miller & Johnson, 2017; Miller, Buhr, Johnson & Hoepner, 2013; Worrall et al., 2011). One such social networking technology is Snapchat. Snapchat is a growing social networking application with appeal as a predominantly digital image-heavy sharing platform. As of September 2018, Snapchat had over 300 million monthly active users. It is used by nearly 20% of all U.S. social media users, who collectively produce 3 billion snaps per day with more than 20,000 photos shared every second (OmnicoreAgency. com). Snapchat holds potential for usage among individuals with communication difficulties in part due to the low-linguistic demands and high degree of visual supports. In a pilot study of Snapchat use among individuals with aphasia at a 3-day weekend, rustic aphasia camp, participants shared images of their activities and interactions at camp. Most snaps were image only, with a small proportion of snaps augmented by additional user-generated text content (Hoepner, Baier, Sather & Clark, 2017). Additionally, researchers identified the importance of staff accessibility for user support to facilitate Snapchat usage. In a subsequent 2-month trial, which took place within the participants' home communities, Baier, Hoepner and Sather (2017) identified multiple facilitative aspects of Snapchat with regard to social exchanges among individuals with aphasia. Positive aspects of Snapchat included contributions to communicative expression through images alone, and the ability to renegotiate identity through sharing and interacting with other Snapchat users. Conversely, there were operational barriers that contributed to negative experiences with Snapchat. Frequent updates to the Snapchat platform create barriers to users who become habituated to a specific layout or operational requirement. Further, users in these studies emphasized, directly and indirectly, the need for incidental and regular support to use Snapchat effectively. Often those supports are small steps that a nearby partner could resolve in a few moments; however, when someone is not present, those small barriers can prevent engagement. These challenges included general device competence (e.g. entering Apple IDs or passwords) and application-specific issues (e.g. viewing stories within the 24-h period).

Such experiences highlight the need for support when using some everyday technologies. Because such supports are not always feasible, there may be a need for other types of dedicated applications to better support users with cognitive-communication impairments. Miller, Buhr, Johnson & Hoepner (2013) developed the AphasiaWeb, an aphasia-specific social networking tool with embedded therapeutic modalities to support individuals with aphasia including written choice and multiple modes of input. They identified multiple episodes in which the technology platform supported social interaction among individuals with aphasia, and largely positive perceptions and experiences among those with aphasia. While they expressed interest in connecting with peers affected by communication impairments on an application specifically designed to scaffold their participation, they also valued the use of universal platforms for connecting with family, friends and new people (Buhr, Hoepner, Miller & Johnson, 2017; Miller, Buhr, Johnson & Hoepner, 2013). As such, finding applications that fit both of those needs is crucial. Further, finding ways to improve accessibility of universal sites through adaptations and training is also necessary.

Brunner, Palmer, Togher and Hemsley (2018) identified multiple themes related to patterns of social media and experiences among individuals with traumatic brain injury (TBI). Interestingly, many individuals with TBI initially pursued social media simply because 'like everyone was on Facebook...everyone was doing it' (Brunner et al., 2018, p. 4). Participants identified benefits related to the reciprocal nature of social media in fostering social connections, and social connections, subsequently, fostering ongoing social media usage. All participants in their study identified 'enhanced connectedness with family and friends' (Brunner et al., 2018, p. 5). Additionally, Facebook has been identified as a means of social support among individuals with mild impairments to cognition following TBI (Eghdam, Hamidi, Bartfai & Koch, 2018). In their study of over 1,300 members in a Swedish public Facebook group for individuals with cognitive fatigue post-brain injury, the authors concluded that participants in the brain-injured group participated and used Facebook similarly to those without brain injuries in Facebook groups. The authors advocate for Facebook as a strong means of communication and social support for those with mild cognitive impairment and indicate the value of Facebook as an easily used medium across users and devices (Eghdam, Hamidi, Bartfai & Koch, 2018). When discussing potential barriers to social media usage among individuals with TBI, Brunner et al. (2018) reported participants identified challenges relating primarily to emotional reactions, communication demands and cognitive fatigue. Interestingly however, these relate to social media as a general platform, rather than specific to a single application or platform. These challenges are not unique to individuals with neurological impairments in comparison to those without; who are newer social media users.

With regard to specific platforms used within everyday technologies, Twitter has the capacity to support increased interactions, communications and relationships among those with and without cognitive-communication impairments. Hemsley, Palmer and Balandin (2014) identify two potential advantages of Twitter use among individuals with disabilities. First, direct benefits to the user include increased ease of access to current information, being a part of the dialogue, and dissemination relating to one's disability. Secondly, increased social media contributions by those with disabilities foster a broader dialogue about the disability (Hemsley, Palmer & Balandin, 2014).

Self-Management Tools

Self-management encompasses a number of tools that support an individual's ability to function independently and successfully. While some of these supports are no-tech or low-tech, technology is becoming increasingly available to address such needs. Self-management is particularly pertinent in the chronic phases of recovery and maintenance. For an excellent description of self-management frameworks in chronic conditions, see the work of Lorig et al. (2012). Hoepner and Olson (2019) also provide an overview of the framework that addresses applications to communication and cognition. Lorig et al. (2012) identify five core skills central to successful implementation of self-management: problem-solving, decision-making, finding and utilizing resources, a partnership between patient and healthcare provider and taking action. As such, successful implementation of self-management tools falls along a continuum of independence, from totally dependent to fully independent. Those on the dependent or semi-independent portions of the continuum rely on a provider or family to support day-to-day use.

Assisted Prompting

Assisted prompting is a technique designed to improve home carryover of exercise and home practice, given support of an assistive technology (AT) device. Early iterations used pagers to deliver reminders (Svoboda & Richards, 2009; Wilson, Emslie, Quirk & Evans, 2001). While universal design for access was relatively poor (i.e. dot matrix text on a small screen with limited or scrolling text), the technique improved follow-through with exercises at home. Considering that dosing and frequency of home practice or exercises are crucial to producing change, this twofold increase in adherence is meaningful. The next generation used television-delivered prompting, which allowed for delivery of prompts for exercises, a reminder about the purpose of those exercises, a video model of how to perform the exercises and prompts to log performance (Lemoncello, Sohlberg, Fickas & Prideaux, 2011; Lemoncello, Sohlberg, Fickas, Albin & Harn, 2011; Sohlberg, Lemoncello & Lee, 2011). While prompts, video models and accountability associated with television-assisted prompting increased follow-through and users valued the ability to follow the direct video model, applications were somewhat limited, in that the person needed to be in front of the television when the prompts and supports were delivered. Newest generations of assisted prompting utilize mobile technologies to deliver prompting and supports. It is worth noting that physical therapy (physiotherapy) studies of adherence programming, where videos of exercises are provided to support follow-through, do not demonstrate better adherence than those with only direct instruction (Lysack et al., 2005; Schoo et al., 2005). This may relate, however, to the way adherence was measured. Surprisingly, those who viewed the video were less accurate but completed exercises more frequently (44% vs. 22%; Lysack et al., 2005). Further, these were individuals without cognitive-communication impairments. Self-monitoring, an element of assisted prompting, has been shown to increase adherence (Goto et al., 2014; Pisters et al., 2010). It may be necessary to include all elements of assisted prompting (i.e. prompt, instructions, video model and prompts to document/self-monitor) in order to achieve a meaningful change to adherence. Further, some elements may be more important for persons with cognitive-communication needs. With the advent of Smart technologies in phones and tablets, assisted prompting can be delivered on mobile devices, wherever the individual is at any given moment. A large-scale study in physiotherapy found that an app-based home exercise programme, coupled with text message prompts and encouragement from the clinician resulted in statistically better follow-through as compared to paper handouts alone (Lambert et al., 2017). The app is associated with www.physiotherapyexercises.com, a free web-based software. Mobile applications to support 'patient' engagement and home exercise programmes are now available commercially (e.g. MedBridge Go). These programmes are presently limited to physical therapy exercise programmes but certainly appear to be a good match for cognitive, communication and swallowing (dysphagia) exercise applications. The application provides written instructions, photographs of the exercise and video demonstrations. Similarly, the *iSwallow* app provides descriptions, rationales and video demonstration for home programmes using swallowing exercises. Paired with other apps that prompt completion of exercises (e.g. Nudge Reminders), such tools have the potential to reduce several barriers to home programme completion. Potential barriers include memory of how to complete the exercises, reminders of purpose/rationale and timing/adherence.

External Memory Aids

External memory aids (EMAs) come in many forms, including no-, low- and high-tech devices such as planners, schedules, reminder apps, timers, memory wallets and captured images. There is a large and diverse body of research on EMAs for persons with TBIs, dementia and mild cognitive impairments but we will focus on those that address principles relevant to selecting and implementing everyday technologies as EMAs. Systematic training is crucial to successful implementation (Lanzi, Wallace & Bourgeois, 2018a). Often, training follows a simple framework identified by Sohlberg and Mateer (1989). While this framework is nearly 20 years old, it remains widely used. The three-phase framework includes acquisition, application and adaptation elements. The acquisition phase includes orientation to the application and/or device, discussion of any previous applications and/or devices that this may replace, and discussions of contexts or purposes for use. The application phase is one of practice and troubleshooting. This may include role-plays or hypothetical implementation of various application and/or device functions alongside of the clinician. The adaptation phase includes transitioning device use to the natural contexts or environments. Gentry et al. (2008) focused specifically on implementation of 'off-the-shelf' calendar/planner devices for persons with TBIs (p. 23). Investigators used one-on-one in-home training and troubleshooting, with modelling and verbal stepwise instructions, along with supportive literature. All participants were able to learn and implement the devices as aids. Client perceptions and preferences for EMAs have also been examined among persons with mild memory impairments (Lanzi, Wallace & Bourgeois, 2018b). Awareness of one's own memory abilities was a factor in device preference, as was attitudes towards the technology. Users also identified that the device needed to be useful in multiple environments, consistent with previous research, which identified the importance of considering environments when applying AT supports (Scherer, Hart, Kirsch & Schulthesis, 2005). Along with those common values, the study identified a number of individual differences, which emphasizes the importance

TABLE 15.2

Potential Off-the-Shelf Devices and EMA Applications

Devices	Applications
Calendars and reminder apps	Prompt completion of daily tasks
Social story or photo album apps	Memory wallets use selected photos and headings to support memory for conversations
Camera function on mobile technologies	Capture images to be used in-the-moment to support recall or augment communication (aka dynamic capture)
Video recording function on mobile technologies	Capture video to support recall of processes
Video playback devices	Playback video to support recall of processes (e.g., YouTube demonstration videos)
Timers/visual timer apps	Support completion of tasks or set parameters for participation. Spaced retrieval, implicit memory training
Voicemail	Messages to self to prompt completion of tasks

of eliciting and considering personal preferences rather than prescribing a specific device and/or application. While the devices themselves change, the principles for selecting ecologically universal devices remain pertinent. Table 15.2 identifies potential devices and applications to serve as EMAs.

Video Modeling: Flourishing with the advent of mobile technologies for recording and viewing videos, video modelling is becoming a widely used medium for self-management. Film study and review has been used for many years in the context of sports. Coaches and players examine film of previous events as they prepared for upcoming events. Better technology has led to the ability to examine mechanics and form at a very specific level. Slowing replay, pausing, overlaid grids and frame-by-frame viewing can allow a baseball batter or golfer to examine their swing, shot put thrower or pitcher to examine their throwing mechanics, and the list goes on and on. Applications like Dartfish and Coach's Eye enable coaches and players to drill down to those miniscule moments. Likewise, these technologies and video capture in general have the potential to augment many aspects of communication and cognition.

In the realm of communication and cognition, video modelling (also known as interpersonal process recall (Youse & Coelho, 2009) or self-coaching (Ylvisaker, 2006) or simply video review). Video modelling can be used by reviewing videos of self or others. Video self-modelling (VSM) capitalizes on the tangible support of directly reviewing one's own actions, followed by guided debriefing regarding successes and challenges. The support of video evidence is crucial, as retrospective negativity bias and memory compromise accuracy with delayed recall (Fiske, 1980; Hoepner & Turkstra, 2013; Matt, Vázquez & Campbell, 1992). Some VSM capitalizes exclusively on positive moments (what went well), so as to provide a successful model to self on how to complete an action, such as how to share information efficiently (Buggey & Ogle, 2012; Buggey, 2007). This approach is true to the original tenants of VSM (Creer & Miklich, 1970). Others use VSM more holistically, capitalizing on both successful moments and opportunities for improvement, with an emphasis on increasing those successful actions (Baker, Lang & O'Reilly, 2009; Cream et al., 2010; Lang et al., 2009; Hoepner & Olson, 2018; Hoepner, 2016; Ortiz, Burlingame, Onuegbulem, Yoshikawa & Rojas, 2012; Prater, Carter, Hitchcock & Ravneberg, 2012). The advent of smart technologies makes collecting and reviewing videos accessible and potentially immediate. VSM has been used to address social skills (Lang et al., 2009), second language acquisition (Ortiz, 2012), speech fluency (Cream et al., 2010), emotional and behavioural disorders (Baker et al., 2009), partner training (Hoepner & Olson, 2018; Magill-Evans, Harrison, Benzies, Gierl & Kimak, 2007; Meharg & Lipsker, 1992) and self-regulation (Hoepner & Olson, 2018; McGraw-Hunter, Faw & Davis, 2006). Video other-modelling may be used to meet the objective of learning from positive models when self-models are inadequate or the person reacts negatively to reviewing their own models. This approach has been examined in the context of partner training (Hoepner, Sell & Kooiman, 2015; Lock, Wilkinson, Bryan, Maxim, Edmundson, Bruce & Moir, 2001; Orange & Colton-Hudson, 1998; Wilkinson, Bryan, Lock & Sage, 2010).

Whatever the application of video modelling, access to video recording and playback features of mobile technologies has made it accessible. The application comes standard on most contemporary mobile devices and is commonly used by people without disabilities.

Experience Sampling and Telehealth Monitoring

Experience sampling methodology (ESM) is a collection of methods designed to better understand individual experiences on a daily basis, utilizing self-report via various sampling schedules and modalities (Larson & Csikszentmihalyi, 2014). Also known as Ecological Momentary Assessment, ESM can be utilized with low- or high-tech data-gathering techniques, and has been used by a variety of populations, including those with health and medical conditions such as mood disorders and anxiety, gastrointestinal impairments and asthma. Additionally, it is used to measure compliance with medications, physical activity and diet regulations (Shiffman, Stone & Hufford, 2008). Recently, ESM has been used with individuals with aphasia, as a means to better understand barriers and facilitators to effective communication and meaningful engagement (Sather, Howe, Nelson & Lagerwey, 2017; Fitzgerald-DeJean, Rubin & Carson, 2012). While ESM has been used primarily as an assessment tool, there is growing application as an intervention tool for behavioural change and support, including use among individuals with mental health impairments in psychotherapy (Riva, Freire & Bassi, 2016), depression (Kramer et al., 2014) and substance abuse (Shiffman, Stone & Hufford, 2008). Data derived from ESM may support a better understanding of one's own behaviours and emotions, such as a review of emotional states, consumption amounts and social interaction. Such data-gathering methodologies may be active, such as requiring the user to input certain responses when prompted. Other methods are passive, where the data-gathering application or tool automatically collects ongoing data without requiring the user to 'push' or send such data, for example, in a FitBit®.

Cornet and Holden (2018) conducted a systematic review of smartphone-based, passive-sensing applications for health and well-being among neurotypicals and those with health conditions. Most frequently captured data include accelerometry, location, audio and usage. Periodically sampled, self-ratings of mental health correlate with clinical mental health measures, as well as detecting stability or deterioration of mental health status. Given the overlap between social isolation and mental health concerns, this monitoring is pertinent to persons with communication disorders who have a higher prevalence of social isolation. Monitoring feedback can be provided to the healthcare team and/or directly to the person being monitored. In studies where feedback was provided to participants (only 40%), participants reported value in feedback that was understandable and applicable. Additional modifications may need to occur to ensure that feedback is accessible to persons with cognitive-communication impairments. Ben-Zeev, Schere, Wang, Xie and Campbell (2015) evaluated the value and application of smartphone utility as behavioural markers for an individual's mental health. They identified significant associations between depression and measures obtained from smartphone applications including speech duration, geospatial activity and sleep duration. Additionally, accelerometry changes were associated with perceived changes in perceptions of loneliness. The authors conclude that smartphone applications may provide extensive value in the transparency and efficiency of mental health assessment and monitoring, far beyond current traditional mental health paradigms.

Some of these data-gathering methodologies are certainly within the consideration of everyday technologies, and may be accessible to those with cognitive-communication impairments. However, one potential downfall is that such everyday technologies often maintain a level of written, operational, visual and/or sequential complexity that renders use infeasible. Regarding apps designed for specific neurologic populations, Giunti, Fernándes, Zubiete and Romero (2018) explored Google Play and Apple App Store to locate apps relevant to mobile health monitoring for individuals with multiple sclerosis (MS). Following application of their pre-identified inclusion and exclusion criteria, only 30 apps of the initial 581 potential apps were identified as potential fits. Unfortunately, most did not include energy management and remote monitoring, and they concluded that available apps failed to meet the needs of individuals with MS. The authors identified the recurring need for industry collaboration with individuals with various health conditions, as well as with key players including healthcare providers and researchers, for ongoing collaboration. In such cases, modified ESM devices may support access to this everyday technology, with simple design strategies with the end user being an individual with cognitive, communication and/or visual impairments (Sather, Howe, Nelson & Lagerwey, 2017). Provision of feedback that is accessible and understandable to persons with cognitive-communication impairments is crucial to supporting use of every-day experience-sampling, health-monitoring devices and applications.

Potential Roles for the Clinician/Rehab Professional

Numerous factors play into the adoption and sustainability of using every-day technologies to assist and augment participation in everyday wants and needs identified by persons with cognitive-communication impairments. Promoting use of technologies likely to be adopted and sustained by end users is dependent upon an awareness of those factors. Figure 15.2 attempts to provide a model for person-driven adoption and sustainability for use of everyday technologies as assistive technology supports. The DARN frame-work is a way to understand readiness for change and adoption of change behaviours (Miller & Rollnick, 2012). Our adaptation maps factors related to adoption and maintenance to the DARN framework. While factors are mapped onto specific elements of DARN, there is inter-dependency across factors and context or environment is relevant across factors. Since the use of everyday technologies as an assistive technology support requires adoption of a device or application, we believe it provides a strong parallel.

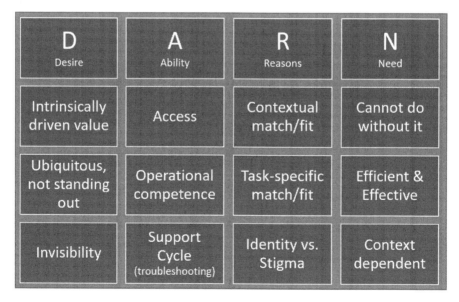

FIGURE 15.2
Person-driven model for adoption and sustainability.

Building the Support Cycle

As has been discussed throughout this chapter, opportunities and applications for everyday technologies exist to support individuals with cognitive-communication impairments. Figure 15.3 depicts our conceptualization of the support cycle, another framework relevant to adoption and sustainability of AT. We feel an understanding of these factors supersedes most device-software app-specific choices. For a summary of how the roles of clinicians intersect with user needs see Takeaways for the Rehabilitation Professional. As illustrated by the previous figures, it is not enough to simply turn the end user with cognitive/communication impairments to the technology and leave them on their own. Rather, even if not modifying the technology there are means through which the (rehabilitation) provider can support the end user. Key to the support cycle is the opportunity for authentic contexts. These may take the shape of, for example, embedded aphasia group or TBI group interventions that foster engagement and interaction while utilizing the technology target. This may also require explicitly or implicitly engaging proxies such as family members, care partners, staff, community, etc. These opportunities are best established prior to the need arising, and these prior-established supports lend to the authenticity of the context, with subsequently increased likelihood of usage. Note that each step within this cycle can be considered a therapeutic target, and can also serve as part of direct intervention. Additionally, note that this process is nonlinear. This is a cycle of constant repetition and need for revisitation. Once an individual has had

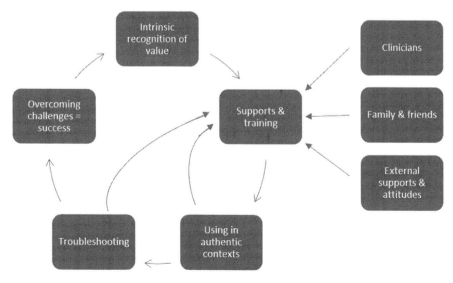

FIGURE 15.3
Support cycle, crucial to sustainability and maintenance.

a success, it is important not to consider the skill or technology 'acquired' but rather to remain vigilant on the need for all aspects of the cycle from presence of supports to authentic contexts and troubleshooting.

Takeaways for the Rehabilitation Professional (or whomever)

1. **Training is crucial:** Clinicians may often overlook the importance of training and underestimate how long it takes for a person with a communication and/or cognitive impairment to reach mastery. Sohlberg and Mateer (1989) propose a three-phase training model: acquisition, application and adaptation. This approach moves from device or application-specific training and hands-on practice to use in authentic contexts. Brunner et al. (2018 discuss a cyclical staging approach to the development and mastery of social media use that addresses motivation and reciprocity in addition to device and application competence. Across two studies where incidental supports were either present or not, Hoepner et al. (2017) and Baier et al., 2017 identified that incidental and ongoing supports for troubleshooting are central to carryover and participation.

2. **Build in a Support Cycle:** Even when training is effective and the user reaches mastery, ongoing supports and troubleshooting remain important. Issues beyond the application or device competence itself can compromise use, including changes and updates to the software. New issues arise that may present substantive barriers if not addressed early. Include multiple support proxies in the support cycle for intentional redundancy and backup. The CCP calls for ongoing 'end-to-end' support throughout digital participation not just solely at the beginning of the experience. It is important to recognize, however, that simply having access to someone to support a potential AT user is not enough to ensure participation. In a survey by Dutton, Blank and Groselj (2013), the authors note that nearly 90% of people who stopped using Internet and 70% of those who refuse to use the Internet had someone who could help them to access it. This reminds us that relying on support from proxies alone is inadequate. Addressing motivation and the potential influence of stigma also play into adoption and carryover.

3. **Be aware of self-stigma:** Evaluate and address the potential implications of self-stigma. Recognize that self-stigma may be context specific. In many ways, the online context increases accessibility for persons with disabilities. Recognize that in-home/private use of technologies may be a facilitating context, whereas public contexts

may evoke more stigma implications. We should consider the role that everyday technologies may have in reducing stigma, as they are less likely to make users stand out.

4. **Identify benefits that eclipse barriers:** Key takeaways from the CCP include ensuring that users identify a benefit, and that the benefit outweighs the perceived barriers to digital activity. Further, the CCP reinforces the need for increased focus on the digital participation experience among individuals with disabilities (CCP, 2010). Included among the items in their call-to-action summary are several relevant to working with individuals with disabilities and supporting their enhanced digital participation. These items include setting up a mentor/support network, ideally in a peer-to-peer model, to provide technical, logistical and experience-based supports throughout the digital journey. Additionally, they call for one's communication and social network to actively engage with the individual embarking on a digital/technology journal (CCP, 2010).

5. **Every individual is different:** While this is intuitive for most of us, it still bears reminding. Evaluating fit for an individual means involving that individual in the process of selecting and vetting everyday technologies. If we prescribe applications or technology, we decrease the odds of adoption and adaptation of that support.

6. **Avoid the pitfall of seeing technology as the panacea:** Technology is merely a tool to support communication, cognition and participation. Yes, it can be a very powerful and effective tool but without training, support and buy-in, it will fail. Further, that tool will continue to change as technologies advance. Therefore, understanding a framework for selecting and implementing a technology is key. Rather than choosing from a list of the latest apps or devices, consider how everyday applications can be repurposed to fit an individual's needs.

References

Alloway, T., Runac, R., Qureshi, M., & Kemp, G. (2014). Is Facebook linked to selfishness? Investigating the relationships among social media use, empathy, and narcissism. *Social Networking*, 3(03), 150.

Baier, C. K., Hoepner, J. K., & Sather, T. W. (2017). Exploring Snapchat as a dynamic capture tool for social exchange among individuals with aphasia. *Aphasiology*, doi: 10.1080/02687038.2017.1409870

Baker, S. D., Lang, R., & O'Reilly, M. (2009). Review of video modeling with students with emotional and behavioral disorders. *Education and Treatment of Children*, 32(3), 403–420.

Ben-Zeev, D., Scherer, E. A., Wang, R., Xie, H., & Campbell, A. T. (2015). Next-generation psychiatric assessment: Using smartphone sensors to monitor behavior and mental health. *Psychiatric Rehabilitation Journal, 38*(3), 218–226.

BIS. (2009). Digital Britain report. http://webarchive.nationalarchives.gov.uk/20100511084737/http://interactive.bis.gov.uk/digitalbritain/category/digital-britain-report

Brown, K., Worrall, L., Davidson, B., & Howe, T. (2010). Snapshots of success: An insider perspective on living successfully with aphasia. *Aphasiology, 24*(10), 1267–1295.

Brunner, M., Palmer, S., Togher, L., & Hemsley, B. (2018). 'I kind of figured it out': The views and experiences of people with traumatic brain injury (TBI) in using social media—self-determination for participation and inclusion online. *International Journal of Language and Communication Disorders, 54*, 221–233.

Buggey, T., & Ogle, L. (2012). Video self-modeling. *Psychology in the Schools, 49*(1), 52–70.

Buckingham, D. (2006). Children and new media. In: Lievrouw, L. A., & Livingston, S. (Eds.), *The handbook of new media update student edition* (75–91). London: Sage Publications Inc.

Buhr, H. R., Hoepner, J. K., Miller, H., & Johnson, C. (2017). Aphasia Web: Development and evaluation of an aphasia-friendly social networking application. *Aphasiology, 31*(9). 999–1020. doi: 10.1080/02687038.2016.1232361

Communications Consumer Panel Policy Report. (2010). Delivering digital participation: The consumer perspective. www.communicationsconsumerpanel.org.uk/FINAL%20DP%20SUMMARY.pdf.

Cornet, V., & Holden, R. (2018). Systematic review of smartphone-based passive sensing for health and wellbeing. *Journal of Biomedical Informatics, 77*, 120–132.

Cream, A., O'Brian, S., Jones, M., Block, S., Harrison, E., Lincoln, M., & Onslow, M. (2010). Randomized controlled trial of video self-modeling following speech restructuring treatment for stuttering. *Journal of Speech, Language, and Hearing Research, 53*(4), 887–897.

Creer, T. L., & Miklich, D. R. (1970). The application of a self-modeling procedure to modify inappropriate behavior: A preliminary report. *Behaviour Research and Therapy, 8*(1), 91–92.

Dobransky, K., & Hargittai, E. (2016). Unrealized potential: Exploring the digital disability divide. *Poetics, 58*, 18–28.

Dutton, W. H., Blank, G., & Groselj, D. (2013). *Cultures of the Internet: The internet in Britain.* Oxford: University of Oxford.

Eghdam, A., Hamidi, U., Bartfai, A., & Koch, S. (2018). Facebook as communication support for persons with potential mild acquired cognitive impairment: A content and social network analysis study. *PLoS One, 13*(1), e0191878. doi:10.1371/journal.pone.0191878

Fiske, S. T. (1980). Attention and weight in person perception: The impact of negative and extreme information. *Journal of Personality and School Psychology, 39*, 889–906.

Fitzgerald-DeJean, D. M., Rubin, S. S., & Carson, R. L. (2012). An application of the experience sampling method to the study of aphasia: A case report. *Aphasiology, 26*(2), 234–251.

Gentry, T., Wallace, J., Kvarfordt, C., & Lynch, K. B. (2008). Personal digital assistants as cognitive aids for individuals with severe traumatic brain injury: A community-based trial. *Brain Injury, 22*(1), 19–24.

Giunti, G., Fernández, E. G., Zubiete, E. D., & Romero, O. R. (2018). Supply and demand in mHealth apps for persons with multiple sclerosis: Systematic search in app stores and scoping literature review. *JMIR mHealth and uHealth, 6*(5), E10512.

Goto, M., Takedani, H., Haga, N., Kubota, M., Ishiyama, M., Ito, S., & Nitta, O. (2014). Self-monitoring has potential for home exercise programmes in patients with haemophilia. *Haemophilia, 20*(2), e121–e127.

Helsper, E. J., & Reisdorf, B. C. (2013). A quantitative examination of explanations for reasons for Internet nonuse. *Cyberpsychology, Behavior, and Social Networking, 16*(2), 94–99.

Hemsley, B., Palmer, S., & Balandin, S. (2014). Tweet reach: A research protocol for using Twitter to increase information exchange in people with communication disabilities. *Developmental Neurorehabilitation, 17*(2), 84–89.

Hoepner, J. K. (2016). Partners as environment: Coaching partners. In: Johnson, P. (Eds.), *A Clinician's Guide to Successful Evaluation and Treatment of Dementia* (pp. 137–153). Gaylord, MI: Northern Speech Services Publishing.

Hoepner, J. K., Baier, C. K., Sather, T. W., & Clark, M. B. (2017). A pilot exploration of Snapchat as an aphasia-friendly social exchange technology at an aphasia camp. *Clinical Archives of Communication Disorders, 1*(1), 1–13. doi: 10.21849/cacd.2016.00087

Hoepner, J. K., & Olson, S. E. (2018). Joint video self-modeling as a conversational intervention for an individual with traumatic brain injury and his everyday partner: A pilot investigation. *Clinical Archives of Communication Disorders, 3*(1), 22–41. doi: 10.21849/cacd.2018.00262

Hoepner, J. K., & Olson, S. E. (2019). Self-management. In: Damico, J., & Ball, M. (Eds.), *The Sage encyclopedia of communication sciences and disorders* (pp. 1672–1674). Thousand Oaks, CA: Sage Publications Inc.

Hoepner, J. K., Sell, L., & Kooiman, H. (2015). Case study of partner training in Corticobasal degeneration. *Journal of Interactional Research in Communication Disorders, 6*(2). 157–186. doi: 10.1558/jircd.v6i2.27178

Hoepner, J. K., & Turkstra, L. S. (2013). Video-based administration of the La Trobe Communication Questionnaire for adults with traumatic brain injury and their communication partners. *Brain Injury, 27*(4), 464–472.

Kent, B., & Smith, S. (2006). They only see it when the sun shines in my ears: Exploring perceptions of adolescent hearing aid users. *Journal of Deaf Studies and Deaf Education, 11*(4), 461–476.

Kramer, I., Simons, C. J., Hartmann, J. A., Menne-Lothmann, C., Viechtbauer, W., Peeters, F.,... & van Os, J. (2014). A therapeutic application of the experience sampling method in the treatment of depression: A randomized controlled trial. *World Psychiatry, 13*(1), 68–77.

Lambert, T. E., Harvey, L. A., Avdalis, C., Chen, L. W., Jeyalingam, S., Pratt, C. A.,... & Lucas, B. R. (2017). An app with remote support achieves better adherence to home exercise programs than paper handouts in people with musculoskeletal conditions: A randomised trial. *Journal of Physiotherapy, 63*(3), 161–167.

Lang, R., Shogren, K. A., Machalicek, W., Rispoli, M., O'Reilly, M., Baker, S., & Regester, A. (2009). Video self-modeling to teach classroom rules to two students with Asperger's. *Research in Autism Spectrum Disorders, 3*(2), 483–488.

Lanzi, A., Wallace, S. E., & Bourgeois, M. S. (2018a). External memory aid preferences of individuals with mild memory impairments. *Seminars in Speech and Language, 39*(3), 211–222.

Lanzi, A., Wallace, S. E., & Bourgeois, M. (2018b). Group external memory aid treatment for mild cognitive impairment. *Aphasiology, 33*, 1–17.

Larson R., & Csikszentmihalyi, M. (2014). The experience sampling method. In: Csikszentmihalyi, M. (Ed.), *Flow and the foundations of positive psychology*. Dordrecht: Springer.

Lemoncello, R., Sohlberg, M. M., Fickas, S., Albin, R., & Harn, B. E. (2011). Phase I evaluation of the television assisted prompting system to increase completion of home exercises among stroke survivors. *Disability and Rehabilitation: Assistive Technology, 6*(5), 440–452.

Lemoncello, R., Sohlberg, M. M., Fickas, S., & Prideaux, J. (2011). A randomised controlled crossover trial evaluating Television Assisted Prompting (TAP) for adults with acquired brain injury. *Neuropsychological Rehabilitation, 21*(6), 825–846.

Lock, S., Wilkinson, R., Bryan, K., Maxim, J., Edmundson, A., Bruce, C., & Moir, D. (2001). Supporting partners of people with aphasia in relationships and conversation (SPPARC). *International Journal of Language and Communication Disorders, 36*(sup1), 25–30.

Lorig, K., Holman, H., & Sobel, D. (2012). *Living a healthy life with chronic conditions: Self-management of heart disease, arthritis, diabetes, depression, asthma, bronchitis, emphysema and other physical and mental health conditions*. Boulder, CO: Bull Publishing Company.

Lysack, C., Dama, M., Neufeld, S., & Andreassi, E. (2005). Compliance and satisfaction with home exercise: A comparison of computer-assisted video instruction and routine rehabilitation practice. *Journal of Allied Health, 34*(2), 76–82.

Magill-Evans, J., Harrison, M. J., Benzies, K., Gierl, M., & Kimak, C. (2007). Effects of parenting education on first-time fathers' skills in interactions with their infants. *Fathering, 5*(1), 42.

Matsuba, M. K. (2006). Searching for self and relationships online. *CyberPsychology and Behavior, 9*(3), 275–284.

Matt, G. E., Vázquez, C., & Campbell, W. K. (1992). Mood-congruent recall of affectively toned stimuli: A meta-analytic review. *Clinical Psychology Review, 12*(2), 227–255.

McGraw-Hunter, M., Faw, G. D., & Davis, P. K. (2006). The use of video self-modelling and feedback to teach cooking skills to individuals with traumatic brain injury: A pilot study. *Brain Injury, 20*(10), 1061–1068.

McMillan, S. J., & Morrison, M. (2006). Coming of age with the Internet: A qualitative exploration of how the Internet has become an integral part of young people's lives. *New Media and Society, 8*(1), 73–95.

Menger, F., Morris, J., & Salis, C. (2016). Aphasia in an Internet age: Wider perspectives on digital inclusion. *Aphasiology, 30*(2–3), 112–132.

Miller, H., Buhr, H., Johnson, C., & Hoepner, J. K. (2013). Aphasia Web: A social network for individuals with aphasia. *In Proceedings of the 15th International ACM SIGACCESS Conference on Computers and Accessibility*, Bellevue, WA, October 21–23, 4. doi: 10.1145/2513383.2513439

Miller, W. R., & Rollnick, S. (2012). *Motivational interviewing: Helping people change*. New York, NY: Guilford Press.

Meharg, S. S., & Lipsker, L. E. (1992). Parent training using videotape self-modeling. *Child and Family Behavior Therapy, 13*(4), 1–27.

Omnicore. (2009). Snapchat by the numbers: Stats, demographics and fun facts. Retrieved October 13, 2018. www.omnicoreagency.com/snapchat-statistics/.

Orange, J. B., & Colton-Hudson, A. (1998). Enhancing communication in dementia of the Alzheimer's type. *Topics in Geriatric Rehabilitation, 14*(2), 56–75.

Ortiz, J., Burlingame, C., Onuegbulem, C., Yoshikawa, K., & Rojas, E. D. (2012). The use of video self- modeling with English language learners: Implications for success. *Psychology in the Schools, 49*(1), 23–29.

Pape, T. L. B., Kim, J., & Weiner, B. (2002). The shaping of individual meanings assigned to assistive technology: A review of personal factors. *Disability and Rehabilitation, 24*(1–3), 5–20.

Parette, P., & Scherer, M. (2004). Assistive technology use and stigma. *Education and Training in Developmental Disabilities, 39*, 217–226.

Pew Research Center. (2014). Older adults and technology use. Retrieved from www. pewin.ternet.org/ 2014/04/03/older-adults-and-technology-use/.

Pisters, M. F., Veenhof, C., de Bakker, D. H., Schellevis, F. G., & Dekker, J. (2010). Behavioural graded activity results in better exercise adherence and more physical activity than usual care in people with osteoarthritis: A cluster-randomised trial. *Journal of Physiotherapy, 56*(1), 41–47.

Prater, M. A., Carter, N., Hitchcock, C., & Dowrick, P. (2012). Video self-modeling to improve academic performance: A literature review. *Psychology in the Schools, 49*(1), 71–81.

Ravneberg, B. (2009). Identity politics by design: Users, markets and the public service provision for assistive technology in Norway. *Scandinavian Journal of Disability Research, 11*(2), 101–115.

Riva, E., Freire, T., & Bassi, M. (2016). The flow experience in clinical settings: Applications in psychotherapy and mental health rehabilitation. In: Harmat, L., Ørsted Andersen, F., Ullén, F., Wright, J., & Sadlo, G. (Eds.), *Flow experience* (pp. 233–247). Cham: Springer.

Rose, D. H., Hasselbring, T. S., Stahl, S., & Zabala, J. (2005). Assistive technology and universal design for learning: Two sides of the same coin. In: Edyburn, D., Higgins, K., Boone, R., & Langone, J. (Eds.), *Handbook of special education technology research and practice* (pp. 507–518). Whitefish Bay, WI: Knowledge by Design.

Sather, T. W., Howe, T., Nelson, N. W., & Lagerwey, M. (2017). Optimizing the experience of flow for adults with Aphasia. *Topics in Language Disorders, 37*(1), 25–37.

Scherer, M. J., Hart, T., Kirsch, N., & Schulthesis, M. (2005). Assistive technologies for cognitive disabilities. *Critical Reviews in Physical and Rehabilitation Medicine, 17*(3), 195–215.

Schoo, A. M. M., Morris, M. E., & Bui, Q. M. (2005). The effects of mode of exercise instruction on compliance with a home exercise program in older adults with osteoarthritis. *Physiotherapy, 91*(2), 79–86.

Shiffman, S., Stone, A. A., & Hufford, M. R. (2008). Ecological momentary assessment. *Annual Review of Clinical Psychology, 4*, 1–32.

Shinohara, K., & Wobbrock, J. O. (2011). In the shadow of misperception: Assistive technology use and social interactions. *In Proceedings of the SIGCHI Conference on Human Factors in Computing Systems*, Vancouver, BC, May 7–12 (pp. 705–714). ACM.

Smith, K. P., & Christakis, N. A. (2008). Social networks and health. *Annual Review of Sociology, 34*, 405–429.

Söderström, S., & Ytterhus, B. (2010). The use and non-use of assistive technologies from the world of information and communication technology by visually impaired young people: A walk on the tightrope of peer inclusion. *Disability and Society, 25*(3), 303–315.

Sohlberg, M. M., Lemoncello, R., & Lee, J. (2011). The effect of choice on compliance using telerehabilitation for direct attention training: A comparison of "Push" versus "Pull" scheduling. *SIG 2 Perspectives on Neurophysiology and Neurogenic Speech and Language Disorders, 21*(3), 94–106.

Sohlberg, M. M., & Mateer, C. A. (1989). Training use of compensatory memory books: A three stage behavioral approach. *Journal of Clinical and Experimental Neuropsychology, 11*(6), 871–891.

Svoboda, E. V. A., & Richards, B. (2009). Compensating for anterograde amnesia: A new training method that capitalizes on emerging smartphone technologies. *Journal of the International Neuropsychological Society, 15*(4), 629–638.

Umberson, D., Crosnoe, R., & Reczek, C. (2010). Social relationships and health behavior across the life course. *Annual Review of Sociology, 36*, 1.

Umberson, D., & Karas Montez, J. (2010). Social relationships and health: A flashpoint for health policy. *Journal of Health and Social Behavior, 51*(1_suppl), S54–S66.

Wielandt, T., McKenna, K., Tooth, L., & Strong, J. (2006). Factors that predict the postdischarge use of recommended assistive technology (AT). *Disability and rehabilitation: assistive technology, 1*(1–2), 29–40.

Wilkinson, R., Bryan, K., Lock, S., & Sage, K. (2010). Implementing and evaluating aphasia therapy targeted at couples' conversations: A single case study. *Aphasiology, 24*(68), 869–886.

Wilson, B. A., Emslie, H. C., Quirk, K., & Evans, J. J. (2001). Reducing everyday memory and planning problems by means of a paging system: A randomised control crossover study. *Journal of Neurology, Neurosurgery and Psychiatry, 70*(4), 477–482.

Worrall, L., Sherratt, S., Rogers, P., Howe, T., Hersh, D., Ferguson, A., & Davidson, B. (2011). What people with aphasia want: Their goals according to the ICF. *Aphasiology, 25*(3), 309–322.

Ylvisaker, M. (2006). Self-coaching: A context-sensitive, person-centered approach to social communication after traumatic brain injury. *Brain Impairment, 7*(03), 246–258.

Youse, K. M., & Coelho, C. A. (2009). Treating underlying attention deficits as a means for improving conversational discourse in individuals with closed head injury: A preliminary study. *NeuroRehabilitation, 24*(4), 355–364.

16

Mobile Technology in Aphasia Rehabilitation: Current Trends and Lessons Learnt

Caitlin Brandenburg

Gold Coast University Hospital

Emma Power

University of Technology Sydney and University of Sydney

CONTENTS

Introduction 294
Aphasia Rehabilitation 294
The Promise of Mobile Technology in Health.. 296
Barriers and Facilitators to Mobile Technology Use by People
with Aphasia.. 298
Factors Related to Aphasia and Related Health Conditions 299
Factors Related to Healthcare Services and Environment 300
    Factors Related to Mobile Technology 301
    Factors Related to the Characteristics of the Person with Aphasia......... 302
How Mobile Technology Is Being Used by People with Aphasia 302
    Social Interaction and Life Participation.. 303
    Aphasia Therapy 303
    Aphasia Therapy Support.. 304
    Alternative and Augmentative Communication 304
    Education and Information.. 305
    Sensors, Tracking and Biofeedback 305
The CommFit App – Theory, Development and Lessons Learnt................ 306
Theory.. 306
    Development and Research 307
Key Learnings.. 309
    Collaborative Design 309
    Support of Participants.. 309
    Commercialisation 310
    Knowledge Translation 310
Conclusion 311
References 311

Introduction

Mobile devices are now a part of daily life for most people in developed countries, and this is set to intensify as these devices increase in functionality and decrease in size. The first review of mobile technology use in aphasia was published in 2013, and since then the technology has developed rapidly, from smartphones to smartwatches to smart rings, each housing an increasing array of sensors. These technologies have significant potential to transform the rehabilitation of aphasia and the experience of living with the condition. However, the new applications for mobile technology are tempered by the impairments characteristic of aphasia and the barriers they cause. The Aphasia White Paper states that 'Nearly thirty years ago, America broke down the barriers for those with physical disabilities by implementing the landmark Americans with Disabilities Act. Now, we must do the same for those with communications barriers' (Simmons-Mackie & Cherney 2018). As participation in our world becomes synonymous with participation in the digital world, removing the barriers to digital inclusion for people with aphasia becomes an imperative.

Aphasia Rehabilitation

Aphasia is an acquired language disorder, occurring as a result of damage to the brain, affecting a person's ability to talk, understand spoken language, read and/or write. It is a highly heterogenous disorder, as it can vary in severity, modality (e.g. talking, understanding, reading and writing), onset (sudden or gradual) and manifestation. Hallowell and Chapey (2008) describe four common parameters that make up most definitions of aphasia:

1. aphasia is neurogenic: it results from damage to the parts of the brain responsible for language;
2. aphasia is acquired: it is not a developmental disability and occurs in people who had previously developed some language ability;
3. aphasia involves language problems: it is a condition that involves the selective impairment of language abilities (talking, understanding, reading and/or writing);
4. aphasia is not a sensory, motor function or intellectual problem: aphasia can be accompanied by these deficits, which may also occur as a result of damage to the brain, but is separate from them.

The spoken communication impairment in aphasia is not a result of being physically unable to form the words, but can co-occur with conditions that affect speech through impaired muscle function (e.g. dysarthria, apraxia).

The most common cause of aphasia is stroke, affecting approximately a third of people following first-time stroke (Maas et al. 2012). Other causes of aphasia include brain tumour, degenerative brain conditions (e.g. dementia), brain infections and traumatic brain injury. Aphasia can manifest very differently between individuals. For example, some people may have what speech pathologists term *non-fluent aphasia*, with halting, effortful speech, characterised by production of few words with minimal connecting words or grammatical elements (e.g. Dog…me…feed) (Worrall et al. 2016). In contrast, people with *fluent aphasia* have flowing speech with near-normal grammatical structure, but which lacks actual content (e.g. Well see he came and did that, but then the other thing happened so I left) (Worrall et al. 2016).

Most importantly, aphasia has a significant effect on a person's quality of life, including their ability to participate fully in meaningful everyday activities and maintain social relationships. A study of over 66,000 hospitalised patients found that aphasia had the most negative affect on a person's health-related quality of life, ahead of cancer and Alzheimer's disease (Lam & Wodchis 2010). Research has shown that 93% of stroke survivors with aphasia had high psychological distress, 58% would like to do more activities and 20% reported having no friends (Simmons-Mackie & Cherney 2018).

Rehabilitation of aphasia must be highly tailored due to the heterogenous nature of the condition, beginning with an in-depth assessment by a speech pathologist. Rehabilitation usually focuses on three main tasks: restoring remaining language function, finding alternative ways of communicating or supporting communication and providing education and interventions to help the person live successfully with aphasia (Brady et al. 2016). Recovery is also highly variable – some people can recover total or near-normal language ability, while others will remain severely impaired for the remainder of their lives (Maas et al. 2012). It is well accepted that recovery of language ability is most rapid in the weeks/months following the stroke or brain injury, and so language therapy often focuses on delivering intensive treatment in this time, with more practice of language skills promoting better language recovery (Doogan et al. 2018). Evidence-based guidelines and best practice statements for aphasia rehabilitation include providing a minimum of 45 min of therapy 5 days a week, and as much as can be tolerated beyond that (Power et al. 2015; Shrubsole et al. 2017). However, audit evidence has shown that most patients do not receive this recommended intensity (SSNAP 2018). As health service resources are limited, technology is a mode by which language therapy can be delivered more intensively to patients, especially after discharge home when sessions with a therapist may only be 1–2 h per week, less than recommended in best practice guidelines. Computer therapy has long been integrated into aphasia therapy to maximise home practice; however, mobile technology has more recently emerged as a therapy tool.

The Promise of Mobile Technology in Health

The mobility and functionality of mobile devices offer unprecedented opportunity to provide health services and support when and where needed (Boulos et al. 2014). Use of computer therapy is documented in evidence-based guidelines for aphasia, but mobile technology has not yet been explicitly included (Shrubsole et al. 2017). The landscape of mobile technology and its use in rehabilitation has had some significant shifts since the first review of mobile technology in aphasia in 2013 (Brandenburg et al. 2013), which this chapter will address.

Mobile technology for the purposes of this chapter includes small, hand-held mobile computing devices incorporating touch screens, such as smartphones, smartwatches and tablet PCs (Brandenburg et al. 2013). These devices feature Internet connectivity and an increasing variety of sensors, including microphones, GPS, accelerometers, barometers, heart rate sensors and gyroscopes. Another key feature is that these devices are easily programmable and customisable using widely available, downloadable applications (apps) and thereby have the capacity to act as any number of devices in tandem (e.g. a voice recorder, a GPS device, a camera, a personal diary, a computer therapy program, and a social networking device). While some definitions of mobile technology include laptops, these devices fulfil the same tasks as desktop computers and are limited in their mobility, so they will not be discussed further here.

Use of mobile technology by the general population is now near ubiquitous in developed countries (Comscore 2017; Ofcom 2018). After a sharp increase in tablet and smartphone ownership between 2010 and 2015, this trend is now beginning to plateau – 58% of U.K. households now own a tablet computer and 78% a smartphone (Ofcom 2018). The new upwards trend in mobile technology is wearable devices, with 20% of U.K. households now owning a fitness tracker or smartwatch device, compared with 3% in 2015 (Ofcom 2018).

However, even as our lives become more integrated with technology, the 'digital divide' still exists for people with disabilities, older people and other vulnerable populations (van Dijk 2012). The term digital divide was originally used in the context of physical difficulties (Warschauer 2003). However, the barriers to technology use for people with cognitive and communication disabilities including aphasia have increasingly been recognised (Kelly et al. 2016). While the 2016 Wireless RERC Survey of User Needs found that ownership of mobile devices by people with disabilities is similar to the rest of the population, a sub-analysis by disability type revealed that those identifying as having difficulty with speech had the lowest ownership rates compared with physical, sensory and cognitive disabilities (Morris, Jones & Sweatman 2016). Research has also shown that people with disabilities also tend to use mobile technology for more traditional uses (e.g. phone calls) rather than functions such as email, Internet, GPS and mobile health monitoring (Jones, Morris & de Ruyter 2018; Morris, Mueller & Jones 2010). Other research has shown that older age, lower education level and presence of disability are the strongest predictors of digital exclusion (Helsper & Reisdorf 2016; Menger, Morris & Salis 2016), and therefore greater attention is required in maximising opportunities for this population.

This divide and challenge is more problematic as the health sector increasingly incorporates mobile technology into services (WHO 2011). There are now some 318,000 health apps, a number which has almost doubled since 2015 (IQVIA 2017) and seems a far cry from the 7,000 referenced in our 2013 review (Brandenburg et al. 2013). While these apps mainly fall into the category of general wellness, health condition management apps have grown at a faster rate and now represent 40% of all health-related apps (IQVIA 2017). In the past 5 years, the legitimacy of these mobile health applications has grown rapidly. Regulatory agencies have now published updated guidance on how mobile apps fit in with their definitions of mobile devices and the level of regulatory scrutiny required, including proof of effectiveness (FDA 2018; TGA 2018). In a high-profile case, 'brain training' app company Lumos Labs was ordered to ensure any future claims of their apps' efficacy backed by 'competent and reliable scientific evidence' including randomised controlled trials (Federal Trade Commission 2016). This type of action has increased the attention paid to mobile health apps as legitimate forms of intervention, which require high-quality research demonstrating their effectiveness (Boulos et al. 2014).

People with disabilities have expressed belief that mobile health (mHealth) will improve their access to healthcare and quality of life (Jones, Morris & deRuyter 2018). People with aphasia have identified more speech therapy and greater autonomy as priorities for their rehabilitation, both of which can be achieved through mobile technology (Wallace et al. 2017; Worrall et al. 2011). A focus group of stroke health professionals and patients (50% of whom had aphasia) indicated that participants valued the role of technology in providing rehabilitation at home and how it can enable additional practice and continuation of therapy after discharge (Brouns et al. 2018). One person with aphasia said about their tablet, 'I'd turn it on then I can do [therapy] myself... and then everyday try, try, try' (Kurland, Wilkins & Stokes 2014).

However, research has indicated that uptake of digital health for rehabilitation (including mobile technology) by stroke health professionals and health services is low (Brouns et al. 2018; Langan et al. 2018). The literature as a whole indicates that mobile technology remains an under-researched and likely underutilised area of aphasia rehabilitation (Menger, Morris & Salis 2016).

Barriers and Facilitators to Mobile Technology Use by People with Aphasia

The enduring digital divide necessitates a closer look at the barriers to mobile technology use for this population, and ways in which use can be supported. Lack of accessible training and support has been identified as one of the main barriers to use of technology in aphasia rehabilitation; however, little research has been done on this topic (Finch & Hill 2014; Kelly et al. 2016; McCall 2012; Parr 2007). Two studies over a decade apart (Egan, Worrall & Oxenham 2004; Kelly et al. 2016) have demonstrated the value of courses for computer skills designed specifically for people with aphasia, with specially designed materials (adapted for individual needs) and small participant–tutor ratios identified as the most helpful elements. In terms of people with aphasia's ability to learn or relearn to use mobile technology specifically, most information comes from brief commentary as part of interventional studies using this technology.

The overall picture is hopeful – research has shown that most patients with aphasia who had limited experience using iPads were able to use them independently after 15 min to 2 h of training, and successfully use them for home practice (Brandenburg et al. 2017b; Kurland, Wilkins & Stoke 2014; Mallet et al. 2019; Stark & Warburton 2018). However, these studies also noted that some patients needed significant support to use the devices and others were never able to use them independently (Guo et al. 2017).

It is critical to identify specific barriers to mobile technology use for people with aphasia (Table 16.1). This is especially important to assist technology developers, as many will be unfamiliar with aphasia (Code et al. 2016) and language deficits are less tangible and visible when considering accessible design. A more detailed exploration of the factors that influence accessibility for this population follows: focusing on four main areas that align with the health condition, environmental and personal factor components of the International Classification of Functioning, Disability and Health (WHO 2001). These are (1) factors related to aphasia and related health conditions (health condition), (2) factors related to healthcare services and environment (environmental factors), (3) factors related to mobile technology (environmental factors) and (4) factors related to the characteristics of the person with aphasia (personal factors).

TABLE 16.1

Summary of Factors Relating to Mobile Technology Access by People with Aphasia

Factors related to aphasia and related health conditions	Aphasic impairments in speaking, understanding spoken language, reading and writing
	Physical impairments
	Other sensory and cognitive impairments
Factors related to healthcare services and the environment	Cost and resources
	Logistical issues
	Access
	Time commitment
	Available evidence of effectiveness
	Change to service model
	Change to clinician role and skills required
	Client suitability
Factors related to mobile technology	Size of device/use of touchscreens
	Privacy and security
	Discoverability
	Reliability
	Predictability
	Accessible design of software
Factors related to the characteristics of the person with aphasia	Confidence
	Motivation
	Expectations
	Family support
	Previous experience
	Demographic factors (age, education level, cultural and linguistic background)

Factors Related to Aphasia and Related Health Conditions

Severity of aphasia has been identified as an important factor in accessibility, including learning to use the technology and using it thereafter (Szabo & Dittelman 2014). As aphasia is highly heterogenous, barriers may differ across individuals. More specifically, difficulty understanding spoken and written language can affect an individual's understanding of a user manual or training video when learning to use the device (Egan, Worrall & Oxenham 2004; Kelly et al. 2016). Impaired written and spoken language can also impact learning as the person may have difficulty writing notes, asking questions or communicating what they do not understand (Egan, Worrall & Oxenham 2004; Kelly et al. 2016). Aphasia can also affect an individual's ability to initially acquire the device and software (e.g. research and purchase a device, look through an app store and select an app), and troubleshoot the technology (e.g. describe a problem over the phone, read a help website) (Menger, Morris & Salis 2016). In terms of sustained use of mobile devices, difficulties with read ng and writing are expected to impact most heavily, as mobile apps usually rely on text and typed input (Menger, Morris & Salis 2016; Roper et al. 2018).

Apart from language deficits, people with aphasia may also experience other deficits related to the damage to their brain, which can affect their ability to use technology. For example, motor deficits resulting from stroke or increased age are likely to cause difficulties with the complex fine motor skills required to tap and swipe a touch screen (Szabo & Dittelman 2014). Presence of hemiplegia may also impact, requiring use of the non-dominant hand. However, some people with motor deficits may actually find the touchscreen to be a facilitator to use, compared with keyboard and mouse input (Palmer et al. 2012). Cognitive deficits may affect ability to learn new skills, recall information or perform complex tasks. Vision impairments, as a result of damage to the brain or increased age, may include presbyopia (inability to focus on close objects), decreased contrast sensitivity and dark/light adaptation and slower recovery from glare (Carter 1994). These have obvious implications for the small screens common in mobile devices, including reading text, viewing picture/video and using touchscreen buttons.

Factors Related to Healthcare Services and Environment

While mobile technology can support self-management of aphasia, aphasia therapy is usually more effective if overseen by a clinician or as part of a rehabilitation programme, and people with aphasia have indicated they prefer this model (Brouns et al. 2018). Healthcare is often slow to change and introduce new services, and this seems to be the case in relation to uptake of mobile devices (Brouns et al. 2018; Langan et al. 2018; Menger, Morris & Salis 2016). A better understanding is needed of the service-related barriers and facilitators to implementing mobile technology in aphasia rehabilitation. Barriers to speech pathologists' uptake of technology include cost, logistical issues, access within the health service (e.g. if software is blocked by firewalls), time commitment, services/resources required and available evidence of effectiveness (Brouns et al. 2018; Chen & Bode 2011; Johnson, Morris & Menger 2014; Kearns, Kelly & Hanafin 2018; Kerr et al. 2018). Some of these issues may be mitigated by the fact that many patients now own and use their own smartphones and tablet PCs, or are willing to purchase them (Brouns et al. 2018).

Another important barrier is that training and supporting the use of mobile technology are not traditionally seen as part of a clinician's role and requires role expansion and possibly additional training (Brandenburg et al. 2013).

Assessment of a client's capability to use mobile technology may need to form part of language assessment, as client suitability was a key concern of speech pathologists (Brouns et al. 2018; Johnson, Morris & Menger 2014). This new role may also include dedicated clinical time to monitor the progress of patients on mHealth programmes and give any necessary feedback/ encouragement (Brouns et al. 2018). Training in using technology and professional development to keep up-to-date on what is available should help support this role shift (Kearns, Kelly & Hanafin 2018). Stroke healthcare professionals have indicated that they are concerned that they may need to field questions about technology-related issues, as there is usually minimal IT support for patients in health services (Brouns et al. 2018), and readily available troubleshooting assistance seems to be a major factor in uptake for this population (Baier, Hoepner & Sather 2018). Service models need modification to allow for mobile technology to be integrated, including technology resources, helpdesk support and appropriate policies and procedures (Hines et al. 2017; Johnson, Morris & Menger 2014).

Factors Related to Mobile Technology

Given the range of impairments associated with aphasia, mobile technology sometimes needs specific adaptation to be suitable for this population. As outlined earlier, the small touchscreens used in these devices can be a barrier, as they require reading of small text and accurate fine motor skills, which may be impaired in people with aphasia (Sarasohn-Kahn 2010). Mobile technology should be designed or adapted for people with aphasia, in collaboration with speech pathologists or people with aphasia and their families, rather than addressing accessibility after the fact. Specific design features for increasing the accessibility of mobile technology for people with aphasia that have been suggested by the literature include multimodal input/output (text-supplemented pictures, symbols, etc.), aphasia-friendly text (large, well-spaced, sans-serif, high contrast font), large buttons, stable interface, simple navigation and visual simplicity (Brandenburg et al. 2013).

Barriers also exist before the person has even accessed the technology. Discoverability is an important factor – as the number of available apps and devices increases, people with aphasia require support to discover and select from the many options. The Aphasia Software Finder is one such service, providing independent guidance on over 100 apps, including number of exercises, available platforms, features and price in a consumer-friendly format (Tavistock Trust for Aphasia n.d.). People with aphasia have also indicated quality of the actual content of apps and whether they meet their needs to be a factor in uptake (Brouns et al. 2018). Another factor is the privacy and security risks of storing health-related information on a mobile device, which needs to be carefully managed (Brouns et al. 2018). However, the need for passwords can be difficult for this population, both due to memory, language and typing difficulty.

Reliability of the technology is an important facilitator to use, as trouble-shooting and access to troubleshooting assistance is a major concern for this population (Brouns et al. 2018). Predictability of the interface is also a factor in technology accessibility – it is the experience of this author as well as others that any unexpected popups (e.g. ads, or re-logon) are a significant barrier to use (Baier, Hoepner & Sather 2018); however, on non-dedicated devices like smartphones this is not always able to be controlled.

Factors Related to the Characteristics of the Person with Aphasia

Barriers related to the person with aphasia and their personal circumstances and characteristics may also affect technology use. This may include things like confidence, motivation, cognition, expectations and family support (Brouns et al. 2018; Chen & Bode 2011; Galliers et al. 2011; McGrenere et al. 2003; Roper et al. 2018; Szabo & Dittelman 2014). It should be noted that while carers can be a supporting factor in using mobile technology, this can be a taxing experience and add to carer burden, and carers in themselves may need support (Menger, Morris & Salis 2016).

A person's previous experience in using mobile technology is a large influencing factor in uptake (Chen & Bode 2011; Galliers et al. 2011; McGrenere et al. 2003; Szabo & Dittelman 2014), with this effect even more relevant if they had used the same software or app before (Roper et al. 2018). As outlined earlier, while people who used mobile technology before acquiring aphasia may retain some of the relevant skills and knowledge for computer literacy, people who need to learn from scratch face significant barriers to learning as a result of their aphasia and related impairments (McGrenere et al. 2003). Other personal factors may also play a role, including age, educational level and linguistic/cultural background (Menger, Morris & Salis 2016).

How Mobile Technology Is Being Used by People with Aphasia

Although there are some significant barriers to use of mobile technology by people with aphasia, it is increasingly being utilised in rehabilitation. A survey of speech pathologists showed that most common uses were for therapy and to increase intensity of practice, followed by use as alternative and augmentative communication (AAC) to give homework and facilitate participation (Johnson, Morris & Menger 2014). Six main categories for mobile technology use in aphasia emerged from review of the academic and non-academic literature, as well as commercially available apps – social interaction and life participation; aphasia therapy; aphasia therapy support; AAC, education and information; and sensors, tracking and biofeedback.

Social Interaction and Life Participation

Rehabilitation priorities of people with aphasia include many focused on social and life participation, including return to pre-stroke life, communication of complex ideas and opinions, and engagement in social, leisure and work activities (Wallace et al. 2017; Worrall et al. 2011). Mobile technology offers new ways to help people with aphasia connect with others and build relationships. Some aphasia experts have commented that social media may help people with aphasia to 'mask' their difficulties, as they are able to use the communication mode that they are strongest in (e.g. using gesture on Skype), and in some forms of social media they may have more time to understand and formulate a response (Kelly et al. 2016).

Very little research has been completed in this area, although anecdotally it is clear that people with aphasia embrace this use of technology. One study examined whether the picture- and video-sharing platform Snapchat was useful in encouraging socialisation for people with aphasia (Baier, Hoepner & Sather 2018). Another study explored social media use after traumatic brain injury and found that participants valued it as a socialisation tool but desired more training and support (Brunner et al. 2019). More work has been done in non-mobile technology, for example, the development of an email system accessible to people with aphasia (Mahmud & Martens 2015), a custom-designed social media platform (Buhr et al. 2017) and use of virtual environments (Galliers et al. 2011; Galliers et al. 2017). People with aphasia are also able to use apps intended for the general population to help manage their condition and support their participation in everyday activities. Examples include using a reminder app for therapy goals, a note-taking app with common phrases for communicating when shopping, and using a public transport app instead of needing to call the information line.

Aphasia Therapy

Another common type of app designed specifically for aphasia are aphasia therapy apps, which are intended to replicate or supplement face-to-face therapy (e.g. Constant therapy, Tactus Language Therapy). Mobile technology can support rehabilitation by increasing treatment intensity and saliency in a cost-effective manner, and enhancing a person's ability to self-manage their rehabilitation. Therapy apps include elements of traditional therapy, including analysis of the user's responses and feedback. There has been less research on the effectiveness of mobile technology-delivered aphasia therapy than computer therapy (Meltzer et al. 2018; Zheng, Lynch & Taylor 2016), but there is a promising selection of literature that indicates its effectiveness (Ameer & Ali 2017; Des Roches et al. 2014; Kurland, Wilkins & Stokes 2014; Stark & Warburton 2018). However, uses for spoken language therapy remain limited, instead focusing on comprehension, reading and writing where the response can be recognised and graded by the app.

While speech recognition has vastly increased in accuracy, an unpublished lab study by the first author testing a number of freely available voice recognition programs showed that it is highly inaccurate for aphasic speech. This is because the speech of people with aphasia is difficult to predict, and does not follow the conventional patterns of speech that this technology relies on. However, this remains a promising avenue as machine learning techniques advance that may allow a speech recognition program to be trained for the individuals' speech pattern.

Aphasia Therapy Support

Another common category of apps is those that support the delivery of aphasia therapy, but do not comprise therapy on their own. This category may include apps, which replace the flashcard and picture stimuli traditionally used by speech pathologists, including functions which allow the person to use the camera to create their own personally relevant therapy materials (McCann & Greig 2012). Some of these apps also provide video stimuli showing the user how to form sounds, words and sentences (e.g. Speech Tutor, VAST therapy) which can be useful for home practice; however, the user must judge on their own if they are successfully following the tutorial. This means that independent practice with feedback is not feasible as a carer or speech pathologist is needed; however, these apps can increase the efficiency of therapy, and have a role in home practice. This category also includes tools for speech pathologists, for example, apps that help count language errors or assist with language assessment (Guo et al. 2017).

Alternative and Augmentative Communication

AAC apps augment or replace human speech as a means of communication, and are the most common types of speech therapy app available commercially. The uptake and benefits of different forms of AAC is the focus of a large body of research in speech pathology, and over the last 5 years, AAC apps have been accepted as a legitimate option alongside more conventional dedicated AAC devices (McNaughton & Light 2013; Moffatt, Pourshahid & Baecker 2015). These apps include text-to-speech functions, and usually work through the user tapping the screen, and the app then says the word aloud. Early AAC apps were very similar to custom-built AAC devices; however, they are increasingly capitalising on the features of mobile technology to enhance their function. For example, some AAC apps now use GPS to locate the user and prioritise which words are displayed based on their location (e.g. 'doctor' if they are in the hospital) (Demmans Epp 2012; Kane et al. 2012). Natural language processing techniques have also allowed AAC mobile apps to develop personalised word sets (Mooney et al. 2018).

As well as traditional AAC, there are other types of augmented communication, which fit in this category, for example, a novel app for communicating with health professionals, which replaces and improves upon traditional paper communication books and works like a 'Health Passport' (Carragher et al. 2018; Rose et al. 2017).

Education and Information

Educational apps for aphasia seek to provide information about aphasia and rehabilitation, and replace traditional brochures or information sheets for client education; however, they are also able to provide multimedia information including videos and sounds (e.g. iSpeech and GeekSLP). These apps can also be interactive, allowing for user choice or even learning quizzes. This category is important as awareness and understanding of aphasia is low, even among health professionals (Cameron et al. 2018; Code et al. 2016), and people with aphasia identify receiving information about their condition as a key priority for rehabilitation (Wallace et al. 2017; Worrall et al. 2011).

Sensors, Tracking and Biofeedback

Sensors, trackers and biofeedback have had extensive attention in the physical rehabilitation space, but less so for language rehabilitation. This category includes simplistic behaviour-tracking apps, which are used to manually log or count behaviours, for example, tracking word-finding difficulties. Mobile devices have a clear advantage for use in this category over non-mobile devices and traditional paper forms, as they are readily available at the time of behaviour. However, there is also an opportunity for automatic tracking of people with aphasia in their everyday environments using device sensors and wearables, which is of interest to speech pathologists who are increasingly interested in capturing real-life language and delivering timely feedback and support in everyday life (Kagan et al. 2008). Automated measurement and feedback can also support generalisation of language tasks from clinic to everyday life and promote self-management. The wide commercial availability of wearable biofeedback devices like the FitBit and smartwatches have led to a rapidly increased social acceptance of this technology in the last 5 years (Ofcom 2018), as well as intensive interest in their applications for physical health and rehabilitation. While computer-based therapy has started to make use of sensors for gesture therapy (Marshall et al. 2013), and GPS has been used in AAC apps, sensor and wearable mobile technology for aphasia has been relatively unexplored, with the CommFit app project remaining one of the key exemplars in this field.

The CommFit App – Theory, Development and Lessons Learnt

The focus in the stroke rehabilitation space has quickly moved from simple apps to wearable devices (which usually pair with apps) to track users in their everyday lives. This is of clear relevance to physical rehabilitation, but is also of use to cognitive and speech/language interventions. In 2009, a team of speech pathologists in Australia set out to harness the potential of mobile technology and the early promise of wearable sensors to create a mobile app for aphasia rehabilitation. This project was later named the CommFit project, short for 'Communicative Fitness'.

Theory

The CommFit mobile app aimed to measure and encourage users to increase their daily talking time, often described as a 'pedometer for language'. The theory behind CommFit was made up of several elements.

- Measurement in real-world contexts
  The project sought to capitalise on the potential of smartphones to allow for remote and automated measurement of a person's behaviour in their everyday life, providing clinicians with an ability to assess and monitor language use outside the clinic. Traditionally, information about a person's communication in everyday life is collected through interview, in-clinic assessment or daily diaries. These methods can be unreliable for people with aphasia as they rely on self-awareness, recall and being able to communicate information accurately.
- Principles of neuroplasticity and increased practice
  The value of increasing talking time in everyday life has its roots in principles of neuroplasticity, or ways in which rehabilitation can maximise recovery of the brain after injury. The act of increasing talking practice capitalises on the 'use it or lose it', 'intensity matters', 'repetition matters' principles and that fact the practice occurs in everyday life contexts fulfils the 'salience matters' principle (Kleim & Jones 2008).
- Biofeedback
  The app aimed to collect and display feedback on a user's speech in a way that was easy for the average user to interpret. It was theorised that this kind of simple, real-time feedback on progress would

be motivating for users to increase their practice. This approach was similar to the use of pedometers and other mobile technologies used to increase physical practice in stroke rehabilitation, using principles of gamification, feedback, self-monitoring and social support (O'Brien et al. 2017; Paul et al. 2016). CommFit also aimed to use some elements of gamification to encourage users to increase their daily score.

- Self-management and independence
  The CommFit app also aimed to promote independence and capacity to self-manage under supervision, empowering users with information about their own progress.

Development and Research

Our programme of work started with a small unpublished project investigating the possibility of using commercially available voice-activated recorders and smartphone apps to measure talk time. These options were found to lack accessibility, accuracy and fitness-for-purpose. It became clear to the research team that a bespoke app needed to be developed for the purpose of measuring and increasing talk time, which was easily accessible for people with aphasia. We conducted a broad-based review of the field of mobile technology use in aphasia, seeking to determine how mobile technology was currently being used in aphasia, and the factors in developing accessible apps (Brandenburg et al. 2013). This review informed the development of CommFit, a smartphone app that used a commercially available BlueTooth headset to pick up speech.

Development was undertaken by a team of aphasia researchers with no experience developing apps, and a team of commercial IT professionals with no experience developing technology for aphasia or disabled populations. Full details of development can be found in Brandenburg et al. (2016). Prior to developing the iPhone app and associated website, preliminary stages involved educating the development team about aphasia, forming and clarifying our seven prioritised design goals and making several key decisions about the direction of the project, for example, selecting the iOS platform and Bluetooth headset. The visual interface of the app was then developed, using a cyclical, iterative design process utilising low-tech mock-ups of appearance and flowcharts/PowerPoint mock-ups for function and navigational elements. A functioning app was then built and subjected to a cycle of testing and redesign, in order to refine and fix bugs. The app/headset was then tested for accuracy in everyday environments by members of the research team and found to be within acceptable levels.

The next stage was testing the app and headset with people with aphasia, both to collect information on talk time and its correlates in this population (Brandenburg et al. 2017a) and to collect formal data on the technology's usability (Brandenburg et al. 2017b). This study showed that CommFit had potential as an assessment of real-world participation in communication for this population. It also gave valuable information of the design of CommFit, which was that the design of the app was accessible, but the BlueTooth headset was difficult to use.

Due to this and also to increase accuracy, we developed a wearable accelerometer device, about 2 cm square, attached with a wire to a battery back. Due to iOS restrictions, the use of this custom-built external hardware necessitated a port of the app to an Android version, shown in Figure 16.1a and b. Further testing occurred with the aim of initiating a larger trial with people with aphasia. We also began to investigate the scale-up and commercialisation of the device with a local engineering company and our university's commercialisation arm. However, significant bugs in the technology remained, beginning a lengthy and expensive process of testing and development.

Ultimately, challenges in remediating these issues, as well as the conclusion of funding and staff movement led to the closure of the CommFit project. However, the project was valuable for researchers working on similar projects, who may benefit from our key learnings and recommendations for future research in this area.

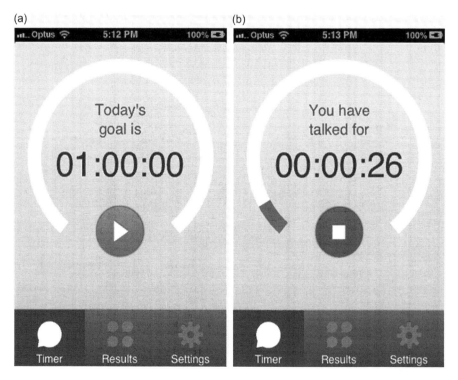

FIGURE 16.1
Screenshots of the CommFit Android app before and while timing.

Key Learnings

Collaborative Design

Our experience, and indeed that of the literature, indicates that there are three key groups necessary for the development of mobile technology (or any technology) for people with aphasia – speech pathologists/aphasia experts, mobile technology developers/experts and people with aphasia/their families. The literature often recommends a process of co-design with people with aphasia (Moffatt 2004; Wilson et al. 2015). As the app we were designing was very specific and designed for a certain task, we did not co-design with people with aphasia, rather, we piloted the first version to get feedback. While this approach was effective, it would have improved the project to explore other ways of enhancing consumer participation (Miller et al. 2017).

The main barrier we experienced during the project was our issues with the technology, namely the accelerometer device and its connectivity with the app. A stronger collaboration with engineering/IT professionals may have mitigated this, including earlier collaboration with academics in these fields rather than reliance on contracted commercial services for the early development. Similar projects working on mobile voice monitoring, which had significant IT and engineering collaboration appear to have been more successful (Mehta et al. 2012). However, when the contractors we worked with had family with disabilities, we found this greatly helped understanding of the project and buy-in.

Support of Participants

Supporting participants with their involvement in the project was a challenging task. Participants were recruited from interstate, and in-person support was not often possible. They were also expected to use the app most of the day on most days, meaning that support could be needed at any time, even at times as early as 6 am in the morning as participants woke and attempted to turn on the app. As participants often had significant impairments, troubleshooting over the phone without being able to see the app was challenging. These difficulties were usually able to be overcome; however, the project was at times demanding for researchers, participants and their families. Other researchers have also noted that they were often contacted to troubleshoot technological issues (Kurland, Wilkins & Stokes 2014), with one group hiring a commercial IT company instead (Szabo & Dittelman 2014) and another hospital-based project providing daily, in-person support visits (Mallet et al. 2019). Other suggestions may include conducting research on mobile technology as part of a larger programme of research to ensure resources and ongoing assistance, for example, intensive aphasia courses. In addition, provision of a custom-designed, aphasia-friendly user manual with liberal use of photos was identified as a supporting factor in use of CommFit. At the very least, prospective researchers should be aware of and plan for how participants will be supported when troubleshooting technology, and ensure sufficient resources. It should also be noted that these issues will continue in the clinical space, with speech pathologists suggesting use of specialist technology services to handle enquiries (Johnson, Morris & Menger 2014).

Commercialisation

It is noted that many of the technologies described in the literature, along with CommFit, do not seem to have made it to market or into wider availability, and of those that did, many were not updated and quickly fell into disuse. It may be useful to analyse this trend and determine degree of use of these technologies post-publication, and how they can be set up for widespread use. Commercialisation is one way of ensuring the longevity of the technology and funding continual updates in an increasingly limited research-funding environment. However, commercialisation partners can have differing goals, i.e. to turn significant profit, whilst researchers may have the goal of making enough money to support the technology but keeping cost to people with aphasia at a minimum. It is suggested that making these goals apparent and keeping open communication can help with finding a model suitable to both parties. We also discovered that the commercialisation process requires knowledge and skills that may warrant the addition of another collaborative group to the three listed above, and one that is growing in the university research sector – commercialisation/business expertise. Researchers should consider early on how and when they will engage with commercialisation partners, whether they have this expertise within their team, and what training is available if they wish to upskill in this area.

Knowledge Translation

The other way of ensuring longevity and clinical use of the technology is through application of knowledge translation (KT) concepts and processes (Graham et al. 2006). KT seeks to use structured processes to ensure the application of research evidence into health practice. In hindsight, it would have been ideal to develop a KT plan from the beginning of the project, and involve practising speech pathologists and health service representatives earlier in the project to increase the likelihood of translation into practice. There have been examples of how to use KT models and implementation strategies in both speech pathology (Shrubsole et al. 2017), and technology in rehabilitation more generally (Levac et al. 2016). In technology design, the approach may be useful to start identifying and designing for potential barriers to implementation throughout the design and testing process. However, KT also seeks a theoretical understanding of how we view technology in healthcare. Greenhalgh et al.'s (2012) work describes a phenomenon where technology has been framed as a panacea for the challenges of healthcare, a commercially driven enterprise to be approached with caution or human-centred phenomena with advantages and disadvantages strongly dependent on the user. Few studies framed technology implementation in health as a change management process, with few identifying a theory of change, and many using this framing only after technologies had failed to implementation fully (Greenhalgh et al. 2012). It is clear from this literature that the stakeholders involved in translating mobile health into practice are not simple 'buyers' and 'sellers', and the process of implementing this change needs careful consideration and planning.

Conclusion

This chapter summarised some of the considerations when designing technology for this population and potential/current uses of this technology in aphasia rehabilitation. We also discussed our experiences developing the CommFit app, which generated some important suggestions for future research. It is apparent that research in mobile technology for this population is highly important. In the words of one person with aphasia, 'It's something that we really have to do because…the way that the world's going…technology is just going so much ahead' (Greig et al. 2008). As researchers and clinicians, we have a responsibility to support that inclusion.

References

Ameer, K & Ali, K 2017, iPad use in stroke neuro-rehabilitation, *Geriatrics*, vol. 2, no. 1, p. 2.

Baier, CK, Hoepner, JK & Sather, TW 2018, Exploring Snapchat as a dynamic capture tool for social networking in persons with aphasia, *Aphasiology*, vol. 32, no. 11, pp. 1336–59.

Boulos, MN, Brewer, AC, Karimkhani, C, Buller, DB & Dellavalle, RP 2014, Mobile medical and health apps: State of the art, concerns, regulatory control and certification, *Online J Public Health Inform*, vol. 5, no. 3, p. 229.

Brady, MC, Kelly, H, Godwin, J, Enderby, P & Campbell, P 2016, Speech and language therapy for aphasia following stroke, *Cochrane Database Syst Rev*, vol. 2016, no. 6., CD000425.

Brandenburg, C, Worrall, L, Copland, D, Power, E & Rodriguez, AD 2016, The development and accuracy testing of CommFit, an iPhone application for individuals with aphasia, *Aphasiology*, vol. 30, no. 2–3, pp. 320–38.

Brandenburg, C, Worrall, L, Copland, D & Rodriguez, AD 2017a, An exploratory investigation of the daily talk time of people with non-fluent aphasia and non-aphasic peers, *Int J Speech Lang Pathol*, vol. 19, no. 4, pp. 418–29.

Brandenburg, C, Worrall, L, Copland, D & Rodriguez, AD 2017b, Barriers and facilitators to using the CommFit smart phone app to measure talk time for people with aphasia, *Aphasiology*, vol. 31, no. 8, pp. 901–27.

Brandenburg, C, Worrall, L, Rodriguez, AD & Copland, D 2013, Mobile computing technology and aphasia: An integrated review of accessibility and potential uses, *Aphasiology*, vol. 27, no. 4, pp. 444–61.

Brouns, B, Meesters, JJL, Wentink, MM, de Kloet, AJ, Arwert, HJ, Vliet Vlieland, TPM, Boyce, LW & van Bodegom-Vos, L 2018, Why the uptake of eRehabilitation programs in stroke care is so difficult—a focus group study in the Netherlands, *Implement Sci*, vol. 13, no. 1, p. 133.

Brunner, M, Palmer, S, Togher, L & Hemsley, B 2019, 'I kind of figured it out': The views and experiences of people with traumatic brain injury (TBI) in using social media-self-determination for participation and inclusion online, *Int J Lang Commun Disord*, vol. 54, no. 2, pp. 221–233.

Buhr, HR, Hoepner, JK, Miller, H & Johnson, C 2017, AphasiaWeb: Development and evaluation of an aphasia-friendly social networking application, *Aphasiology*, vol. 31, no. 9, pp. 999–1020.

Cameron, A, McPhail, S, Hudson, K, Fleming, J, Lethlean, J, Tan, NJ & Finch, E 2018, The confidence and knowledge of health practitioners when interacting with people with aphasia in a hospital setting, *Disabil Rehabil*, vol. 40, no. 11, pp. 1288–93.

Carragher, M, O'Halloran, R, Johnson, H, Taylor, N, Torabi, T & Rose, M 2018, People with aphasia and health professionals report difficulty communicating with one another: Can a novel eHealth intervention help? *Aphasiology*, vol. 32, no. sup1, pp. 34–6.

Carter, TL 1994, Age-related vision changes: A primary care guide, *Geriatrics*, vol. 49, no. 9, pp. 37–42.

Chen, C & Bode, R 2011, Factors influencing therapists' decision-making in the acceptance of new technology devices in stroke rehabilitation, *Am J Phys Med Rehabil*, vol. 90. no. 5, pp. 415–25.

Code, C, Papathanasiou, I, Rubio-Bruno, S, Cabana Mde, L, Villanueva, MM, Haaland-Johansen, L, Prizl-Jakovac, T, Leko, A, Zemva, N, Patterson, R, Berry, R, Rochon, E, Leonard, C & Robert, A 2016, International patterns of the public awareness of aphasia, *Int J Lang Commun Disord*, vol. 51, no. 3, pp. 276–84.

Comscore 2017, The 2017 U.S. mobile app report, www.comscore.com/ USMobileAppReport2017.

Demmans Epp, C, Djordjevic, J, Wu, S, Moffatt, K & Baecker, RM 2012, Towards providing just-in-time vocabulary support for Assistive and Augmentative Communication. *In ACM International Conference on Intelligent User Interfaces (IUI)*, Lisbon, Portugal, pp. 33–6.

Des Roches, CA, Balachandran, I, Ascenso, EM, Tripodis, Y & Kiran, S 2014, Effectiveness of an impairment-based individualized rehabilitation program using an iPad-based software platform, *Front Hum Neurosci*, vol. 8, p. 1015.

Doogan, C, Dignam, J, Copland, D & Leff, A 2018, Aphasia recovery: When, how and who to treat? *Curr Neurol Neurosci Rep*, vol. 18, no. 12, pp. 90.

Egan, J, Worrall, L & Oxenham, D 2004, Accessible Internet training package helps people with aphasia cross the digital divide, *Aphasiology*, vol. 18, no. 3, pp. 265–80.

FDA 2018, Mobile medical applications, U.S. Food and Drug Administration, U.S. Department of Health and Human Services, www.fda.gov/medicaldevices/digitalhealth/mobilemedicalapplications/default.htm.

Federal Trade Commission 2016, Lumosity to pay $2 million to settle FTC deceptive advertising charges for its "Brain Training" Program, www.ftc.gov/news-events/press-releases/2016/01/lumosity-pay-2-million-settle-ftc-deceptive-advertising-charges.

Finch, E & Hill, AJ 2014, Computer use by people with aphasia: A survey investigation, *Brain Impairment*, vol. 15, no. 2, pp. 107–19.

Galliers, J, Wilson, S, Marshall, J, Talbot, R, Devane, N, Booth, T, Woolf, C & Greenwood, H 2017, Experiencing EVA Park, a multi-user virtual world for people with aphasia, *ACM Trans Access Comput*, vol. 10, no. 4, pp. 1–24.

Galliers, J, Wilson, S, Muscroft, S, Marshall, J, Roper, A, Cocks, N & Pring, T 2011, Accessibility of 3D game environments for people with aphasia: An exploratory study. *In The Proceedings of the 13th International ACM SIGACCESS Conference on Computers and Accessibility*, Dundee, Scotland, UK, pp. 139–46.

Graham, ID, Logan, J, Harrison, MB, Straus, SE, Tetroe, J, Caswell, W & Robinson, N 2006, 'Lost in knowledge translation: Time for a map?', *J Contin Educ Health Prof*, vol. 26, no. 1, pp. 13–24.

Greenhalgh, T, Procter, R, Wherton, J, Sugarhood, P & Shaw, S 2012, The organising vision for telehealth and telecare: Discourse analysis, *BMJ Open*, vol. 2, no. 4, p. e001574.

Greig, CA, Harper, R, Hirst, T, Howe, T & Davidson, B 2008, Barriers and facilitators to mobile phone use for people with aphasia, *Top Stroke Rehabil*, vol. 15, no. 4, pp. 307–24.

Guo, YE, Togher, L, Power, E, Hutomo, E, Yang, YF, Tay, A, Yen, SC, Koh, GC 2017, Assessment of aphasia across the International Classification of Functioning, Disability and Health using an iPad-based application, *Telemedicine and e-Health*, vol. 23, no. 4, pp. 313–26.

Hallowell, B & Chapey, R 2008, Introduction to language intervention strategies in adult aphasia, In: R Chapey (ed.), *Language Intervention Strategies in Aphasia and Related Neurogenic Communication Disorders* (5th ed., pp. 3–19), Lippincott Williams & Wilkins, Baltimore.

Helsper, EJ & Reisdorf, BC 2016, The emergence of a "digital underclass" in Great Britain and Sweden: Changing reasons for digital exclusion, *New Media Soc*, vol. 19, no. 8, pp. 1253–70.

Hines, M, Brunner, M, Poon, S, Lam, M, Tran, V, Yu, D, Togher, L, Shaw, T & Power, E 2017, Tribes and tribulations: Interdisciplinary eHealth in providing services for people with a traumatic brain injury (TBI), *BMC Health Serv Res*, vol. 17, no. 1, p. 757.

IQVIA 2017, The growing value of digital health, IQVIA Institute for Human Data Science, www.iqvia.com/institute/reports/the-growing-value-of-digital-health.

Johnson, L, Morris, J & Menger, F 2014, Facilitating the use of technology with people with aphasia: What are the challenges for SLTs. *In Poster session at British Aphasiology Society Research Update Meeting*, Newcastle upon Tyne.

Jones, ML, Morris, J & de Ruyter, F 2018, Mobile healthcare and people with disabilities: Results from a preliminary survey. In K Miesenberger & G Kouroupetroglou (eds), *Computers Helping People with Special Needs* (pp. 457–463). Lecture Notes in Computer Science, vol 10897. Springer, Cham.

Kagan, A, Simmons-Mackie, N, Rowland, A, Huijbregts, M, Shumway, E, McEwen, S, Threats, T & Sharp, S 2008, Counting what counts: A framework for capturing real-life outcomes of aphasia intervention, *Aphasiology*, vol. 22, no. 3, pp. 258–80.

Kane, S, Linam-Church, B, Althoff, K & McCall, D 2012, What we talk about: Designing a context-aware communication tool for people with aphasia. *In Proceedings of the 14th International ACM SIGACCESS Conference on Computers and Accessibility*, Boulder, CO, USA, pp. 49–56.

Kearns, Á, Kelly, H & Hanafin, R 2018, Speech and language therapists' perspectives of ICT use in aphasia rehabilitation, *Aphasiology*, vol. 32, no. sup1, pp. 109–10.

Kelly, H, Kennedy, F, Britton, H, McGuire, G & Law, J 2016, Narrowing the "digital divide"—facilitating access to computer technology to enhance the lives of those with aphasia: A feasibility study, *Aphasiology*, vol. 30, no. 2–3, pp. 133–63.

Kerr, A, Smith, M, Reid, L & Baillie, L 2018, Adoption of stroke rehabilitation technologies by the user community: Qualitative study, *JMIR Rehabil Assist Technol*, vol. 5, no. 2, p. e15.

Kleim, JA & Jones, TA 2008, Principles of experience-dependent neural plasticity: Implications for rehabilitation after brain damage, *J Speech Lang Hear Res*, vol. 51, no. 1, pp. S225–39.

Kurland, J, Wilkins, AR & Stokes, P 2014, iPractice: Piloting the effectiveness of a tablet-based home practice program in aphasia treatment, *Semin Speech Lang*, vol. 35, no. 1, pp. 51–63.

Lam, JM & Wodchis, WP 2010, The relationship of 60 disease diagnoses and 15 conditions to preference-based health-related quality of life in Ontario hospital-based long-term care residents, *Med Care*, vol. 48, no. 4, pp. 380–7.

Langan, J, Subryan, H, Nwogu, I & Cavuoto, L 2018, Reported use of technology in stroke rehabilitation by physical and occupational therapists, *Disabil Rehabil Assist Technol*, vol. 13, no. 7, pp. 641–7.

Levac, D, Glegg, SMN, Sveistrup, H, Colquhoun, H, Miller, PA, Finestone, H, DePaul, V, Harris, JE & Velikonja, D 2016, A knowledge translation intervention to enhance clinical application of a virtual reality system in stroke rehabilitation, *BMC Health Serv Res*, vol. 16, no. 1, p. 557.

Maas, MB, Lev, MH, Ay, H, Singhal, AB, Greer, DM, Smith, WS, Harris, GJ, Halpern, EF, Koroshetz, WJ & Furie, KL 2012, The prognosis for aphasia in stroke, *J Stroke Cerebrovasc Dis*, vol. 21, no. 5, pp. 350–7.

Mahmud, AA & Martens, J-B 2015, Iterative design and field trial of an aphasia-friendly email tool, *ACM Trans Access Comput*, vol. 7, no. 4, pp. 1–36.

Mallet, K, Shamloul, R, Pugliese, M, Power, E, Corbett, D, Hatcher, S, Shamy, M, Stotts, G, Zakutney, L, Dukelow, S & Dowlatshahi, D 2019, RecoverNow: A patient perspective on the delivery of mobile tablet-based stroke rehabilitation in the acute care setting, *Int J Stroke*, vol. 14, no. 2, p. 1.

Marshall, J, Roper, A, Galliers, J, Wilson, S, Cocks, N, Muscroft, S & Pring, T 2013, Computer delivery of gesture therapy for people with severe aphasia, *Aphasiology*, vol. 27, no. 9, pp. 1128–46.

McCall, D 2012, Steps to success with technology for individuals with aphasia, *Semin Speech Lang*, vol. 33, no. 3, pp. 234–42.

McCann, CG, & Greig, L. 2012, From single words to sentences: The novel use of video stimuli in verb therapy. *Paper Presented to 15th International Aphasia Rehabilitation Conference*, Melbourne, Australia, October.

McGrenere, J, Davies, R, Findlater, L, Graf, P, Klawe, M, Moffatt, K, Purves, B & Yang, S 2003, Insights from the aphasia project: Designing technology for and with people who have aphasia. *Paper Presented to Proceedings of the 2003 Conference on Universal Usability, Vancouver*, British Columbia, Canada.

McNaughton, D & Light, J 2013, The iPad and mobile technology revolution: Benefits and challenges for individuals who require augmentative and alternative communication, *Augment Altern Commun*, vol. 29, no. 2, pp. 107–16.

Mehta, DD, Zañartu, M, Feng, SW, Cheyne II, HA & Hillman, RE 2012, Mobile voice health monitoring using a wearable accelerometer sensor and a Smartphone Platform, *IEEE Trans Biomed Eng*, vol. 59, no. 11, pp. 3090–6.

Meltzer, JA, Baird, AJ, Steele, RD & Harvey, SJ 2018, Computer-based treatment of poststroke language disorders: A non-inferiority study of telerehabilitation compared to in-person service delivery, *Aphasiology*, vol. 32, no. 3, pp. 290–311.

Menger, F, Morris, J & Salis, C 2016, Aphasia in an Internet age: Wider perspectives on digital inclusion, *Aphasiology*, vol. 30, no. 2–3, pp. 112–32.

Miller, CL, Mott, K, Cousins, M, Miller, S, Johnson, A, Lawson, T & Wesselingh, S 2017, Integrating consumer engagement in health and medical research – an Australian framework, *Health Res Policy Syst*, vol. 15, no. 1, p. 9.

Moffatt, K 2004, Designing technology for and with special populations: An exploration of participatory design with people with aphasia, M.Sc. Thesis, University of British Columbia, www.cs.ubc.ca/labs/imager/th/2003/Moffatt2004 /moffatt2004.pdf.

Moffatt, K, Pourshahid, G & Baecker, R 2015, Augmentative and alternative communication devices for aphasia: The emerging role of "smart" mobile devices, *Univers Access Inf*, vol. 16, pp. 115–28.

Mooney, A, Bedrick, S, Noethe, G, Spaulding, S & Fried-Oken, M 2018, Mobile technology to support lexical retrieval during activity retell in primary progressive aphasia, *Aphasiology*, vol. 32, no. 6, pp. 666–92.

Morris, J, Jones, M & Sweatman, M 2016, Wireless technology use by people with disabilities: A national survey, *J Tech Persons Disabil*, vol. 4, p. 101.

Morris, J, Mueller, J & Jones, M 2010, Toward mobile phone design for all: Meeting the needs of stroke survivors, *Top Stroke Rehabil*, vol. 17, no. 5, pp. 353–61.

O'Brien, MK, Shawen, N, Mummidisetty, CK, Kaur, S, Bo, X, Poellabauer, C, Kording, K & Jayaraman, A 2017, Activity recognition for persons with stroke using mobile phone technology: Toward improved performance in a home setting, *J Med Internet Res*, vol. 19, no. 5, p. e184.

Ofcom 2018, Communications market report, www.ofcom.org.uk/__data/assets/ pdf_file/0022/117256/CMR-2018-narrative-report.pdf.

Palmer, R, Enderby, P, Cooper, C, Latimer, N, Julious, S, Paterson, G, Dimairo, M, Dixon, S, Mortley, J, Hilton, R, Delaney, A & Hughes, H 2012, Computer therapy compared with usual care for people with long-standing aphasia poststroke: A pilot randomized controlled trial, *Stroke*, vol. 43, no. 7, pp. 1904–11.

Parr, S 2007, Living with severe aphasia: Tracking social exclusion, *Aphasiology*, vol. 21, no. 1, pp. 98–123.

Paul, L, Wyke, S, Brewster, S, Sattar, N, Gill, JMR, Alexander, G, Rafferty, D, McFadyen, AK, Ramsay, A & Dybus, A 2016, Increasing physical activity in stroke survivors using STARFISH, an interactive mobile phone application: A pilot study, *Top Stroke Rehabil*, vol. 23, no. 3, pp. 170–7.

Power, E, Thomas, E, Worrall, L, Rose, M, Togher, L, Nickels, L, Hersh, D, Godecke, E, O'Halloran, R, Lamont, S, O'Connor, C & Clarke, K 2015, Development and validation of Australian aphasia rehabilitation best practice statements using the RAND/UCLA appropriateness method, *BMJ Open*, vol. 5, no. 7, p. e007641.

Roper, A, Grellmann, B, Neate, T, Marshall, J & Wilson, S 2018, Social networking sites: Barriers and facilitators to access for people with aphasia, *Aphasiology*, vol. 32, no. sup1, pp. 176–7.

Rose, M, Carragher, M, Taylor, N, Johnson, H, Torabi, T & O'Halloran, R 2017, The Aphasia App: A novel technology-based approach to improving healthcare communication for people with post stroke aphasia and healthcare professionals, *Int J Stroke*, vol. 12, p. 57.

Sarasohn-Kahn, J 2010, How smartphones are changing health care for consumers and providers, www.chcf.org/wp-content/uploads/2017/12/PDF-HowSmartphonesChangingHealthCare.pdf.

Shrubsole, K, Worrall, L, Power, E & O'Connor, DA 2017, Recommendations for post-stroke aphasia rehabilitation: An updated systematic review and evaluation of clinical practice guidelines, *Aphasiology*, vol. 31, no. 1, pp. 1–24.

Simmons-Mackie, N & Cherney, LR 2018, Aphasia in North America: Highlights of a white paper, *Arch Phys Med Rehabil*, vol. 99, p. e117.

SSNAP 2018, SSNAP National Results- Clinical Audit July-September 2018, King's College London, www.strokeaudit.org/results/Clinical-audit/National-Results.aspx.

Stark, BC & Warburton, EA 2018, Improved language in chronic aphasia after self-delivered iPad speech therapy, *Neuropsychol Rehabil*, vol. 28, no. 5, pp. 818–31.

Szabo, G & Dittelman, J 2014, Using mobile technology with individuals with aphasia: Native iPad features and everyday apps, *Semin Speech Lang*, vol. 35, no. 1, pp. 5–16.

Tavistock Trust for Aphasia, n.d. Aphasia Software Finder, www.aphasiasoftwarefinder.org/.

TGA 2018, Regulation of software as a medical device, Therapeutic Goods Administration, Department of Health, Australian Government, www.tga.gov.au/regulation-software-medical-device.

van Dijk, JAGM 2012, The evolution of the digital divide: The digital divide turns to inequality of skills and usage, In: J Bus, M Crompton, M Hildebrandt, & G Metakides (eds), *Digital Enlightenment Yearbook 2012* (pp. 57–78), IOS Press, Amsterdam.

Wallace, SJ, Worrall, L, Rose, T, Le Dorze, G, Cruice, M, Isaksen, J, Kong, APH, Simmons-Mackie, N, Scarinci, N & Gauvreau, CA 2017, Which outcomes are most important to people with aphasia and their families? An international nominal group technique study framed within the ICF, *Disabil Rehabil*, vol. 39, no. 14, pp. 1364–79.

Warschauer, M 2003, *Technology and Social Inclusion: Rethinking the Digital Divide*, MIT Press, Cambridge, MA.

WHO 2001, *International Classification of Functioning, Disability and Health*, World Health Organisation, Geneva.

WHO 2011, *mHealth: New Horizons for Health through Mobile Technologies: Second Global Survey on eHealth*, World Health Organisation Global Observatory for eHealth, Geneva.

Wilson, S, Roper, A, Marshall, J, Galliers, J, Devane, N, Booth, T & Woolf, C 2015, Codesign for people with aphasia through tangible design languages. *Codesign*, vol. 11, no. 1, pp. 21–34.

Worrall, L, Rose, T, Brandenburg, C, Rohde, A, Berg, K & Wallace, S 2016, Aphasia in later life, In: AN Pachana (ed.), *Encyclopedia of Geropsychology* (pp. 1–7), Springer, Singapore.

Worrall, L, Sherratt, S, Rogers, P, Howe, T, Hersh, D, Ferguson, A & Davidson, B 2011, What people with aphasia want: Their goals according to the ICF, *Aphasiology*, vol. 25, no. 3, pp. 309–22.

Zheng, C, Lynch, L & Taylor, N 2016, Effect of computer therapy in aphasia: A systematic review, *Aphasiology*, vol. 30, no. 2–3, pp. 211–44.

17

Technology Acceptance, Adoption, and Usability: Arriving at Consistent Terminologies and Measurement Approaches

Lili Liu
University of Waterloo and
University of Alberta

Antonio Miguel Cruz
University of Alberta and
Glenrose Rehabilitation Hospital

Adriana Maria Rios Rincon
University of Alberta

CONTENTS

Introduction 320
Acceptance, Adoption, and Usability of Technologies: Distinguishing
between Concepts and Theories 321
    The Chicken or Egg Paradox as it Relates to the Concepts of
    Acceptance, Adoption, and Usability of Technologies 321
    Attitudes, Behaviours, and Behavioural Changes: The Roots of the
    Theories and Theories of Acceptance, Adoption, and Usability of
    Technologies 323
    Theories of Acceptance, Adoption, and Usability of Technologies 324
Measuring and Testing Technology Acceptance, Adoption and Usability 327
A General Overview about how to Conduct Technology Acceptance
Usability Studies 328
    Methods for Measuring Technology Acceptance and Testing Usability.... 330
    Choosing a Method for Measuring Technology Acceptance and
    Usability Testing 332
Technology Acceptance and Usability Studies: Examples 333
    Online Consumer Guideline for Locator Technologies 333
    The Locator Device Project (GPS Study) 334

Rehabilitation Therapists' Acceptance of New Technologies for
Rehabilitation 335
Summary 336
Declaration of Conflict of Interest 336
Acknowledgement 336
References 336

Introduction

As the evolution of everyday technologies grows exponentially, so must we re-conceptualize assistive and related technologies in healthcare (Liu, 2018). It is no longer assumed that customized technologies cost more to create because the process of creating these one-off products, such as the use of 3-D printers, is becoming more affordable. More than ever, the boundaries between technologies that are 'assistive' or 'health-related', and everyday technologies, such as the Internet of Things (IoT) are blurred (Liu, 2018). Today, we see commercial products, such as smartphones, equally useful to people for everyday purposes (phone calls, photos, social media, etc.) as to those who need support for managing their health conditions (reminders to take medications, communications with health providers, operating objects in one's living space with limited mobility).

In recent years, it has become evident that the concepts of technology acceptance, adoption and usability have become a focus of researchers, educators and health service providers. The early concept of 'technology abandonment', previously associated with rehabilitation assistive devices, now has a more general meaning, and can be applied to everyday innovations available to the general public, in the context of 'commercialization' of products. With exponential growth in technologies and innovations, some commercial products are 'abandoned' or replaced before a manufacturer can even upgrade a model.

We are now faced with the challenge of how health researchers and service providers can assess technology acceptance, predict whether technology will be adopted and test the usability of technologies in a world where everyday technologies can also be used for health applications. Inconsistent terminologies in the assistive technology field 'hampers understanding and collaboration, and service transitions' (Scherer, 2017, p. 1). The purpose of this chapter is to provide structure and consistency in how we can address the concepts of acceptance, adoption, and usability. We use the terms technology, system and innovation interchangeably.

This chapter addresses the following questions: (1) What do the concepts *technology acceptance, technology adoption,* and *usability* of technologies mean? (2) Why are certain technologies, or innovations, better accepted and adopted than others? (3) How should one determine or measure acceptance and adoption, and test usability of technologies?

Acceptance, Adoption, and Usability of Technologies: Distinguishing between Concepts and Theories

The Chicken or Egg Paradox as it Relates to the Concepts of Acceptance, Adoption and Usability of Technologies

According to Scherer (2017), technology acceptance, adoption and usability have traditionally been of primary concern to product designers, engineers and manufacturers although adoption is also a concern of those in the marketplace. Providers and users of these products, on the other hand, tend to focus more on realization of benefit and functional gain from use as well as their useworthiness. Satisfaction with use and the process of getting the product are key concerns of clinic directors and product vendors. Several studies on acceptance, adoption, and usability of various types of technologies have used these three terms interchangeably; however, they are not the same. In this section, we will offer clarification of these three concepts.

Unlike the chicken or egg paradox where either the chicken or egg could come first, we propose that *acceptance* precedes adoption, and in turn, *adoption* precedes usability (see Figure 17.1). Note that the concept of usability is related to the two preceding concepts, as depicted by the dotted lines. If a product is perceived to be usable, acceptance and adoption (or actual use) would occur.

According to Nielsen (1993, p. 24), a technology is accepted when 'the [technology] is good enough to satisfy all the needs and requirements of the users and other potential stakeholders'. A technology is accepted when it has *social* and *practical acceptability* (Nielsen, 1993, p. 24). Acceptability occurs when a complex system of *attitudes* and *individuals' beliefs* take place and these beliefs, in turn, provoke *a specific behavioural change in individuals*. An example of this is the use of seat belts in vehicles. At the beginning, people had a negative attitude towards the use of seat belts. Due to external factors such as regulations and statistics collected by the transit agencies, which showed that seat belt use saved lives (Pickrell & Ye, 2012), people began to change their attitude towards its use, and believing that the seat belt could really save their lives. This change of attitude led to the establishment of a well-founded belief that belts increase safety on roads. Nowadays, it is rare (1%) to see a driver who does not use a seat belt; an indication that a behaviour change towards the use of the seat belt has occurred (Kidd, Mccartt & Oesch, 2014).

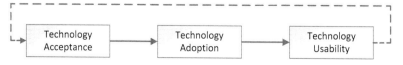

FIGURE 17.1
Relationship between the concepts of acceptance, adoption and usability of technologies.

Technology adoption refers to the consistent process of an individual's decision to integrate, or not to integrate, a technology into his or her life. The decision process consists of five steps: (1) *awareness* (an individual becomes aware of a technology (or an innovation[1]) existence), (2) *persuasion* (individual gains enough knowledge about the technology's features), (3) *decision* (individual adopts or rejects the technology), (4) *implementation* (individual acts on his or her decision) and (5) *confirmation* (individual re-evaluates whether to continue or discontinue with the technology adoption decision) (Rogers, 1995) cited by Straub (2009).

Usability is a concept associated to the adoption or *actual use* of a technology. A fundamental premise for technology usability is its *usefulness* (whether the system can be used to achieve a desired goal). However, usability should be understood as a multidimensional concept. For example, according to the International Organization for Standardization (ISO) 9241-11:2018,[2] usability is defined as 'the extent to which a system, product or service can be used by specified users to achieve *specified goals* with *effectiveness, efficiency* and *satisfaction* in a specified context of use' (ISO 9241-11, 2018, p. 6). Three key dimensions can be identified in the ISO's usability definition, namely: *effectiveness, efficiency and satisfaction*. According to ISO, *effectiveness* refers to the level of *'accuracy* and *completeness* with which users achieve their specified goals' (ISO 9241-11, 2018, p. 9). Within the context of ISO definition of usability to achieve specified goals means that users 'achieve the intended outcome' (ISO 9241-11, 2018, p. 3). *Efficiency* refers to 'resources used in relation to the results achieved' (ISO 9241-11, 2018, p. 10). *Satisfaction* is understood as the 'extent to which the user's physical, cognitive and emotional responses that result from the use of a [technology] meet the user's needs and expectations' (ISO 9241-11, 2018, p. 11).

Nielsen (1993) also describes usability as a multidimensional concept with five attributes: *learnability, efficiency, memorability, errors* and *satisfaction*. *Learnability* refers to how easy it is to learn the technology, so once a user learns to use the technology, he or she can rapidly start to use the technology and perform the necessary related tasks or work. *Efficiency* means that a user should achieve a high level of productivity with minimum required resources (i.e., money, time, and effort). Of course, it assumed that a user would have learned to use the technology first. *Memorability* refers to how easy it is to remember how to use the technology, i.e., when a user stops to use the technology for period of time, and returns to the product, the user does not have to spend a lot of time to re-learn. The *error* attribute of the usability concept refers to the technology. Ideally, it should be free of error, or in a more realistic scenario, has a low error rate. More importantly, catastrophic errors must not occur. Finally, *satisfaction* means that the technology should be pleasant to use; in other words, when a user uses the technology, he or

---

[1] According to Rogers (1995, p. 11), an innovation is an 'idea, practice or object that is perceived as new by an individual or other unit of adoption'.
[2] A multipart standard from the ISO covering ergonomics of human–computer interaction.

TABLE 17.1

Comparison between Nielsen's and ISO 9241-11's Definitions of Usability

Usability Attribute	Nielsen (1993)	ISO 9241-11 (2018)
Effectiveness		X
Efficiency	X	X
Satisfaction	X	X
Learnability	X	
Memorability	X	
Errors	X	X

ISO defines accuracy under the framework of usability as 'the extent to which an actual outcome matches an intended outcome' (ISO 9241-11, 2018, p. 9), which is the definition of error.

she is pleased when using it (Nielsen, 1993). In conclusion, technology with a high level of usability is technology that is *learnable, effortless, memorable, free of errors* and *attractive* in characteristics. Table 17.1 compares Nielsen's and ISO 9241-11's definition of usability and shows they complement each other, and have in common, the attributes of efficiency, satisfaction and free of errors.

Attitudes, Behaviours, and Behavioural Changes: The Roots of the Theories and Theories of Acceptance, Adoption and Usability of Technologies

An individual decides to accept, adopt and ultimately use a particular technology because factors have provoked behavioural changes in this individual. Although there exist specific theories that explain acceptance and adoption of technologies (we will explain them below), all of these are based on two root theories that explain why an individual chooses to use or not use a technology. These theories are the *Theory of Planned Behaviour* (Ajzen, 1991), and its predecessor, *Theory of Reasoned Action* (Fishbein & Ajzen, 1975). The main postulate of these theories relies on the assumption that 'since much human behavior is under *volitional control*, most behaviors can be accurately predicted from an "appropriate measure" of the *individual's intention* to perform the behavior in question' (Fishbein, 1980). In turn, an individual's intention to perform the behaviour is determined by certain individual's reactions to perform the target behaviour (Fishbein & Ajzen, 1975) (see Figure 17.2a). In general terms, one can say that these individual's reactions can be broken into *beliefs* and *attitudes*. According to Fishbein and Ajzen (1975, p. 12), attitudes are favourable or unfavourable evaluations of an object, whereas the term belief is the information that an individual has about an object. In other words, beliefs are an *individual's cognition* that link and object to certain attributes, whereas attitudes are *feelings and evaluations* that a person has about an object. Beliefs influence a person's attitude towards the target behaviour. There are two kinds of beliefs, including an *individual's* and *normative nature* beliefs. The last kind of belief refers 'to certain referents think the person

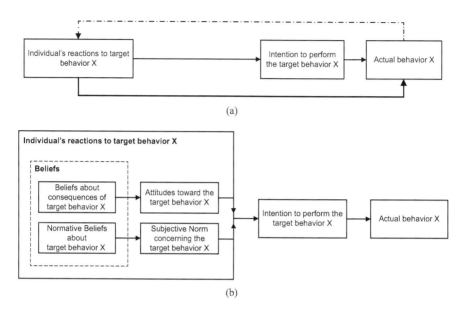

FIGURE 17.2
General conceptual framework for the prediction of specific intentions and behaviours:
(a) Simplified and (b) expanded.

should or should not to perform the behavior in question' (Fishbein & Ajzen, 1975). An individual may or may not be *motivated* to comply with a given referent, thus, the combination of individuals' motivations and the normative beliefs lead to *normative pressures*. This is what has been defined as *subjective norm*, i.e., 'the person's perception that most people who are important to him or her think he or she should or should not perform the behavior in question' (Fishbein & Ajzen, 1975). Thus, ultimately a person's behavioural intention is determined by two main factors: one's subjective norm and one's attitude towards the behavioural intention. In turn, the actual behaviour (the overt behaviour) is determined by a person's behavioural intention (conation) to perform the overt behaviour under study (Figure 17.2b).

Theories of Acceptance, Adoption, and Usability of Technologies

The most common theories used to explain acceptance and adoption of technologies are the *Technology Acceptance Model* (in its versions TAM and TAM2) (Davis, 1989), the *Combined Technology Acceptance Model* and *Theory of Planned Behaviour models* (C- TAM TPB) (Taylor & Todd, 1995), the *Innovation Diffusion Theory (IDT)* (Rogers, 1995), the *Social Cognitive Theory (SCT)* (Compeau & Higgins, 1995) and the *Motivational Model (MM)* (Davis, Bagozzi & Warshaw, 1992). Recently, the Unified Theory of Acceptance and Use of Technology, in its versions UTAUT (Venkatesh, Morris, Davis & Davis, 2003) and UTAU2 (Venkatesh, Thong & Xu, 2012) which integrates previous models with the behavioural intention perspectives and usage of technologies (i.e., TAM-TAM2, TPB, C- TAM TPB, IDT, SCT and MM) have emerged as dominant models to explain the behavioural intention to use technologies and the actual use of technologies.

Figure 17.3a,b show the conceptual framework of the UTAUT and UTAUT2 models, respectively. The original UTAUT model theorized four constructs

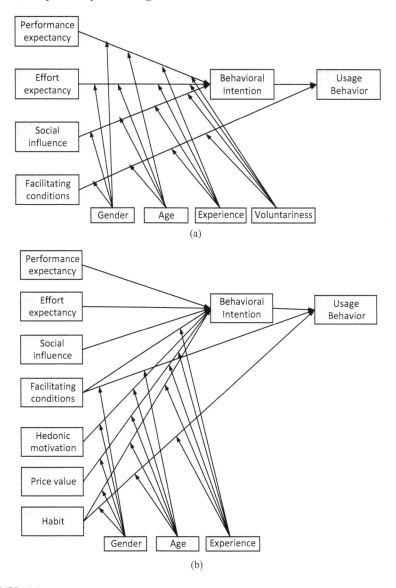

(a)

(b)

FIGURE 17.3
The UTAUT models: (a) UTAUT and (b) UTAUT2. (*Source:* Modified from Venkatesh, Thong & Xu, 2012, p. 160 and Venkatesh, Morris, Davis & Davis, 2003, p. 447.)

that play a role as direct predictors of the behavioural intention to use a given technology. According to Venkatesh, Morris, Davis and Davis (2003), *performance expectancy, effort expectancy* and *social influence* are direct determinants on behavioural intention to use the technology under study, whereas *facilitating conditions* and *behavioural intention* to use the technology are the two determinants of the *use behaviour* (in this context, the *overt behaviour of using* the technology is under study). Performance expectancy is defined 'as the degree to which an individual believes that using the system or technology will help him or her to attain gains in job' (Venkatesh, Morris, Davis & Davis, 2003). *Effort expectancy* has been defined 'as the degree of ease associated with the use of the system or technology under study' (Venkatesh, Morris, Davis & Davis, 2003). The last construct that has a direct impact on behavioural intention to use the technology under study is *social influence*, which is defined 'as the degree to which an individual perceives that important others believe he or she should use the new system' (Venkatesh, Morris, Davis & Davis, 2003).

The UTAUT2 is a modified version of the UTAUT. It was modified to include the consumer's use context. The UTAUT2 is basically the same as UTAUT with three new constructs added. These constructs are: *hedonic motivation* defined 'as the fun or pleasure derived from using a technology' (Venkatesh, Thong & Xu, 2012, p. 161), the *price value* defined as the 'consumers' cognitive tradeoff between the perceived benefits of the applications and the monetary cost for using them' (Venkatesh, Thong & Xu, 2012, p. 161) and *habit* defined as 'the extent to which people tend to perform behaviors automatically because of learning' (Venkatesh, Thong & Xu, 2012, p. 161).

Although Venkatesh, Morris, Davis and Davis (2003) assert that the constructs used in the UTAUT and UTAUT2 models are independent of any particular theoretical perspective, it is evident that UTAUT and UTAUT2 models are, in essence, a variation of the Theory of Reasoned Action (Fishbein & Ajzen, 1975) (Figures 17.2 and 17.3a,b). The variation consist of two aspects. First, Venkatesh et al. (2003) theorized that the attitude towards using a technology is not a direct determinant of the intention to use it and secondly, each of the determinants specify the role of four key moderators: *gender, age, voluntariness* and *experience*. Thus, in the UTAUT and UTAUT2 models, a person's behavioural intention to use a technology is determined by two main factors: the subjective norm (social influence construct) and his or her beliefs towards the behavioural intention to use the technology in question (performance and effort expectancy constructs). In turn, the actual use of technology is determined by a person's behavioural intention to use the technology and the facilitating condition belief.

At the beginning of this section we asserted that acceptance precedes adoption, and in turn, adoption precedes usability. A technology would be accepted only when an individual's system of beliefs and the subjective norms positively influence the indivudial's intention to use a certain technology. The technology can be adopted only when individuals make the

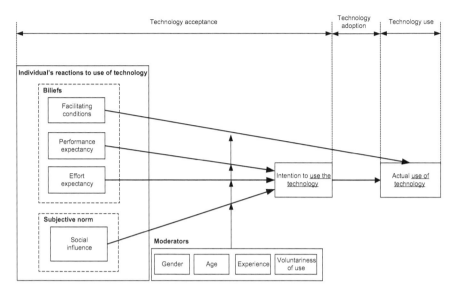

FIGURE 17.4
Conceptual framework for the prediction of intentions and use of technologies (UTAUT model). (Modified from Venkatesh, Morris, Davis & Davis, 2003, p. 447.)

decision to use the technology, in other words, a behavioural change has occurred. Finally, usability can be measured only when an individual uses the technology. According to Figure 17.4, acceptance, adoption and usability are captured in the UTAUT model.

Measuring and Testing Technology Acceptance, Adoption, and Usability

There are approaches to measure technology acceptance and test usability. Nielsen (1993) in his book, *Usability Engineering*, identifies nine different methods for measuring and testing usability, whereas Rohrer (2014) identifies 20 methods mapped across three dimensions, i.e., *Attitudinal-beliefs* versus *behavioural*, *qualitative* versus *quantitative* and *context of use*. The approaches would depend on whether the nature of a measure is *direct* or *indirect*. Direct methods measure the actual use of a technology through metrics such as users' performance or users' behavioural patterns while they are interacting with the technology. Indirect methods measure users' opinions about their experience with a technology, e.g., through questionnaires or interviews (Nielsen, 1993). Technology acceptance would be measured using an indirect approach. The attitudinal versus behavioural dimension of measuring usability refers to whether one wants to understand or measure individuals' stated beliefs (attitudinal beliefs) or to understand or measure what individuals' do (behavioural). It may be assumed that studies about attitudinal beliefs of the usability are associated to 'what people think', and the behavioural ones are associated with what 'people actually do'. When one conducts a study about individuals' attitudinal beliefs, it is preferable to say that one is conducting a *technology acceptance study*. On the contrary, when one does a study about use behaviours it is preferable to say that one is examining the actual *usability of a technology*.

The qualitative and quantitative approaches to describing usability refer to how data is collected and measured. In the qualitative approach, we use *participant observation, interviews, focus groups, document review* and *audio-visual materials*. In the quantitative approach, we use actual *performance measures, surveys* and *questionnaires* (e.g., five-point Likert scale). Qualitative methods are useful to respond to questions like: *Why is there an usability issue and how to fix it?* Quantitative methods are useful to respond to a question such as: *How many errors occurred?* Or, *how long does it take to perform a certain task?* The context of measuring usability refers to how and whether participants in the study are using the technology. Rohrer (2014) identifies three contexts: (1) *natural or near-natural* use of the product (when users test the technology in their homes, workplaces or other environments), (2) *scripted* study (more controlled environments such as laboratories), and (3) *not using the product* during the study (perceptions and expectations before using the technology). When usability is measured about a technology with actual users in a specific context using direct methods of measurement, one can say that usability is *tested* (Nielsen, 1993, p. 165).

The application of the usability methods according to the approaches and contexts mentioned can be combined; for example, one study can measure usability using the behavioural component through a quantitative approach in laboratory settings.

A General Overview about how to Conduct Technology Acceptance Usability Studies

Usability tests, in general, consist of five steps: (1) usability *test plan*, (2) *preparation of the test*, (3) *introduction to the users to the usability test*, (4) *usability test itself* and (5) *debriefing session* (Nielsen, 1993). Table 17.2 summarizes the main features of each usability step according to Nielsen (1993).

The measurement of technology acceptance generally begins with the selection of a theoretical framework (see Section on 'Theories of acceptance, adoption, and usability of technologies), the development of a technology acceptance questionnaire and the administration of the questionnaire to

TABLE 17.2

Usability Test Steps

Usability Step	Main Features
Usability test plan	Typical sections of a usability test plan are: • The goal of the usability test • The place and the time in which the usability test will take place • The number of sessions (e.g., one or five sessions), and the time each test session is expected to last (e.g., 1 h per session) • The number of equipment that will be needed and the software needed to be installed to conduct the usability test • The number of experimenter(s) • The sample size of users required • The tasks that will be conducted and the testing protocol (e.g., the criteria to determine when a task is completed, whether users will be allowed to use any aid (e.g., manual), whether the experimenter is allowed to provide prompts (verbal or physical) to users • Data collection and analyses procedures • Budget • Pilot test on the usability of test procedure
Usability test preparation	Under controlled environment usability tests, the experimenter should make sure that: • The test room is ready for the usability test • The technology being tested is in the starting state that was specified in the test and in the plan • All test materials, instructions and questionnaires are available
Introduction to users	• The purpose of the test is explained to the users • The person who is in charge of the experiment should mention that he or she has no personal interest in the technology being tested • The test results will be useful to improve the features of the technology being tested • A statement that the information collected from the users and test itself is confidential and the participation in the test is voluntary and that the user may stop at any time. • User should be invited to ask any clarifying questions before the start of the usability test
The usability test	• Usability data is collected through direct methods (e.g., thinking aloud, eye tracking, performance and observation) • During the test, the experimenter(s) must abstain from making any comments to the users • In the case where more than one person is in the room during the testing usability session, one person should be designated as the person who provides instructions and speaks during the usability test
The debriefing session	• Occurs after the test is conducted • The indirect methods of collecting data can be individual application of questionnaires either structured or semi-structured, focus groups can also be used • Questionnaires should be administered before any further discussion about the usability test, doing so avoids bias the experimenter might introduce • After the application of the questionnaires, users are asked for comments (e.g., suggestions for improving the technology)

potential users or actual users of the technology under study. The development of the questions and the levels of the scale (e.g., a seven-point Likert scale is more difficult to respond to than a three-point Likert scale) are critical elements when one develops an acceptance questionnaire. Thus, the research team must take into account the characteristics of the respondents in aspects such as age, cognitive skills and years of education.

Methods for Measuring Technology Acceptance and Testing Usability

A comprehensive explanation of methods for measuring technology acceptance and testing usability is beyond the scope of this chapter; however, the most common methods are described here.

Performance Measures. This is a direct method of measuring and testing usability. This is a method used for evaluating whether usability goals have been achieved. The usability goals are assessed through metrics that measure the user performance while users are engaged with the technology being tested. The usability test is run by having a group of test users who perform a predefined set of tasks while the experimenter is collecting data such as performance time and number and types of errors (Nielsen, 1993). The performance measurements can be conducted either in a laboratory setting or by observing users in their natural work environment. Typical quantifiable usability performance measurements are time users take to complete a specific task, number of users' errors, frequency of use of the manuals or the help system and amount of 'dead' time when a user is not interacting with the system (Nielsen, 1993, p. 194).

Thinking Aloud. This is a direct method of measuring usability. In this method, a user verbalizes his or her thoughts while interacting with the technology being tested. Studies on usability that used the thinking aloud protocol have shown that users performed 9% faster and make only about 20% of the errors made by users who were working silently (Nielsen, 1993, p. 194). Another advantage of this approach is that low-sample sizes are adequate to conduct this method (Nielsen, 1993, p. 174). Five users are enough for identifying up to 85% of usability problems when testing a technology using the thinking aloud approach (Nielsen, 2000).

Thinking Aloud – Constructive Interaction. This is considered a direct method of measuring usability and is a variation of the thinking aloud method. In the constructive interaction method two test users together use the technology being tested. This method is considered much more natural and engaging than standard thinking aloud tests 'since people normally verbalize when they are trying to solve a problem together' (Nielsen, 1993, p. 198). The method does have the disadvantage that, in some cases, users cannot work together. Therefore, the selection and pairing of users should be thoughtfully done when using this method.

Thinking Aloud – Retrospective Testing. This is a direct method of measuring usability and another variation of the thinking aloud method. This method is also called *retrospective think aloud*. Using a video recording of a user test session, the experimenter can ask participants to provide additional comments when the session is completed. By doing so, the users watch the video replay of their actions (Usability, 2018). The disadvantage of this method is that each test can take twice as long to complete (Nielsen, 1993, p. 199).

Eye-Tracking. This is a direct method of testing usability. In this method, an eye tracking device and a software are configured to measure where users' eyes are focused while performing tasks or interact naturally with the technology being tested. This method is particularly suited for measuring usability of websites, software applications, physical products or environments (e.g., smart homes) (Rohrer, 2014). The software generates data about users' actions in the form of *heat maps* (i.e. colour scale moving from blue to red) or *saccade pathways* (i.e. a combination of circles and lines, a red circle is the area of focus, the red line indicates the flight) (Usability, 2018).

Observation. This is a direct method of measuring usability consisting in the experimenter or observer visiting several users in their natural environment, and observing them while doing their tasks using the technology under study. The observer makes notes and may video record the users for further analysis. The main disadvantage of this method is that the presence of the observer may affect the user behaviour. Therefore, the observer must endeavour to 'not to interfere with the users' work' (Nielsen, 1993, p. 207).

Logging the Actual Use. This is considered a direct method of measuring usability, as the technology being tested automatically collect data about the patterns of use (e.g., time, frequency of use) (Nielsen, 1993). One disadvantage of this method is that it only shows what users do, but not why or how they do it (Nielsen, 1993). One solution is to apply a variation of this method that consists of performing weekly phone calls to users and asking them standard questions about their experience while using the technology being tested and logging the responses onto a database (Liu, Miguel-Cruz, Ruptash, Barnard & Juzwishin, 2017).

Interviews and Questionnaires. These methods are indirect methods of measuring technology acceptance and testing usability. As mentioned (in Section on 'Theories of acceptance, adoption, and usability of technologies'), these methods can be used to obtain information related to users' beliefs and attitudes towards the use of the technology being examined (Nielsen, 1993, p. 209). In this method, the experimenter should apply the interviews and questionnaires to users shortly after using the technology, otherwise the reliability of the responses decreases as the time increases (Nielsen, 1993). However, in technology acceptance studies, the questionnaires may be administered before the participants use a technology and again after participants have used the technology (Liu, Miguel-Cruz, Ruptash, Barnard & Juzwishin, 2017). Semantic differential and Likert scale questions are used in acceptance and usability questionnaires. Questionnaires in a single page or two sides of a single sheet of paper with short questions have demonstrated

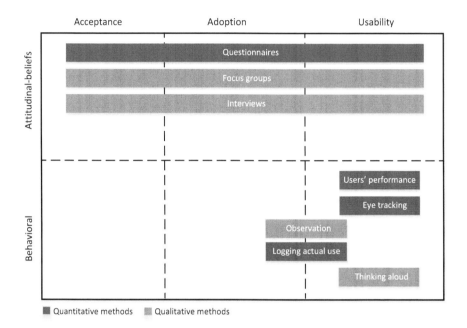

FIGURE 17.5
Methods for measuring technology acceptance, adoption and usability.

to have the best reliability and validity measures (Nielsen, 1993). Interviews include open-ended questions where users are encouraged to comment about the technology being studied. Interview methods are best suited in exploratory usability studies (Nielsen, 1993).

Focus Groups. This method is an indirect method of measuring usability. In this method, a group of users are interviewed at the same time about the usability of the technology being tested. The use of affirmative statements or open-ended questions is the most common practice while a focus group is conducted (Portney & Watkins, 2008). This method is more useful than the interviews when it is desirable to obtain multiple responses on a specific topic about usability. The main advantage of this method is that a focus group with three to five participants is more than enough to obtain information needed about the usability of a technology (Letts, Wilkins, Law, Stewart, Bosch & Westmorland, 2007; Rohrer, 2014) (Figure 17.5).

Choosing a Method for Measuring Technology Acceptance and Usability Testing

As a rule of thumb, if very few users are available, the best methods for usability testing are thinking aloud, observation and focus groups. On the contrary, if an experimenter has the possibility to test the technology with a large number of users, then performance measurement, questionnaires and usage logging are the best options for usability testing (Nielsen, 1993). Our recommendation is, whenever possible, it is best to combine methods. The use of a combination of direct and indirect methods is ideal, as direct methods give us answers to 'how much and how the technology was used', and the indirect methods give us the answers to 'why and how this happens'. For example, combining logging the actual use, questionnaire and focus groups, or combining performance measures, a questionnaire and focus groups are good practices for testing usability (Nielsen, 1993).

On the other hand, in technology acceptance studies, the statistical analysis performed on data, called path analysis, demands larger sample sizes. The sample size rational for this type of research depends on the level of significance and the number of constructs included in the analyses. More information about the calculations of sample sizes for path analysis can be found in the reference (Hair, Hult, Ringle & Sarstedt, 2014).

Technology Acceptance and Usability Studies: Examples

Online Consumer Guideline for Locator Technologies

The first example is a study we conducted (Rios-Rincon et al., 2018) to assess the usability and acceptance of a web-based consumer guidelines of features of commercially available locator technologies by caregivers of persons who have dementia and are at risk of wandering and vendors of these technologies. This website was created by the research team as an online guideline of locator technologies for caregivers of persons who have dementia and at risk for wandering. This allows vendors to describe their products, and consumers to access this information when looking for an acceptable locator device for their relatives with dementia. The study used a combination of methods. First, for measuring the website usability, a direct method, the 'Thinking Aloud' was used with two vendors and three caregivers. Each participant was placed in front of a computer where the web-based consumer guideline (www.tech.findingyourwayontario.ca) for locator technologies was available for participants to interact with (see Figure 17.6). Each participant (caregiver or vendor) had up to 10 min to freely surf the website. A researcher instructed the participants to verbalize their thoughts about the website presentation, navigation, content and anything else they wanted to comment about. After this time, participants were asked to perform a second task. Vendors were asked to add a product on the website, and caregivers to look for a specific product. Dialogue spoken was recorded and transcribed verbatim for content analysis. Analysis of the thinking aloud method revealed the website usability issues, which allowed the research team to improve the design of the website. Next,

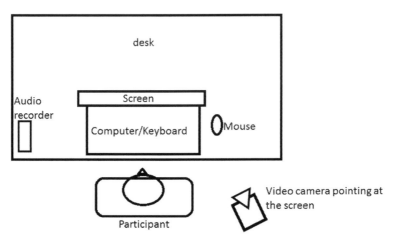

FIGURE 17.6
Usability test setup.

once the website was improved, the research team conducted a technology acceptance study using an indirect method, i.e. an online questionnaire. A total of 23 caregivers of individuals living with dementia accessed the website and, after using it, were invited to respond to a six-item online Likert scale questionnaire covering constructs of performance expectancy, effort expectancy and social influence. Items were scored on a Likert scale, ranging from 'strongly disagree (1)' to 'strongly agree (5)'. The questionnaire we developed for this study was short and easy to understand by older adults as we knew it was likely that the main caregiver of an individual living with dementia was a spouse who is also an older adult. Results indicated that the information from the website was easy to understand and useful.

The Locator Device Project (GPS Study)

In the second example (Liu et al., 2017), we aimed 'to examine the acceptance of Global Positioning System (GPS) used to help people with dementia, who are at risk for wandering in their communities' (Liu, Miguel-Cruz, Ruptash, Barnard & Juzwishin, 2017, p. 99). Although Liu et al. (2017) called this study 'an acceptance study', this study can be considered an actual usability study. The study used a combination of methods, with a strong theoretical-based rational, and the technology was tested and used in real context for a prolonged period of time. The study used the UTAUT as theoretical framework. The GPS technology was tested in 45 dyads consisting of people living with dementia, and their caregivers. The wearable GPS devices were used for an average of 5.8 months over a 1-year period. The GPS technology was used in community settings in rural and in urban areas. Three types of devices were used, 'a simplified cell phone that could be worn on a lanyard or belt, another was a pair of insoles, and the third was a watch' (Liu, Miguel-Cruz & Juzwishin, 2018, p. 638). Liu et al. (2017) used a combination of methods to determine the usability of the GPS: (1) pre- and post-paper-based quantitative questionaires to understand what factors affected the use of the GPS devices; (2) seven focus groups of 1.5 h duration with 15 caregivers and 9 stakeholders (e.g., Grande Prairie Royal Canadian Mounted Police, the Calgary Police Service, Home Care Case Management, Rehabilitation, and Primary Care Network, Social Work) were conducted; and (3) logging the actual use, i.e., 'client-caregiver dyads were contacted on a weekly basis by phone to respond to a structured questionnaire based on their experience using the GPS' (Liu, Miguel-Cruz, Ruptash, Barnard & Juzwishin, 2017, p. 102). The study concluded that 'the GPS provided caregivers peace of mind and reduced anxiety in dyads when clients got lost'. and 'that dyads would continue to use the GPS devices if they were able to do so' (Liu, Miguel-Cruz, Ruptash, Barnard & Juzwishin, 2017, p. 119).

Rehabilitation Therapists' Acceptance of New Technologies for Rehabilitation

The third example is a study in which we aimed to examine what factors affect the acceptance behaviour and use of new technologies for rehabilitation by therapists at a large rehabilitation hospital in Canada (Liu, Miguel Cruz, Rios Rincon, Buttar, Ranson & Goertzen, 2015). The study used a single indirect method for measuring technology acceptance, with a strong theoretical-based rational. In doing so, a self-administered 45-item paper-based questionnaire was created by adapting scales with high levels of internal consistency in prior research using the UTAUT. Items were scored on a seven-point Likert scale, ranging from 'strongly disagree (1)' to 'strongly agree (7)'. The target population was all occupational therapists and physical therapists involved with the provision of therapeutic interventions at the hospital. Therapists could participate in the study regardless of their gender, age and experience with the use of the targeted technologies. We distributed packages including the information letter, informed consent form and the questionnaire to the potential participants through clinic managers at the hospital. The questionnaire was returned to two different locations anonymously. The research model was tested using Partial Least Squares (PLS) technique. Results showed that performance expectancy construct did matters in the behavioural intention to use new technologies in rehabilitation, whereas effort expectancy and social influence constructs did not. Behavioural intention and facilitating condition constructs did matter in the current use of new rehabilitation technologies by occupational and physical therapists.

Summary

In this chapter, we proposed that technology acceptance precedes adoption, which precedes actual use that would continue as long as the product is considered to have usability. Usability attributes as described by Nielsen (1993) continue to be referred to in today's standards for consumer products. The concepts of acceptance, adoption and usability can be operationally defined and quantitatively measured within the context of theories, the most recent would be Technology of Acceptance Model and now, the UTAUTs. We demonstrated that these concepts can be examined directly (e.g., behaviourally), or indirectly (e.g., attitudes or beliefs of users). Finally, we provided three examples from our work that illustrate how we determined acceptance, adoption and tested usability of technologies for rehabilitation practitioners, and people living with dementia, including their care partners. We hope that this chapter contributes to consistency in terminologies used by researchers, educators and health service providers in the area of everyday technologies in health.

Declaration of Conflict of Interest

The authors report no conflicts of interest.

Acknowledgement

Research funding was provided from AGE-WELL NCE for the online consumer guideline for locator technologies, Alberta Innovation and Advanced Education for the Locator Device Project, and the Glenrose Rehabilitation Hospital Foundation for the technologies for rehabilitation study.

References

Ajzen, I. (1991). The theory of planned behavior. *Organizational Behavior and Human Decision Processes, 50*(2), 179–211.

Compeau, D., & Higgins, C. (1995). Application of social cognitive theory to training for computer skills. *Information Systems Research, 6*(2), 118–143.

Davis, F. (1989). Perceived usefulness, perceived ease of use, and user acceptance of information technology. *MIS Quarterly*, *13*(3), 319–339.

Davis, F., Bagozzi, R., & Warshaw, P. (1992). Extrinsic and intrinsic motivation to use computers in the workplace. *Journal of Applied Social Psychology*, *22*(14), 1111–1132.

Fishbein, M. (1980). A theory of reasoned action: Some application and implications. In: H. Howe & M. Page Licoln (eds), *Symposium on motivation* (pp. 65–116). Lincoln, NE: University of Nebraska Press.

Fishbein, M., & Ajzen, I. (1975). *Belief, attitude, intention and behavior: An introduction to theory and research*. Reading, MA: Addison-Wesley.

Hair, J., Hult, G., Ringle, C., & Sarstedt, M. (2014). *A primer on partial least squares structural equation modelling (PLS-SEM)*. Los Angeles, CA: Sage.

ISO 9241-11. (2018). ISO 9241, Ergonomics of human-system interaction. In: *Usability: definitions and concepts* (pp. 1–28). ISO. Retrieved November 26, 2018, from www. iso.org/obp/ui/#iso:std:iso:9241:-11:ed-2:v1:en:fn:1.

Kidd, D.G., Mccartt, A. T., & Oesch, N. J. (2014). Attitudes toward seat belt use and in-vehicle technologies. *Traffic Injury Prevention*, *15*, 10–17. doi: 10.1080/15389588.2013.792111

Letts, L., Wilkins, S., Law, M., Stewart, D., Bosch, J., & Westmorland, M. (2007). Guidelines for critical review form: Qualitative studies (version 2.0). Retrieved from https://srs-mcmaster.ca/wp-content/uploads/2015/05/Guidelines-for-Critical-Review-Form-Qualitative-Studies.pdf.

Liu, L. (2018). Occupational therapy in the Fourth Industrial Revolution. *Canadian Journal of Occupational Therapy*, *85*(4), 272–283. doi: 10.1177/0008417418815179

Liu, L., Miguel-Cruz, A., & Juzwishin, D. (2018). Caregivers as a proxy for responses of dementia clients in a GPS technology acceptance study. *Behaviour and Information Technology*, *37*, 634–645.

Liu, L., Miguel Cruz, A., Rios Rincon, A., Buttar, V., Ranson, Q., & Goertzen, D. (2015). What factors determine therapists' acceptance of new technologies for rehabilitation – a study using the Unified Theory of Acceptance and Use of Technology (UTAUT). *Disability and Rehabilitation*, *37*(5), 447–455.

Liu, L., Miguel-Cruz, A., Ruptash, T., Barnard, S., & Juzwishin, D. (2017). Acceptance of Global Positioning System (GPS) technology among dementia clients and family caregivers. *Journal of Technology in Human Services*, *35*, 99–119.

Nielsen, J. (1993). What is usability. In: J. Nielsen (ed.), *Usability engineering* (p. 30). Mountain View, CA: AP Professional.

Nielsen, J. (2000). Why you only need to test with 5 users. Retrieved December 2, 2018, from www.nngroup.com/articles/why-you-only-need-to-test-with-5-users/.

Pickrell, T., & Ye, T. (2012). Seat belt use in 2012—overall results. Report no. DOT HS–811–691. Washington, DC: National Highway Traffic Safety Administration.

Portney, L., & Watkins, M. (2008). *Foundations of clinical research: Application to practice* (3rd edn). Upper Saddle River, NJ: Prentice-Hall, Inc.

Rios-Rincon, A., Neubauer, N., Conway, C., Juzwishin, D., Mihailidis, A., & Liu, L. (2018). *Usability of an online consumer guideline for locator technologies*. Vancouver: CAOT.

Rogers, E. (1995). *Diffusion of innovations* (4th edn). New York, NY: Free.

Rohrer, C. (2014). When to use which user-experience research methods. Retrieved November 27, 2018, from www.nngroup.com/articles/which-ux-research-methods/.

Scherer, M. (2017). Technology adoption, acceptance, satisfaction and benefit: Integrating various assistive technology outcomes. *Disability and Rehabilitation: Assistive Technology*, *12*(1), 1–2.

Straub, E. (2009). Understanding technology adoption: Theory and future directions for informal learning. *Review of Educational Research*, *79*(2), 625–649.

Taylor, S., & Todd, P. (1995). Understanding information technology usage: A test of competing models. *Information Systems Research*, *6*(2), 144–176.

Usability. (2018). Running a usability test. Retrieved November 29, 2018, from www.usability.gov/how-to-and-tools/methods/running-usability-tests.html.

Venkatesh, V., Morris, M., Davis, G., & Davis, F. (2003). User acceptance of information technology: Toward a unified view. *Mis Quarterly*, *27*(3), 425–478.

Venkatesh, V., Thong, J., & Xu, X. (2012). Consumer acceptance and use of information technology: Extending the unified theory of aceptance and use of technology. *MIS Quarterly*, *36*(1), 157–178.

18

Artificial Intelligence

Hadi Mat Rosly
International Islamic University Malaysia

Maziah Mat Rosly
University of Malaya

CONTENTS

Introduction: Evolution of Artificial Intelligence 339
Overview of AI Technology 341
The Challenges in Healthcare Services and Innovative Advancement 342
Application of AI in Clinical Diagnosis 343
Application of AI in Patient Treatment and Management 345
AI in Autonomous Intervention and Innovative Assistance 348
Conclusion 350
References 351

Introduction: Evolution of Artificial Intelligence

Artificial Intelligence (AI) is a field of computer science that focuses on creating machine-based algorithmic programs to replicate human cognition, such as reasoning, understanding and learning. The composition of this complex algorithm produces 'intelligent machines' or more popularly known as 'smart technology'. The primary function of AI is to perform tasks, such as pattern recognition, data analysis, workflow planning, control manipulation and problem-solving, autonomously. AI development is a highly complex and specialised field of expertise, but has shown considerable increase of interest by researchers and company ventures. More and more companies, such as Google, Facebook, Apple, Amazon and Microsoft, are investing their resources into establishing intelligent system, which indicate robust growth in AI products and applications in the near future (Brynjolfsson, Rock & Syverson 2017). Unlike its initial misconception of having a narrow application, AI is being extensively used in various fields such as manufacturing, business, education and medical and has now become an essential part in advancing technology (Bostrom 2015). With so much reliance on AI-embed machines or tools, experts and analysts are convinced that AI is no longer the future but presently relevant.

One of the most iconic examples of AI technology includes the utilisation of Siri by Apple product. Siri is a voice-activated personal assistant that provides user-friendly interactions to assist on requests for information, navigation, planning and communication. Siri uses natural language recognition AI system to navigate through smart devices and utilises its applications. A similar concept was applied for healthcare diagnosis under the name Watson by IBM product. A more recent breakthrough in AI has shown phenomenal achievements in surpassing human capabilities. The AlphaGo, an AI engineered to play the board game 'Go', has successfully won matches with the world champion Go player. Using advanced search tree with deep neural network technique, the AlphaGo goes through recursive gameplay simulation against itself, to develop multiple counter-play strategies (Fortunato et al. 2017). AlphaGo has even shown to develop its own move sets, unknown to many players, yet effective against all the strategies developed by humans passed through generations. Nonetheless, the AlphaGo is constricted within the game rule, which is a highly controlled environment. Such environment is unattainable in a real-world application. Another famous example is the fully autopilot AI system in Tesla and Google cars, capable of providing features such as self-driving, regulating navigation and predicting traffic events simultaneously. In medicine, particularly surgery, the da Vinci Surgical System is a robotic-powered AI-enhanced technology that translates hand coordination into smaller, precise movements of tiny instruments during surgical procedure. It has brought minimally invasive surgery to more than 3 million patients worldwide, rapidly improving post-surgical recovery and reducing mortality or morbidity-related complications. Such achievements are accomplished by integrating AI analysis, prediction and control manipulation into complex machinery equipped with multiple sensors to monitor its environment and movements.

The prospect of AI has led to a major paradigm shift in many professional fields, especially in business, media and production line, which thrives from this progress. However, it has yet to shift the flow of healthcare sectors, mainly due to safety and ethical concerns. AI would certainly fill the inadequacy in healthcare services, by assisting in tasks such as healthcare management, clinical diagnosis and intervention, providing early detection and prevention. With AI's data aggregation and pattern recognition, it can perform clinical diagnosis to infer pathological symptoms from physical assessments or medical records. Clinical diagnosis using AI can be applied as a supporting tool to reduce potential human errors, as well as home-based diagnosis via online system for emergencies. In addition to that, AI can also perform mundane tasks such as managing medical records and scheduling plans, which reduce the workload of healthcare practitioners, allowing them to put more focus into providing quality and efficient services. A more extensive application of AI in healthcare includes the usage of intelligent machineries like servicing robots, autonomous rehabilitation systems, surgical robots and autonomous wheel chairs. These highly intelligent machineries will not only lessen the workload of healthcare practitioners but also maximise the service quality and efficiency. Alternatively, intelligent machineries can even be extended as home-based solution to long-term recovery in rehabilitation intervention and health monitoring system. Additionally, using AI predictive tools, early detection of genetic disease can be achieved, allowing for early intervention to minimise the complications and potential recurrence. The versatility AI has delivered will definitely improve healthcare facilities and services, whilst granting high-quality healthy living for both the patient and healthcare members.

Overview of AI Technology

Researchers have offered many different techniques to enhance AI algorithm (i.e. fuzzy logic, search tree, classifier, expert system, artificial neural network (ANN), genetic algorithm, reinforced learning and deep learning. Some of the more advanced AI technology utilises a combination of different techniques to further enhance the precision, accuracy and efficiency of cognitive replication. Fuzzy logic technique, a rudimentary form of AI introduced back in 1960s, was used to attain partiality in logic by clustering data. Expert system, on the other hand, is a rule-based algorithm designed to replicate human decision-making skill in a specific field of expertise. Both of these techniques are sub-categories of traditional AI techniques, which were criticised for its brittle performance, a false output caused by error in parameters selection (Bostrom 2015). Expert system was demonstrated in rehabilitation to replicate physiotherapeutic interventive response towards patient motor reaction (Akdoğan, Taçgın & Adli 2009). Another technique called genetic algorithm, utilises fitness function to select the most optimised parameters to generate the desired outcome. As the number of iterations increase, the function converges closer to its optimum solution. A cyclic convergence represents the function attaining its local optimum.

A more popular technique was later introduced, changing the view of AI altogether and has successfully garnered the attention of researchers and business investors. This technique is known as ANN, which utilises multiple layers of pattern recognition algorithm for better proficiency in generating true positive and true negative output. Unlike other complex systems, ANN does not require prior knowledge input from experts. From the foundation of ANN, AI algorithm evolved further into deep learning and reinforced learning techniques. These techniques offered better performance in replicating complex tasks. The advancement of neural networks proposed by researchers, have changed the pace of AI development. However, intricate processes are required to train an AI algorithm prior to field application. This process involves setting up the primary parameters and feeding it with large data samples of a specific diagnosis. The algorithm will perform several iterative processes, by discarding failed diagnostic parameters and retaining the successful ones for the next iteration. The diagnostic output will then be evaluated by a group of experts for validation of its performance and accuracy. To further validate the performance and accuracy analysis, new data samples were fed into the AI algorithm. During performance testing, researchers occasionally feed outlier data samples to test the sensitivity of the system. True positive output will validate the reliability of the AI analysis. As more samples are collected and fed into the AI, the algorithm becomes more accurate and reliable. This continuous process of learning is the source of AI's reliability in diagnostic and prediction analysis and control.

The Challenges in Healthcare Services and Innovative Advancement

Malpractice, misinterpretation and human errors are the biggest concern in healthcare work environment that need to be addressed. Ongoing reports estimate approximately 40,500 fatalities occurred in United States due to diagnosis error with 65% of it, due to medical malpractice and miscommunication (Winters et al. 2012; Amin, Agarwal & Beg 2013) Furthermore, a survey has reported that the majority of victims involved in medical malpractices suffer the consequences of an easily preventable disease, should accurate diagnosis and early intervention were initiated (Jao & Hier 2010). This occurrence is inevitable due to the heavy workload healthcare practitioners are burdened with. Large patient to healthcare practitioner ratio is hazardous, with long hours of service causing fatigue-induced errors. In countries like Taiwan, there are 357.9 nurses for every 100,000 patients; a ratio that is half compared to the United States (Liao et al. 2015). This has led to an average of 20%–32% of junior nurses resigning, citing stress and high workload as factors in Taiwan. These numbers are higher compared to other professions, which are only estimated to be at 9% (MacPhee, Ellis & McCutheon 2006). Another report in Isfahan, Iran, claimed that approximately 35% of nurses would opt for switching occupation, mainly due to stress and being overburdened with heavy workload (Mosadeghrad 2013). According to a logbook recorded by American Nurses Association (ANA), approximately 40% of nurses work more than the recommended hours of 8 h a day and 40 h a week (Rogers et al. 2004). These reasons contribute to the high frequency of errors in healthcare service, which has contributed to long-term illnesses, catapulted by fatigue, musculoskeletal disorders and possibly higher morbidity due to a weakened immune system. Studies reported that long hours of working in the healthcare sector are one of the major contributors to long-term illnesses, especially musculoskeletal disorders in the lower-back region (Andersen et al. 2012; Triolo 1989; Tullar et al. 2010). With all these challenges apparent in the healthcare sector, AI is offered as a solution to reduce their workload, whilst also increasing the efficiency and quality of healthcare service.

Nonetheless, society is still sceptical with the accuracy and reliability of AI, especially in terms of human–machine intervention and interaction. Concerns are raised with reported cases of fatalities caused by automation failure, where some are seemingly secondary to negligence in standard operating procedures and maintenance protocols. Unlike the production line, which only revolves around material production with minimal human interaction and supervision, the healthcare working environment requires dynamic human contact. This necessitates human-like features such as awareness, ethics and emotional intelligence prior to incorporating the system into healthcare. Additionally, new protocols may be required to ensure safety is maintained throughout. This includes routine maintenance, system updates for security measures and occasional protocol supervision from experts. The challenges posed in integrating AI system into healthcare services include society's confidence in trusting non-human interaction and diagnoses. This also includes security and privacy concerns regarding patients' personal records stored in a global network databank, the capitals required for large purchases of intelligent machineries, allocating large areas to facilitate each equipment and adapting to a sudden paradigm shift of workflow in a constantly busy facility. Fully automated AI machine-powered tools have yet to gain the confidence of society to fully entrust their lives.

Application of AI in Clinical Diagnosis

The utilisation of AI in health assessments, most notably in diagnosis, is the basis of AI application in healthcare. Current scenario for physician-based care, demonstrated limited ability for them to distinguish positive predictive symptomatic diagnosis, which may lead to false-positive and false-negative results. Several studies involving simulation and application observations demonstrated that incorporating an AI-based decision support system has helped improve diagnostic accuracy (Barinov et al. 2018; Bhavaraju 2018). The workflow schemes involve a dynamic machine learning AI, based on a scoring system. Traditionally, the core mechanics of simple AI diagnosis in healthcare involve input, computational analysis and decisive output application. The input aspects comprise collecting available data related to patient biography, presenting symptoms, clinical signs and laboratory findings into a pool of categories, where the computational analysis further aggregates the data into a more meaningful finding. The computational analysis consists of machine-based cognition, where the algorithms were engineered to provide a replication of human intellect, such as reasoning, understanding and learning. This is the basis of AI, which infers series of data into appropriate output presentation for a possible diagnosis. Algorithms are a series of programming languages designed for autonomous machine learning, also known as the AI core, replicating human intellectual cognition. The physical component of AI in output can also include medical devices and robots for delivering appropriate care.

Early iterations of AI-based decision support system provide meaningful increase in sensitivity but a large decrease in specificity of accurate disease diagnosis. Specificity, also called the true negative rate, is defined as the extent to which a diagnostic test is specific for a particular condition, disease or trait; in other words, to correctly reject a patient without a condition. On the other hand, sensitivity is the extent to which actual diseases are detected, creating fewer rooms for false negative or false positives. As AI algorithmic dynamics and complexity progress, newer AI-based decision support system offers substantial improvement in both sensitivity and specificity, whilst providing possible available differential diagnosis within the description provided. However, higher specificity in AI-supported diagnostic decisions is more sought after, as a highly sensitive test rarely overlooks an actual positive disease identification. AI has been used successfully in cancer-related diseases, showing promise in areas related to tumour biopsies, histopathological descriptions, tracking tumour development and predicting prognosis.

AI systems have traditionally been used as an aid for the detection of early- or late-stage diseases, by combining a series of data-driven predictive model of patient presentation, as a decision support tool. This conceptual framework has evolved with the current attention to big data analysis, which is impossible to achieve through individual physician interpretation. Big data are extremely large data sets that can be used to reveal patterns, trends and associations, especially relating to human behaviour and interactions, which are far more complex than traditional data-processing analysis. The power of big data integrated into AI has gained widespread attention in the domain of health, in particular, due to its ability to predict possible outcomes from minute to major warning signs. We have seen how the same collection of data have allowed consumer marketing companies, be able to predict, with a startling degree of accuracy, which of their customers are pregnant, along with their range of due dates.

Incidentally, by working through the search activities of a user in a search engine, AI boosted by big data analysis has also demonstrated the ability to indicate if they had been diagnosed with cancer. By combining these algorithms with big data sets from users' search logs, researchers are now able to offer early diagnoses of pancreatic cancer between 5% and 15% of cases, returning almost no false positives (Paparrizos, White & Horvitz 2016). It is important to note that pancreatic cancer symptoms are incredibly difficult to detect in its early stages, with high mortality rates if presented at the later stages. Big data combined with complex AI algorithms, can provide potential for early diagnosis, thus giving early treatment intervention and improving survival rates. In relation to atypical presentations of specific illnesses, such as dementia (Egger & Rijntjes 2018), there is a growing need for AI combined with computer-aided big data analyses. The current scenario of medicine and health is bound by sub-specialisation diversity, coupled with rapidly increasing amount of new knowledge on the disease pathogenesis. As a result, the speed of patient disease diagnosis can be significantly reduced through the ongoing support of big data AI algorithms. With the homogenisation of underlying symptoms, clinical signs, biological imaging, epidemiological characteristics, molecular genetics and economic data allow for more appropriate generation of prevention and treatment decision support.

The downside to AI-based diagnosis and support system in healthcare services involves high equipment price and frequent maintenance costs. The complexity of AI algorithms may also require longer technical support, should breakdowns or processing errors occur. Additionally, one can expect that complex AI-based algorithms require higher human expertise, which may be limited in availability. There are also aspects of AI dynamics that are limited in comparison to human understanding, such as emotional intelligence, ethical conduct and spiritual relations. Current stance on the use of computerised or AI-dependent clinical decision support in healthcare system is fairly conservative (Koutkias & Bouaud 2018). This position stance is in view of the limited scale of existing guidelines, which is somewhat static. Approach to AI-based clinical decision support has been limited due to both the lack of evidence for all interventions and the cost of human authoring processes. This approach does not account for the perpetually evolving practice of medicine, with certain dynamics that are still beyond machine-based comprehension. The evolution of medical practice strives by learning from past practices in order to make future decisions, but is somehow paradoxical because it raises concerns about the suitability of such a decision in human ethics. Of course, in due time, these somewhat rather abstract aspects can be conceptualised algorithmically in AI-based decision support. Future AI-supported interventions can be applied in healthcare services in the form of automatically regulated equipment maintenance, patient-specific healthcare management and rehabilitation training. However, one would wonder, whether AI can completely take over human-based approaches in healthcare settings.

Application of AI in Patient Treatment and Management

The basic concept in understanding the potential applications of AI in patient treatment and management lie in the computational learning process called deep learning. This deep learning technique is a subset of machine-based learning derived from neural networks used in analysing and modelling for any disease-specific pattern recognition (Dilsizian & Siegel 2018). It carries a synonymous meaning to AI, often used interchangeably, but carries a more complex approach to utilising the techniques in software and statistical programming. The application of deep learning AI machines in medicine, can deliver promising effective and efficient healthcare delivery system in a large-scale setting. Significant reach for savings in medical cost could benefit from highly accurate predictive treatment comparisons against the more conventional techniques. The results of such comparisons can assist in delivering effective treatment and its subsequent management, by shifting any inappropriate treatment delivery to more appropriate patient subgroups. This cost-efficacy analysis approach can be helpful in efforts made to cut down on expensive and unnecessary preventive treatment measures, whilst reducing potential drug or treatment-related side effects.

Newer AI-based tools can now automatically calculate optimum dose of drug response treatment, allowing the patient to benefit from cost-efficient healthcare with minimal side effects. Major diseases and illnesses such as diabetes mellitus, hypertension, asthma or cancer may benefit tremendously from this AI application, by reducing potential errors, detecting any irregularities earlier, provides ease of use and encourages higher compliance (Dankwa-Mullan et al. 2018). This innovative approach transforms AI complexity into relevant health advances, by providing automated health status screening, clinical decision support, predictive risk stratification and patient self-management information support. Large public primary healthcare centres can combine these AI-based systems with an online web-based service that connects various different clinics nationally, ensuring complete information transfer and accurate treatment continuity. However, the health structural dynamics is somewhat fragile, being solely dependent on the storing system and vulnerable to technical issues such as system processing errors or emergency blackouts.

Mobile health management has been an increasingly popular solution to improving patient treatment and management delivery. This concept of treatment delivery focuses on allowing the patient to be the owner of their own data, where they can easily share it with different stakeholders. For instance, in the DataBox project (Brinker et al. 2018), patient's own data can be transferred, displayed and stored online where it aims to replace the conventional and inefficient method of paper-based documentation. This approach can ease better archival, organisation and availability of data, which reduces treatment errors, duplicates and allows production of complex AI algorithms for large data sets. It also allows patients to travel anywhere with ease, ensuring continuous reach for medical treatment that transcends beyond borders or countries, providing translated information and optimised contact forms. This is especially useful in areas where sensitive and direct documentation is required by healthcare practitioners, such as ensuring tuberculosis treatment completion, highly communicable disease prevention or drug-related addiction management practices. The disadvantage to this data-storing system revolves around the ethical considerations surrounding leakage of information and abuse of information.

Wearables technology, which includes smartwatches, wristbands, hearing aids, electronic chips, subcutaneous sensors, electronic footwear or clothing constitutes some examples. It uses sensors, apps or remote monitoring that could provide continuous clinical information for physicians with ease. It is an integral part of patient data collection, allowing physiological measurements, recording hemodynamic parameters or alerting scheduled appointments and treatments. These flexible electronics are now increasingly miniaturised, allowing physical ease of carriage and comfort during wear. Sensors integrated in these wearable devices typically contain microprocessors and sensors that are interfaced with a form of data communication detection technology, which includes smartphones, wireless cloud stores and online communication networks. The configuration of these gadgets with AI algorithms can generate real-time medical data that is more comprehensive in profiling. Patient data can be wirelessly transmitted to the medical service or another wearable device, within a closed-loop therapeutic system (Yetisen et al. 2018). Continuous health status measurements such as physical activity levels, blood profiles (i.e. cholesterol, blood sugar or uric acid measurements) and physiological readings (i.e. blood pressure and heart rate) help promote pursuits to a healthier lifestyle.

As the age of digital information progresses further, advanced analytics based on multi-modal data, constituting the 'digital health' continues to provide greater standardisation of health protocols (Mazzanti et al. 2018). There are calls for digitalising patient information and data storage through use of a 'tagging system', by identifying each individual through a barcode. This can be permanently encrypted in the form of a tattoo or wristband or microchips (Yetisen et al. 2018). However, this approach has some many ethical guidelines to consider before being fully feasible. Online reporting of symptoms and signs can now be issued through a website, within a structured format that helps filter cases by urgency (Tenhunen et al. 2018). This approach helps streamline patients' preliminary health concerns, directing them to appropriate point of care, within a timely manner. Emergency cases can be notified efficiently to relevant centres, transforming the workflow system into a more organised and well-controlled healthcare delivery structure. It also prevents oversaturation of healthcare centres during emergency crisis or if outbreaks and epidemics were to occur.

Healthcare delivery in treatment and management models continue to evolve and the opportunities for further improvements with the involvement of technology multinationals, such as Google, Facebook, Instagram or Microsoft, is rapidly promoted (Wong & Bressler 2016). With the involvement of AI and medicine in association with leading technological-savvy companies, the future of AI in healthcare looks very promising. Precise personalised care for any patient leads to better health information on their needs and preferences, disease progression, drug response and tolerance of treatments. This ultimately leads to better patient understanding, organised information transfer and archival, compliance to treatment and better health prospects.

AI in Autonomous Intervention and Innovative Assistance

AI-enhanced autonomous machineries are machine with the ability of performing simple to complex task with minimal supervision. Researchers have offered many variations of autonomous machineries, which include autonomous rehabilitation system and intelligent robots. Intelligent robots have shown promising feature in replicating human actions with greater power output, speed and accuracy. Boston Dynamic has demonstrated an AI-embed robot capable of replicating high-speed movements, such as running on unstable terrains, performing summersault and dexterous prehensile activities (Raibert et al. 2008). These robots undergo several iterations of attempts in order to successfully replicate the desired actions. The training process for AI robots begins from virtual simulation and later re-trained within an actual environment using real actuators and sensors. Intelligent robots can assist in carrying heavy load, such as transporting patient or equipment. For patients with tetraplegia who have difficulty in performing fine hand movements, an intelligent wheelchair robot was offered as solution instead of the conventional joystick-controlled wheel chair. The basis of this application was taken from the self-driving vehicle, where features such as autopilot and regulating navigation for the patient to move around are applied on a motor-powered wheelchair (Matsumotot, Ino & Ogsawara 2001). Navigation can be done via minimal body movements like eye coordination or nodding (Matsumotot, Ino & Ogsawara 2001). A widespread application of this intelligent machineries can reduce the frequency of healthcare practitioner to personally handle or steer the patients for relocation. Delegating heavy-duty labour to robots helps in reducing risk of accidents, occupational hazards and long-term fatigue, as well as promotes better quality healthcare services by prioritising management and intricate duties.

Another application of AI for autonomous assistance is in the rehabilitation field. Autonomous rehabilitation system has brought attention among physiotherapists as a solution to efficient rehabilitation recovery process for neurological disabilities in patients. Medical reports revealed that the recovery process of neurological disorder takes a long period of time to complete even with a dose-potent rehabilitation intervention. Despite that, only a small number of successful full recovery has been reported. Researchers suggested applying autonomous system as a supplementary rehabilitation intervention, which may increase the chances of full recovery. In the current preliminary development stage, autonomous rehabilitation system demonstrated promising result in providing a dose-potent rehabilitation intervention (Prange et al. 2009; Choi et al 2009; Mehrholz et al. 2015; Grimm & Gharabaghi 2016). The autonomous rehabilitation system responds to muscle tone resistance, spasticity and reflexes whilst guiding the patient through the course of a rehabilitation regimen. A simple event-based system switches from passive, passive-active and active intervention according to the rehabilitation regimen assigned by the physiotherapist. Due to the distinctive nature of the system, there are factors disregarded throughout the rehabilitation regimen process. Factors such as initiative, pain, muscle tone condition and progression are omitted as they are difficult to interpret even among expert physiotherapists. Therefore, a more intelligent system is proposed to compute the patient's behaviour and adapt their movements through the intervention process. AI-boosted autonomous system increases the efficiency and effectiveness of rehabilitation intervention by promoting a progressive and neurological condition-sensitive training. This concept is achievable by extracting both the physical feedback from muscle dynamics and electrical response from electromyogram (EMG) signals as the inputs. Using this information, the AI understands the behaviour of the patient by computing their muscle reflexes with the intended neurological movements. Following various iterations, researchers have offered many techniques to interpret intention and neurological activity from biological electrical emission known as bio signals. This application was demonstrated in the interpretation of electroencephalogram activity for seizure diagnostic using k-class nearest neighbour classifier (Fergus et al. 2015) and high performance and accuracy interpretation of movements from EMG signals using artificial neuro-fuzzy inference system (Bandou et al. 2017). Bio signalling interpretation provides an in-depth analysis of the patient's neurological behaviour, which facilitates autonomous rehabilitation system in providing proficient interventive measures.

With the synergic combination of AI diagnosis and automation, an optimal intervention can be achieved without physiotherapists' constant supervision. Optimal intervention can be described as a dynamic regime that changes intensity, difficulty and techniques based on the patient output, recovery and initiative. Both of these factors can be analysed from the muscle tone feedback and EMG signals produced during the rehabilitation training. This analysis will also support future studies in understanding neurological recovery progression and improve the intervention plan. Additionally, AI can also increase the difficulty level of rehabilitation training as deemed necessary. This includes increasing the difficulty level of a game in exergaming, changing task-oriented rehabilitation training and increasing the machineries' resistance and feedback. The challenges many healthcare facilities may experience from the utilisation of autonomous rehabilitation system are high maintenance cost and large space to facilitate the equipment. Like most exercise equipment, each equipment is designed for specific extremity and muscle development. This raises more concerns on healthcare commitment in facilitating necessary equipment for all neurological disorders.

AI is notably utilised in prediction analysis, as seen in social trending and marketing analysis for businesses, environmental and control simulation during early stage of research studies. Healthcare facilities could gain advantages in improving quality of service delivery and treatment management by combining AI with various professional experts. AI prediction analyses can be a powerful tool to mitigate potential threats, such as a potential pandemic, biohazardous outbreaks and genetic hereditary diseases. Forecasting diseases help minimise pandemic outbreaks and potential complications through early intervention. Genetic hereditary disease prediction will be a very useful tool for this purpose. Prediction diagnostics require more extensive medical and personal records than contemporary diagnostic. This includes the patient's present and past physical body conditions, genetics, lifestyle and familial medical records. But the data required can be reduced with a more narrowed scope of disease prediction. Researchers have demonstrated this ability in predicting cardiovascular diseases from a smaller series of data, which includes sex, cardiogram, pain description, age, blood pressure, sugar levels, heart rate and lifestyle factors (Masethe & Masethe 2014). The algorithm will increase the weightage to a more meaningful parameter, and this will heavily influence the prediction sensitivity. However, because of this, it may pose critical challenges if the information fed is inaccurate. It is difficult to obtain substantial information gathered within an extended time frame via verbal interviews and written records. Incomplete data can influence the outcome of a prediction heavily, causing a false negative or false positive prediction. As a result, predictive AI will have a high frequency of false negative and false positive prediction rates due to incomplete records. A false negative or positive prediction can pose critical ramifications in preventive medical intervention, such as double mastectomy in prevention of breast cancer. The challenges of predictive diagnostic AI revolve around the accuracy of the information given. Nevertheless, a reliable predictive diagnosis would certainly bring a remarkable impact in reducing health issues, which will subsequently reduce the workload of a healthcare practitioner.

Conclusion

The creation of super intelligent AI in medicine might be the biggest event in human history, which will either trigger an intelligence exponential or leave human intellect behind. Indeed, AI is lacking human emotional quotient needed for empathy, which may potentially pose risks in two devastating scenarios. This can include AI that is programmed to maximise positive outcome during crises (i.e. genetic selection to minimise potential threats in the future) or develop a destructive method to achieve its goal (i.e. contain a disease pandemic by mass human eradication). These scenarios are examples of a philosophical dilemma called the 'trolley problem', a philosophical question that has been debated for years regarding decision made by sacrificing the few to save the many. Regardless, AI features in machines have been the subject of controversy among critics, due to reports of inconsistencies, accidents, plausible loss of human control (i.e. cases of unsupervised learning algorithm astray from its true purposes), and breach of security. It is important to align the goals of humanity with AI advancements for public safety. The ethical concern that we must consider is, whether machines will act as a superior tool to replace human resources or simply as an assistive technology to improve efficiency. Nonetheless, adaptability has always been humanity's greatest features. We simply need to change the flow of actions to adapt the situation. It is our duty to attain the most cost-efficient solution to our everyday problems, which includes enhancing the quality of our healthcare services.

References

Amin, S.U., Agarwal, K. and Beg, R., 2013. Data mining in clinical decision support systems for diagnosis, prediction and treatment of heart disease. *International Journal of Advanced Research in Computer Engineering and Technology (IJARCET)*, 2(1), pp. 218–223.

Akdoğan, E., Taçgın, E. and Adli, M.A., 2009. Knee rehabilitation using an intelligent robotic system. *Journal of Intelligent Manufacturing*, 20(2), p. 195.

Andersen, L.L., Clausen, T., Mortensen, O.S., Burr, H. and Holtermann, A., 2012. A prospective cohort study on musculoskeletal risk factors for long-term sickness absence among healthcare workers in eldercare. *International Archives of Occupational and Environmental Health*, 85(6), pp. 615–622.

Bandou, Y., Fukuda, O., Okumura, H., Arai, K. and Bu, N., 2017, November. Development of a prosthetic hand control system Based on general object recognition analysis of recognition accuracy during approach phase. *In 2017 International Conference on Intelligent Informatics and Biomedical Sciences (ICIIBMS)*, Okinawa, Japan, pp. 110–114, IEEE.

Barinov, L., Jairaj, A., Becker, M., Seymour, S., Lee, E., Schram, A., Lane, E., Goldszal, A., Quigley, D. and Paster, L., 2018. Impact of data presentation on physician performance utilizing artificial intelligence-based computer-aided diagnosis and decision support systems. *Journal of Digital Imaging*, 32(3), pp. 408–416.

Bhavaraju, S.R., 2018. From subconscious to conscious to artificial intelligence: A focus on electronic health records. *Neurology India*, 66(5), p. 1270.

Brinker, T.J., Rudolph, S., Richter, D. and von Kalle, C., 2018. Patient-centered mobile health data management solution for the German health care system (The DataBox Project). *JMIR Cancer*, 4(1), e10160.

Bostrom, N., 2015. The control problem. Excerpts from superintelligence: Paths, dangers, strategies. In: S. Schneider (ed.), *Science Fiction and Philosophy: From Time Travel to Superintelligence*, John Wiley & Sons: Hoboken, NJ, Inc., p. 308–330.

Brynjolfsson, E., Rock, D. and Syverson, C., 2017. Artificial intelligence and the modern productivity paradox: A clash of expectations and statistics. In: *Economics of Artificial Intelligence*. University of Chicago Press: Chicago, IL, pp. 23–57.

Choi, Y., Gordon, J., Kim, D. and Schweighofer, N., 2009. An adaptive automated robotic task-practice system for rehabilitation of arm functions after stroke. *IEEE Transactions on Robotics*, 25(3), pp. 556–568.

Dankwa-Mullan, I., Rivo, M., Sepulveda, M., Park, Y., Snowdon, J. and Rhee, K., 2018. Transforming diabetes care through artificial intelligence: The future is here. *Population Health Management*, 22(3), pp. 229–242.

Dilsizian, M.E. and Siegel, E.L., 2018. Machine meets biology: A primer on artificial intelligence in cardiology and cardiac imaging. *Current Cardiology Reports*, 20(12), p. 139.

Egger, K. and Rijntjes, M., 2018. Big data and artificial intelligence for diagnostic decision support in atypical dementia. Der Nervenarzt.

Fergus, P., Hignett, D., Hussain, A., Al-Jumeily, D. and Abdel-Aziz, K., 2015. Automatic epileptic seizure detection using scalp EEG and advanced artificial intelligence techniques. *BioMed Research International*, 2015, pp. 1–17.

Fortunato, M., Azar, M.G., Piot, B., Menick, J., Osband, I., Graves, A., Mnih, V., Munos, R., Hassabis, D., Pietquin, O. and Blundell, C., 2017. Noisy networks for exploration. *arXiv Preprint arXiv*, 1706, p. 10295.

Grimm, F. and Gharabaghi, A., 2016. Closed-loop neuroprosthesis for reach-to-grasp assistance: Combining adaptive multi-channel neuromuscular stimulation with a multi-joint arm exoskeleton. *Frontiers in Neuroscience*, 10, p. 284.

Jao, C.S. and Hier, D.B., 2010. Clinical decision support systems: An effective pathway to reduce medical errors and improve patient safety. In: *Decision Support Systems*, pp. 121–138. doi: 10.5772/39469

Koutkias, V., Bouaud, J. and Section Editors for the IMIA Yearbook Section on Decision Support, 2018. Contributions from the 2017 literature on clinical decision support. *Yearbook of Medical Informatics*, 27(01), pp. 122–128.

Liao, P.H., Hsu, P.T., Chu, W. and Chu, W.C., 2015. Applying artificial intelligence technology to support decision-making in nursing: A case study in Taiwan. *Health Informatics Journal*, 21(2), pp. 137–148.

MacPhee, M., Ellis, J. and McCutheon, A.S., 2006. Nurse staffing and patient safety. *Canadian Nurse*, 102(8), pp. 18–23.

Masethe, H.D. and Masethe, M.A., 2014, October. Prediction of heart disease using classification algorithms. *In Proceedings of the World Congress on Engineering and Computer Science*, San Francisco, CA, Vol. 2, pp. 22–24.

Matsumotot, Y., Ino, T. and Ogsawara, T., 2001. Development of intelligent wheelchair system with face and gaze based interface. *In Proceedings 10th IEEE International Workshop on Robot and Human Interactive Communication. ROMAN 2001* (Cat. No. 01TH8591), Bordeaux, Paris, France, pp. 262–267, IEEE.

Mehrholz, J., Pohl, M., Platz, T., Kugler, J. and Elsner, B., 2015. Electromechanical and robot-assisted arm training for improving activities of daily living, arm function, and arm muscle strength after stroke. *Cochrane Database of Systematic Reviews*,11, pp. 1–128.

Mazzanti, M., Shirka, E., Gjergo, H. and Hasimi, E., 2018. Imaging, health record, and artificial intelligence: Hype or hope? *Current Cardiology Reports*, 20(6), p. 48.

Mosadeghrad, A.M., 2013. Occupational stress and turnover intention: Implications for nursing management. *International Journal of Health Policy and Management*, 1(2), p. 169.

Paparrizos, J., White, R.W. and Horvitz, E., 2016. Screening for pancreatic adenocarcinoma using signals from web search logs: Feasibility study and results. *Journal of Oncology Practice*, 12(8), pp. 737–744.

Prange, G.B., Jannink, M.J.A., Groothuis-Oudshoorn, C.G.M., Hermens, H.J. and Ijzerman, M.J., 2009. Systematic review of the effect of robot-aided therapy on recovery of the hemiparetic arm after stroke. *Journal of Rehabilitation Research and Development*, 43(2), pp. 171–184.

Rogers, A.E., Hwang, W.T., Scott, L.D., Aiken, L.H. and Dinges, D.F., 2004. The working hours of hospital staff nurses and patient safety. *Health Affairs*, 23(4), pp. 202–212.

Tenhunen, H., Hirvonen, P., Linna, M., Halminen, O. and Hörhammer, I., 2018. Intelligent patient flow management system at a primary healthcare center-the effect on service use and costs. *Studies in Health Technology and Informatics*, 255, pp. 142–146.

Triolo, P.K., 1989. Occupational health hazards of hospital staff nurses: Part I: Overview and psychosocial stressors. *AAOHN Journal*, 37(6), pp. 232–237.

Tullar, J.M., Brewer, S., Amick, B.C., Irvin, E., Mahood, Q., Pompeii, L.A., Wang, A., van Eerd, D., Gimeno, D. and Evanoff, B., 2010. Occupational safety and health interventions to reduce musculoskeletal symptoms in the health care sector. *Journal of Occupational Rehabilitation*, 20(2), pp. 199–219.

Raibert, M., Blankespoor, K., Nelson, G. and Playter, R., 2008. Bigdog, the rough-terrain quadruped robot. *IFAC Proceedings Volumes*, 41(2), pp. 10822–10825.

Winters, B., Custer, J., Galvagno, S.M., Colantuoni, E., Kapoor, S.G., Lee, H., Goode, V., Robinson, K., Nakhasi, A., Pronovost, P. and Newman-Toker, D., 2012. Diagnostic errors in the intensive care unit: A systematic review of autopsy studies. *BMJ Quality and Safety*, 21(11), pp. 894–902.

Wong, T.Y. and Bressler, N.M., 2016. Artificial intelligence with deep learning technology looks into diabetic retinopathy screening. *JAMA*, 316(22), pp. 2366–2367.

Yetisen, A.K., Martinez-Hurtado, J.L., Ünal, B., Khademhosseini, A. and Butt, H., 2018. Wearables in medicine. *Advanced Materials*, 30, p. 1706910.

Index

A

Actor-network theory, xi
Adolescent, 73, 213
Algorithms, 54
Alone together, 5
Alzheimer's, 31
Amazon, 339
Amazon's Echo, 127
Anxiety, 59
Aphasia, 36, 89, 293
Apple, 339
App stores, 229, 264
Apraxia, 295
Ataxia, 77
Artificial Intelligence, 54, 57, 127, 132, 339
Assistive Technology, 71, 115, 138, 259
Augmented reality, 237, 271
Autism, 35

B

Balancing, 63, 242, 247
Behavioural therapies, 63
Biofeedback, 305
Blindness, 76
Brain tumour, 295
Brief Stimulation Events, 73

C

Cancer, 295
Cardiovascular, 242
Caregivers, 35, 72, 127, 217
Cerebral Palsy, 62
Childhood, 12, 111
Children, 39, 54
Cognition Technologies, 271
Cognitive behavioural therapy, 220
Cognitive-Communication Deficits, 89
Communication, 129, 194

CommFit, 306
Computers, 3
Consent, 43
Consumer, 43
Consumer motivation, 123
Cybersecurity, 39

D

Dance, 59
Degenerative retinopathy, 77
Dementia, 32, 89
Depression, 59
Digital images, 90
Digital network environment, 62
Digital photography, 89, 126
Disability, 18
Dosage calculations, 109
Drones, 129
Dysarthria, 295
Dyslexia, 110, 125
Dyscalculia, 111

E

e-book, 124, 274
Elderly, 40, 54
e-mail, 195
Emerging technologies, 127
Encryption, 39
Engineering, 309
Epistemology, 6
Ethics, 31
Everyday communications, 271
Exercise, 56
Exergaming, 53
External memory aids, 280

F

Facebook, 36, 278, 339
Fear, 59

Feedback-based technology, 143
First technology arrangement, 79
Fitbit, 36
Fitness, 53
Focus groups, 198, 296

G

Games, 53, 151
Gamification, 54, 145, 236
Gaming consoles, 3
General Practitioner, 113
Google, 116, 128, 339
Google Play, 283
GPS, 128, 154, 237, 296, 334

H

Health and Well-being, 130
Hospitalisations, 62

I

Independent living, 127
Infant, 59
Informed consent, 109
Instant messaging, 4
Intellectual disabilities, 71
Intensive care unit, 4
International Classification of
          Functioning, 12
Internet of things, 237
iPads, 263
iTunes, 229
IT professionals, 309

K

Kindle, 124

L

Language disorder, 175
Learning Disabilities, 109
LEGO®, 13
Leisure, 71
Life participation, 303

M

Machine learning, 127
Matching person and technology, 259
mHealth, 31, 118, 213, 296
Microswitch, 75
Microsoft Xbox, 242
Mobile applications, 34, 304
Mobile instant interviewing, 4
Mobile technology, 213, 293
Mobility, 128
Motor impairments, 72
Motor co-ordination, 63
Motor learning, 146

N

Neurological, 144
Neuropathic pain, 61
Nintendo, 237
Nintendo Wii, 147

O

Obesity, 59
Occupational therapists, 181
Ontology, 6
Orthopaedic, 144

P

3D printing, 131, 217, 320
Paradigm, 219
Paediatric Rehabilitation, 11
Parkinson's disease, 62, 235, 244
Pedometer, 153
Photographs, 89, 309, 320
Physical disabilities, 54
Physiotherapists, 181
Play, 12, 185
Playstations, 237
Post traumatic stress disorders, 62
Privacy, 31, 38
Problem-solving, 23
Public policy, 135

Q

Qualitative, 196
Quantitative, 160, 328

R

Randomized controlled trials (RCT), 220
Refugees, 4
Relaxation, 38
Reminiscence Therapy, 89
Remote monitoring, 4
Research and development, 140
Robotics, 12, 129
Robots, 341

S

Safeguarding, 40
Samsung Gear VR, 153
Self-esteem, 38
Self-stigma, 274, 286
Service development, 135
Sexual function, 38
Science, technology, engineering and
    math, 12
Skype, 188
Smartphone apps, 158
Smartphones, 3, 32, 39, 130, 196, 223, 320
Smart technology, 339
Smart rings, 294
Smartwatches, 3, 130, 294
Social constructivism, 6
Social media, 132, 193, 195, 320
Speech pathologists, 36, 181, 300
Spina bifida, 220
Spinal cord injury, 62
STEM, 12
Storytelling, 89
Stress management, 38
Stroke, 62, 295
Student technology accommodations
    resources, 267

T

Tablets, 3, 39, 151, 272
Talking maps, 197

Teachers, 224
Technology solutions, 71
Telephone calls, 71
Telehealth, 176, 188
Television device, 71
Tesla, 128, 340
Texting, 195
Text messages, 71
Training, 139
Traumatic brain injury, 35, 89, 260, 277
Treadmill walking, 155

U

Uber, 125
User behaviour, 124

V

Video calls, 195
Video conferencing, 175, 187
Video games, 54, 62
Virtual reality, 55, 151, 235
Visual impairments, 19
Voice recognition, 127

W

Wheelchair, 60
World Health Organisation, 64, 133, 260
World Wide Web, 118

X

Xbox, 237
Xbox Kinect, 151

Y

YouTube, 140
Young adults, 213, 273
Young children, 175

Printed and bound by CPI Group (UK) Ltd, Croydon, CR0 4YY

17/10/2024

01775682-0015